# NEW DEVELOPMENTS IN
# CERVICAL CANCER SCREENING
# AND PREVENTION

# New Developments in Cervical Cancer Screening and Prevention

EDITED BY

## Eduardo Franco

Department of Oncology
McGill University
Montreal, Quebec, Canada

AND

## Joseph Monsonego

Department of Cyto-Colposcopy
Institut Alfred Fournier
Paris, France

FOREWORD BY

## Albert Singer

**Blackwell
Science**

© 1997 by
Blackwell Science Ltd
Editorial Offices:
Osney Mead, Oxford OX2 0EL
25 John Street, London WC1N 2BL
23 Ainslie Place, Edinburgh EH3 6AJ
350 Main Street, Malden
  MA 02148 5018, USA
54 University Street, Carlton
  Victoria 3053, Australia

Other Editorial Offices:
Blackwell Wissenschafts-Verlag GmbH
  Kurfürstendamm 57
  10707 Berlin, Germany

Zehetnergasse 6
  A-1140 Wien
  Austria

First published 1997

Set by Semantic Graphics, Singapore
Printed and bound in Great Britain
at the University Press, Cambridge

The Blackwell Science logo is a
trade mark of Blackwell Science Ltd,
registered at the United Kingdom
Trade Marks Registry

A catalogue record for this title
is available from the British Library

ISBN 0-632-04765-8

DISTRIBUTORS

Marston Book Services Ltd
PO Box 269
Abingdon
Oxon OX14 4YN
(*Orders:* Tel: 01235 465500
          Fax: 01235 465555)

USA
Blackwell Science, Inc.
Commerce Place
350 Main Street
Malden, MA 02148-5018
(*Orders:* Tel: 800 759 6102
          617 388 8250
          Fax: 617 388 8255)

Canada
Copp Clark Professional
200 Adelaide St, West, 3rd Floor
Toronto, Ontario M5H 1W7
(*Orders:* Tel: 416 597 1616
          800 815 9417
          Fax: 416 597 1617)

Australia
Blackwell Science Pty Ltd
54 University Street
Carlton, Victoria 3053
(*Orders:* Tel: 3 9347 0300
          Fax: 3 9349 5001)

Library of Congress
Cataloging-in-publication Data

New developments in cervical cancer
  screening and prevention / edited by
  Eduardo Franco and Joseph Monsonego.
      p.       cm.
  Includes bibliographical references
  and index.
  ISBN 0-632-04765-8
  1. Cervix uteri—Cancer—Diagnosis—
  Congresses.   2. Cervix uteri—Cancer—
  Prevention—Congresses.   3. Medical
  screening—Congresses.
  I. Franco, EduardoLuiz Fabiano.
  II. Monsonégo, Joseph.
  [DNLM: 1. Cervix Neoplasms—
  prevention & control—congresses.
  2. Cervix Neoplasms—epidemiology—
  congresses.   3. Mass Screening—
  congresses.   4. Cytodiagnosis—congresses.
  5. Papovaviridae Infections—prevention
  & control—congresses.
  WP 480 1997]
  RC280.U8N49   1997
  362.1′9699466—dc21
  DNLM/DLC
  for Library of Congress            96-37506
                                        CIP

# Contents

## Section 5: Automation in Cytology

## Section 6: Human Papillomavirus Testing

**Section 7: Adjunct Screening Tests**

**Section 8: Prevention and Therapy by Immunization**

**Section 9: Summary of Presentations and Consensus**

# Foreword

The 60 papers that were presented on nine topics, covered the whole scientific and clinical experience of cervical cancer. What was most exciting in this three-day meeting in Geneva was that a free discussion developed concerning many of the important aspects of cervical cancer research. In particular, the epidemiology evidence that was presented unequivocally supports an aetiological role for HPV infection. Furthermore, with this in mind, valid and objective tests using viral markers can be confidently predicted to indicate disease, therefore helping not only research into the natural history of the disease but also clinical management.

Notwithstanding these achievements in highlighting the aetiological factor, the reality of the situation in respect of cervical cancer worldwide, is depressing. Close to half a million women develop the disease annually, of whom one-third will die and there are probably in excess of this number who are undiagnosed. Ninety per cent of them will be in the developing world where resources are scarce and where the sophisticated techniques in diagnosis that were discussed in Geneva would seem inappropriate or extremely difficult to introduce. However, the Costa Rican study of a high-risk population gave some hope for the future and it presented a challenge to all the participants in Geneva to work out ways by which new technologies can be geared towards reducing the enormous toll in human suffering that is the woman with cervical cancer.

The future as seen in Geneva looks optimistic. Although there will be difficulties as mentioned above in transference of technologies, the ultimate goal will be to develop some form of vaccination or immunization against the viral cause of cervical cancer. Before this comes about much work needs to be expended in this field of basic science. There also needs to be a significant investment and effort aimed at sexual health education. Human behaviour both in men and women is extremely difficult to alter but it is only by this education that this can be influenced in the direction of a more responsible form of behaviour; the experience already gained with HIV proves that it is not impossible. However, the overriding impression in Geneva was that there were still many years of endeavour and hard work ahead before the worldwide problem of cervical cancer can even begin to be resolved.

Albert Singer
*University of London*

# The Rationale:
# Cervical Cancer Control

Cytological screening for detection of precursors of cancer of the uterine cervix has been one, and possibly the most successful, of public health measures introduced so far for the prevention of cancer.

Papanicolaou and Traut published their monograph in 1943. Since then, it has been shown that the appropriate policies and management of CIN could lead to effective and successful prevention of cervical cancer: a steady decline in mortality has been observed. Nevertheless, even in many developed countries, the impact has been far less than might be expected. For the past 10–15 years, the decline of the disease has been very small. We still observe a substantial proportion of cases of invasive cervical cancer in patients who are regularly screened, particularly young women. This is cause for alarm.

There is no evidence that Pap smear screening can lead to the complete eradication of the disease in any of the populations studied so far. Part of the failure has been organizational, either the inability to reach high-risk women, lack of adequate quality control, or follow-up procedures. The suggestion is that we have already reaped most of the benefits from an otherwise outstanding screening approach. Several attempts to change this technique have been made including the latest modifications introduced by the Bethesda system, which most likely will have no impact on cervical cancer rates.

The time has come for us to improve cervical cancer screening strategies. In the current climate of financially stretched health resources and given the extended three–five yearly screening intervals adopted by some European countries, the effectiveness of national screening programmes is likely to suffer with the inevitable return of cervical cancer rates that we could consider as part of a distant past.

But how can we improve on Pap cytology screening? Automation and use of monolayer systems should be one of possible answers, improving quality control of smears, reducing false-negative rates, improving the interobserver reproducibility in recognizing borderline cytological changes (ASCUS) and small cell lesions. In view of the enormous impact that these new technologies may have on the effectiveness of cervical cancer screening, the development of comparative trials should be considered in the future.

New and innovative molecular techniques such as HPV DNA testing should also be used in the secondary triage of minor cervical smear abnormalities and as an adjunct to cervical cytology in primary screening with an aim at finding an adequate interval between Pap smears.

Future and ongoing studies clarify the various outstanding issues in cervical cancer screening. The time has come, however, for clinicians to learn and assess the benefits of the various emerging technologies.

## Acknowledgements

EUROGIN would like to extend grateful thanks to the following companies for their valuable support: 3M Pharmaceuticals, Cytyc Corporation, Digene Diagnostic, AutoCyte Roche, Neopath, NSI, Medscand and Pasteur Vaccins.

Joseph Monsonego

# Introduction

On June 17–19, 1996, the European Research Organization on Genital Infection and Neoplasia (EUROGIN) and the World Health Organization's (WHO) Division of Noncommunicable Diseases jointly convened a workshop of experts to review new concepts and technological developments in cervical cancer screening and prevention. The workshop was held at WHO's headquarters in Geneva, Switzerland.

EUROGIN is a non-profit scientific organization chartered in Paris, France, whose objectives are to promote and develop research, training, and information on genital infections and on genital cancers and their precursor lesions. In April 1994, EUROGIN organized the 2nd International Congress on Papillomavirus in Human Pathology. A consensus conference, which took place during that meeting, published its recommendations as a monograph on cervical cancer screening. The June 1996 meeting was convened to update and to expand on the discussions and deliberations from the 1994 meeting, considering that the last two years have seen a wealth of scientific and technological developments concerning the aetiology, prevention, and prognosis of cervical cancer. The meeting was co-convened by J. Monsonego, Executive Secretary of EUROGIN, and by M. Tsechkovski and V. Koroltchouk, from WHO. H. ZurHausen was the Chairman of the meeting, with A. Singer serving as Vice-Chairman and E. Franco as General Rapporteur.

With WHO's priorities on cancer control as backdrop, 32 speakers presented more than 60 papers distributed in nine sessions on the following topics: epidemiology of cervical cancer and HPV infection (rapporteur: E.L. Franco), natural history of cervical cancer and its implications on screening policy (rapporteur: K. Syrjänen), cervical cancer screening programmes (rapporteurs: C. De Wolf and J. Patnick), advantages, limitations, and optimization of cytology (rapporteur: A. Ferenczy), automated screening devices (rapporteur: E. McGoogan), human papillomavirus (HPV) testing (rapporteur: F.X. Bosch), adjuvant tests to cytology (rapporteur: A. Singer), development of HPV vaccines (rapporteur: N. Muñoz), and public health aspects (rapporteur: A. Meheus). A summary of the meeting presentations has been published as a WHO technical document.

This book contains the unabridged major papers given in the Geneva meeting, with most of them having been updated during the summer of 1996. It contains 53 chapters organized in 9 sections as follows: (i) epidemiology and public health aspects of cervical cancer; (ii) natural history and management of cervical cancer precursors; (iii) the cervical cytology paradigm; (iv) cytology screening programmes; (v) automation in cytology; (vi) HPV testing; (vii) adjunct screening tests; (viii) prevention and therapy by immunization; (ix) summary of presentations and consensus.

The authors of the individual chapters are among the most influential basic and clinical scientists shaping our knowledge on the aetiopathogenesis and management of cervical cancer and its precursor lesions. Some may be tempted to view the list of contributors as perhaps somewhat overrepresenting European and North American experiences. This would be a mistaken assumption, however, as research on cervical cancer control has truly lost its international boundaries; many studies nowadays are conducted as multicentre investigations which simultaneously collect standardized information from populations in both developed and developing countries in all continents. Some of the chapters present results obtained from large-scale studies in Latin America, Africa, and Asia, regions which are overburdened by the lion's share in cervical cancer morbidity and mortality world-wide.

We would like to express our deep gratitude to Dr Eliane Duarte, for assistance with the preliminary phase of the editorial process, and to Ms Candida Pizzolongo (Montreal) and Ms Jacqueline Villaros and Veronique Varallo (Paris) for secretarial assistance. We are also grateful to the members of EUROGIN's Executive Committee for unconditional support and valuable opinions. All session rapporteurs named above also contributed important suggestions along with their summary reports. Finally, we were fortunate to have worked with the competent staff of Blackwell Science and in particular with Dr Stuart Taylor, our senior managing editor, and Julie Elliott who worked hard to harmonize the diversity of writing styles and publish the book within such a tight production schedule.

Eduardo Franco
Joseph Monsonego

# Section 1
# Epidemiology and
# Public Health Aspects of
# Cervical Cancer

# 1: Human Papillomavirus and Cervical Cancer: Epidemiological Evidence

## N. Muñoz

## Summary

The epidemiological evidence linking human papillomavirus (HPV) to cervical cancer is reviewed. It is concluded that over 90% of cervical cancers can be attributed to certain HPV types. HPV 16 accounts for the highest proportion (50%), followed by HPV 18 (12%), HPV 45 (8%) and HPV 31 (5%). The recognition of this fact has far-reaching implications for the primary and secondary prevention of this malignancy. Prophylactic and therapeutic HPV vaccines are now under development and HPV typing is being integrated into screening programmes in pilot studies in a few developed countries. In developing countries, well-conducted conventional screening programmes remain the best approach for the control of cervical cancer until a safe and efficient HPV vaccine can be used in the general population.

## Introduction

Until 5 years ago, critical assessments of the epidemiological evidence linking HPV to cervical cancer concluded that it was highly suggestive but not conclusive of a causal association [1,2]. Since then, a series of well-designed epidemiological studies using accurate hybridization assays to assess HPV exposure have been reported. These studies were important contributors to the overall assessment of certain types of HPV as carcinogenic to humans carried out by an interdisciplinary expert group convened by the International Agency for Research on Cancer (IARC) [3]. They comprise an impressive and largely

*Correspondence*: Dr N. Muñoz, Unit of Field and Intervention Studies, International Agency for Research on Cancer, 150 Cours Albert Thomas, F-69372 Lyon Cédex 08, France.

consistent set of case series, case-control studies and some cohort investigations that will be reviewed below.

## Case series

Prevalences of HPV DNA ranging from 22% to 100% have been reported in over 30 series of cervical intraepithelial neoplasia (CIN) and cervical cancer [3]. This broad range in HPV prevalence is due to variation in the hybridization method used (with or without amplification), the different tumour specimens (cervical swabs, lavages, biopsies or surgical specimens) and tissue preservation (fresh, frozen or fixed).

The IARC has coordinated an international prevalence survey of HPV in cervical cancer that can be regarded as the prototype of this type of studies. Over 1000 frozen biopsies from histologically confirmed cervical cancers were collected from 22 countries around the world using a standard protocol. They were tested in a central laboratory using a polymerase chain reaction (PCR)-based assay capable of detecting more than 25 HPV types. HPV DNA was detected in 93% of the tumours and the use of additional HPV detection methods suggests that fewer than 5% of cervical cancers are probably truly HPV-negative tumours. The most common HPV types detected were HPV 16 in 49.2%, HPV 18 in 11.7%, HPV 45 in 8% and HPV 31 in 5% of the specimens. HPV 16 was the predominant type in all countries except Indonesia, where HPV 18 was more common. A clustering of HPV 45 was apparent in western Africa, while HPV 39 and 59 were detected almost exclusively in Latin America. HPV 16 was the most common type detected in squamous cell carcinomas but HPV 18 predominated in adenocarcinomas [4].

The knowledge of the distribution of the various HPV types associated with cervical cancer in the different geographical areas is essential to the development of HPV vaccination strategies to curb the burden of cervical cancer.

## Case-control studies

### High-grade CIN lesions (CIN II–III)

Considering that low-grade CIN or CIN I lesions are cytologically or histologically indistinguishable from the morphological signs of HPV-productive infection, CIN I could be regarded as an insensitive marker of HPV exposure and not as a disease outcome. Thus, only high-grade CIN lesions will be considered in this review.

Table 1.1 summarizes the results of six case-control studies combining a good epidemiological design and a PCR-based hybridization assay [5–9].

**Table 1.1** Polymerase chain reaction-based case-control studies on cervical intraepithelial neoplasia (CIN) II–III.

| Study area (author) | Case (no.) | Controls (no.) | HPV prevalence | | | Adjusted OR (95% CI) | HPV AF (%) | Adjustment for: |
|---|---|---|---|---|---|---|---|---|
| | | | HPV | Cases | Controls | | | |
| Spain | 157 (CIN III) | 193 | Any HPV<br>HPV 16 | 70.7<br>49.0 | 4.7<br>0.5 | 56.9 (24.8–130.6)<br>295.5 (44.8–1946.6) | 72.4<br>59.6 | Age, study area, NSP, AFSI, *Chlamydia trachomatis* |
| Colombia (Bosch *et al.*, 1993) [5] | 125 | 181 | Any HPV | 63.2 | 10.5 | 15.5 (8.2–29.4) | 60.3 | Age, NSP, AFSI, smoking, *Chlamydia trachomatis* |
| Portland, USA (Schiffman *et al.*, 1993) [6] | 50 (CIN II–III) | 433 | Any HPV<br>HPV 16/18 | 90.0<br>62.0 | 17.7<br>2.9 | 42.0 (15.3–124.3)<br>180.0 (49.0–630.0) | 87.9<br>83.8 | Age, NSP |
| New Mexico, USA (Becker *et al.*, 1994) [7] | 176 (CIN II–III) | 311 | Any HPV<br>HPV 16 | 93.8<br>52.4 | 42.1<br>8.6 | 20.8 (10.8–40.2)<br>9.9 (5.4–18.3) | 89.0<br>44.0 | Age, NSP, AFSI, ethnicity |
| Norway (Olsen *et al.*, 1995) [8] | 98 (CIN II–III) | 221 | Any HPV<br>HPV 16 | 90.8<br>65.3 | 15.4<br>6.3 | 72.8 (27.6–191.9)<br>182.4 (54.0–616.1) | 92.0<br>92.0 | Age, NSP, AFSI, smoking, OC use, parity, E, genital warts |
| Taiwan (Liaw *et al.*, 1995) [9] | 39 (CIN III) | 261 | Any HPV<br>High-risk | 91.7<br>58.3 | 9.2<br>0.8 | 122.3 (38.5–388.9)<br>1279.9 (185.5–8829.8) | 91.0<br>58.0 | Age at screening |

HPV, Human papillomavirus; OR, odds ratio; CI, confidence interval; AF, attributable fraction; NSP, number of sexual partners; AFSI, age at first sexual intercourse; OC, oral contraceptive; E, education.

In the IARC studies in Spain and Colombia, an early version of the L1 consensus primer system was used with a generic probe detecting a narrower spectrum of HPV types [10], while in the studies in the USA and Taiwan an improved version of the L1 consensus primer system with a more sensitive generic probe and 25 HPV type-specific probes were used [6,7,9]. In the study in Norway nested general primers were used [8].

Comparing the results of the six studies summarized in Table 1.1, it is clear that HPV DNA prevalence among cases is higher (>90%) in those studies using highly sensitive PCR-based assays than in those using the early versions of these assays (63–70%). In comparing the prevalence of HPV DNA among controls we shall take into account the age structure as well as the source of control patients, in addition to the accuracy of the hybridization techniques. Thus, the higher prevalences in Portland, USA and Norway than in Spain and Colombia are probably explained by the younger age of the study populations as well as the more sensitive PCR assays in the former studies, while the higher prevalence of HPV DNA in New Mexico than in the Portland study is probably determined by the nature of the control group (women referred to a colposcopy clinic). Thus, selection bias cannot be totally excluded in the study carried out in New Mexico.

As mentioned before, the PCR assay used in the studies in Spain and Colombia was less sensitive than the PCR-based assay used in the other studies; thus, the odds ratios (ORs) and attributable fractions (AF) given in Table 1.1 for Spain and Colombia are probably underestimates of the true ORs and AFs.

The adjusted OR for HPV DNA (any type) ranged from 16 in Colombia to 122 in Taiwan and for HPV 16 from 10 in New Mexico to 296 in Spain. The OR for high-risk HPV types (HPV 16, 18, 31, 45) was 1280 in Taiwan.

The fraction of high-risk CIN attributable to HPV ranged from 60% in Colombia to 92% in Norway.

## Invasive cervical cancer

Table 1.2 summarizes four case-control studies fulfilling the inclusion criteria; in all of them, PCR-based assays were used.

In Spain and Colombia, Muñoz *et al.* [11] conducted two population-based case-control studies including women with invasive squamous cell cervical cancer and population controls randomly selected from the populations under study. HPV detection was done using PCR methods based on the L1 region consensus primers as described above [10].

In Brazil and China, hospital-based case-control studies were carried out and two different PCR assays were used. In Brazil, a PCR-based assay using a general primer which amplifies a small region of L1 gene and various type-specific probes was employed [12].

**Table 1.2** Polymerase chain reaction (PCR)-based case-control studies on invasive cervical cancer.

| Study area (author) | Cases (no.) | Controls (no.) | HPV prevalence | | | Adjusted OR (95% CI) | HPV AF (%) | Adjustment for: |
|---|---|---|---|---|---|---|---|---|
| | | | HPV | Cases | Controls | | | |
| Spain | 250 | 238 | Any HPV | 69.0 | 4.6 | 46.2 (18.5–115.1) | 67.5 | Age, study area, NSP, AFB, E, screening history |
| | | | HPV 16 | 45.8 | 3.1 | 14.9 (5.0–49.5) | 30.1 | |
| Colombia (Muñoz et al., 1992) [11] | 186 | 149 | Any HPV | 72.4 | 13.3 | 15.6 (6.9–34.7) | 66.0 | Age, NSP, AFB, E, screening history |
| | | | HPV 16 | 50.6 | 9.2 | 5.5 (2.4–12.9) | 29.3 | |
| Brazil (Eluf-Neto et al., 1994) [12] | 199 | 255 | Any HPV | 84.0 | 17.0 | 37.1 (19.6–70.4) | 86.0 | Age, SES |
| | | | HPV 16 | 53.8 | 5.3 | 74.9 (32.5–173.0) | 79.7 | |
| China (Peng et al., 1991) [13] | 101 | 106 | HPV 16/33 | 34.7 | 1.4 | 32.9 (7.7–141.1) | 31.0 | Age, I, R, AFM, smoking |

HPV, Human papillomavirus; OR, odds ratio; CI, confidence interval; AF, attributable fraction; NSP, number of sexual partners; AFB, age at first birth; E, education; SES, socio-economic status; I, income; R, residence; AFM, age at first marriage.

The PCR assay used in the Chinese study did not include a consensus primer that amplifies a broad spectrum of HPV types, but only primers for HPV 16 and 33; thus, it is not directly comparable with the other three studies [13].

The four case-control studies summarized in Table 1.2 give consistent results. The higher HPV DNA prevalence among cases from Brazil than among cases from Spain and Colombia is probably test-related. Among controls higher HPV prevalences are observed in the high-risk countries for cervical cancer (Brazil and Colombia) than in the low-risk countries (Spain and China). The adjusted ORs for HPV DNA (any type) ranged from 16 in Colombia to 46 in Spain and those for HPV 16 from 6 in Colombia to 75 in Brazil. The fraction of cervical cancer attributable to HPV ranged from 66% in Colombia to 86% in Brazil.

No formal case-control studies on cervical adenocarcinoma have been reported.

Case-control studies suffer from inherent temporal ambiguity concerning exposure and disease outcome. Thus, the higher prevalence of HPV DNA among cases than among controls could be interpreted in two ways:

1 If we assume that single measurement of HPV DNA is a good marker of chronic persistent infection with HPVs, HPV DNA detected at recruitment of cases and controls could be regarded as a marker of an HPV infection that preceded the cancer development.

2 HPV DNA could be more readily detected in tumoral cells than in normal cells or could be a marker of an opportunistic infection with HPV.

Direct evidence in support of the first possibility can only be derived from long-term follow-up studies and a few such studies will be reviewed below. However, indirect evidence may be obtained from the trend of HPV DNA prevalence by time since last sexual intercourse, because sexual transmission is the major route of transmission. Data from our studies in Spain and Colombia show a stable high rate of HPV DNA positivity both in women with cervical cancer who reported being sexually active at the time of the interview and in women who had their last sexual intercourse many years before entry into the study [5,10].

The possibility of enhanced detectability in tumoral cells is unlikely because the HPV DNA prevalence in precursor lesions (CIN II–III) is as high as in invasive cervical cancer. Against the argument of HPV being an opportunistic infection there is a great deal of laboratory data indicating that DNA and transcripts of specific HPV types are usually detected in tissue specimens from cervical cancer and its precursor lesions, and that high-risk HPV are able to immortalize human cells and their oncoproteins interfere with the functions of negative cellular regulators [3].

## Cohort studies

Although several cohort or follow-up studies have been reported, only those having as end-point CIN II–III, using Southern blot or PCR-based hybridization assays for HPV DNA detection and fulfilling basic design criteria will be considered here.

Three studies from the USA have been reported. In the first one, a cohort of 241 cytologically normal women recruited from a sexually transmitted disease (STD) clinic were followed every 4 months for an average of 25 months. HPV DNA was detected using dot blot and Southern blot. HPV DNA positivity increased the risk of developing CIN II–III. The adjusted relative risk was 11.0 (95% confidence interval (CI) = 3.7–31.0) [14].

In a second study, 206 women (173 with low-grade squamous intraepithelial lesions (SIL) and 33 with high-grade SIL) who participated in an intervention trial were followed every 2 months for 6 months. HPV DNA 16 was detected at study entry and at each follow-up examination by Southern blot. Using multivariate modelling and adjusting for age, race, smoking, oral contraceptive use and plasma levels of micronutrients, HPV 16 was found to be related to progression to high-grade SIL with a relative risk of 1.19 and 95% CI = 1.03–1.38 [15].

In the third study, 70 women with a histological diagnosis of dysplasia were followed at 3-month intervals for 15 months. These women were enrolled in a double-blind randomized trial to assess the efficacy of β-carotene for the treatment of CIN. HPV DNA was detected by both Southern blot and a PCR-based assay. Persistent SIL was associated with persistent HPV infection and especially with persistent high viral load (OR = 4.1; 95% CI = 1.4–12.3), detected by Southern blot. ORs were adjusted for the randomized group [16].

In the Netherlands a cohort of 342 women with abnormal cytology (with Papanicolaou (Pap) class 3b or lower, i.e. CIN III or lower) were followed up every 3–4 months for an average follow-up period of 16 month [17]. During the follow-up visits the following examinations were performed: cytology, colposcopy without biopsy and HPV DNA testing for 27 HPV types using an accurate PCR technique. Nine (3.0%) of the 298 women with an original cytological diagnosis of Pap 3a (CIN I–II) progressed to CIN III (diagnosed by colposcopy and histology) and all of them were HPV DNA-positive for high-risk types at enrolment and during the follow-up. The authors reported that the progression rate was higher among women positive for high-risk HPV types than among women with low-risk HPV or negative for HPV.

Two retrospective cohort studies based on archival cytological or histological slides have been reported.

In the UK, a cohort of 93 untreated women with cervical abnormalities was identified from a randomized control trial undertaken some years ago. The patients were followed every 4 months by colposcopical and cytological examinations for a median period of 26 months. HPV 16 and 18 were detected in the baseline biopsy sections by a PCR-based assay. HPV 16 and/or 18 were detected in 47 women (51%) and their presence was associated with an increased risk of progression (OR = 2.3; 95% CI = 1.2–4.3) [18].

In Sweden, smears from 30 women with invasive cervical cancer (18 squamous cell carcinomas and 12 adenocarcinomas) and from 58 with carcinoma-*in-situ* positive for HPV DNA were compared with smears of a control group of women. For the cases, the smears were taken 1.5–7 years before the diagnosis of cancer. HPV DNA was detected with a nested PCR-based assay, in 67% of the smears preceding the cancer in case women and in 11% of control women (OR = 16; 95% CI = 6.8–38.0) [19].

Results from the above studies suggest that persistent infection with high-risk HPV types precedes the development of CIN II–III and predicts a high risk of developing it. The main limitation of this study design is that in most settings follow-up is interrupted at stages CIN II–III for treatment of these lesions and therefore the role of HPV in the progression to invasive cancer cannot be investigated. In addition, it is known that a certain proportion of CIN II–III lesions regress spontaneously.

Various other cohort studies are in progress in Colombia, Costa Rica, India, the USA and UK but results have not yet been reported.

## Conclusions

The epidemiological data reviewed above indicate that the association between certain HPV types and cervical cancer fulfil the accepted criteria of causality proposed by Sir Bradford Hill:

1   It is very strong, with ORs over 15 in all methodologically sound case-control studies using reliable methods for HPV DNA detection. The strength of the association rules out the possibility that it can be explained by chance, bias or confounding.

2   It is consistent, as equally strong associations have been found both in high- and low-risk countries for cervical cancer.

3   There is a dose–response relationship with viral load. High levels of HPV DNA appear to carry a higher risk of cervical neoplasia than low levels.

4   Results from a few cohort studies indicate that infection with certain HPV types precedes the development of CIN II–III lesions.

5   The association is specific for certain HPV types called high-risk HPV types. Out of the 30 HPV types that infect the uterine cervix, HPV 16 accounts for the highest proportion of cervical cancer, followed by HPV 18.

6   The epidemiological evidence is supported by a great number of laboratory investigations indicating a carcinogenic potential of the HPV types implicated in cervical neoplasia [3].

These conclusions have been endorsed by an international multidisciplinary group which met recently in Lyons to evaluate the carcinogenicity of HPV [3].

Results from the reviewed case-control studies and the IARC international prevalence survey of HPV DNA in invasive cervical cancer indicate that over 90% of these tumours can be attributed to certain HPV types. The fact that only a small minority of the persistent HPV infections progress eventually to cancer indicates that there should be other factors or cofactors that increase the progression to malignancy. Thus, if we consider the small fraction of cervical cancers in which HPV DNA has not been detected as truly HPV-negative cases we conclude that HPV is neither a necessary nor a sufficient cause of cervical cancer. Two types of cofactors may be of importance:

1  Host factors that would modulate the effect of HPV, such as genetic factors (human leukocyte antigen or major haplotypes), genetic or induced immunosuppression, endogenous hormonal factors, reflected in the associations with high parity detected in our studies [12,20,21] as well as early age at first sexual intercourse that could be regarded as a surrogate of early age at first HPV infection.

2  Exogenous factors. In our studies in Spain, Colombia and Brazil, only long-term use of oral contraceptives emerged as a cofactor among HPV-positive women [12,21]. However, our observations need to be confirmed in other populations and in larger studies. Our ongoing multicentre study, in which a larger number of women with HPV-positive invasive cervical cancer will be compared with HPV-positive control women, will produce valuable information on the role of cofactors.

Our studies also suggest that the above cofactors probably influence more the progression from persistent HPV infection to CIN III than from CIN III to invasive cervical cancer. In fact, a comparison of the risk factors identified for CIN III and invasive cancer in Spain and Colombia did not reveal any risk factor that was consistently different between CIN III and invasive cancer to suggest a role in the progression of CIN III to invasive cancer [22].

Finally, the role of aetiological factors independent from HPV has not been considered, as it is still uncertain whether the small proportion of cervical cancer negative for HPV DNA is truly negative or falsely negative, but might become HPV-positive when more sensitive methods of HPV DNA detection are available. In any case, if a subgroup of HPV-negative cervical cancer is finally identified, it would probably account for fewer than 5% of cervical cancers.

## Implications

The knowledge that certain types of HPV account for over 90% of cervical cancer has far-reaching implications for the primary and secondary prevention of this malignancy. Prophylactic and therapeutic HPV vaccines are now under development and a few phase I trials are underway with therapeutic vaccines [23]. Preliminary results suggest that HPV testing may be of great use in predicting high-grade CIN whenever the cytology fails [24].

## References

1 Muñoz N, Bosch FX, Kaldor JM. Does human papillomavirus cause cervical cancer? The state of the epidemiological evidence. *Br J Cancer* 1988; **57**: 1–5.
2 Muñoz N, Bosch FX. Current views on the role of human papillomavirus in the genesis of cervical neoplasia. *Papillomavirus Rep* 1991; **2**: 57–60.
3 IARC. *Monographs on the Evaluation of the Carcinogenic Risk of Chemicals to Humans*, vol. 64. *Human Papillomaviruses*. Lyon: International Agency for Research on Cancer, 1995.
4 Bosch FX, Manos MM, Muñoz N *et al.* Prevalence of human papillomavirus in cervical cancer: a worldwide perspective. *J Nat Cancer Inst* 1995; **87**: 796–802.
5 Bosch FX, Muñoz N, de Sanjosé S *et al.* Human papillomavirus and cervical intraepithelial neoplasia grade III/carcinoma *in situ*: a case-control study in Spain and Colombia. *Cancer Epidemiol Biomarkers Prevent* 1993; **2**: 415–422.
6 Schiffman M, Bauer H, Hoover R *et al.* Epidemiologic evidence showing that HPV infection causes most cervical intraepithelial neoplasia. *J Nat Cancer Inst* 1993; **85**: 958–964.
7 Becker TM, Wheeler CM, McGough NS *et al.* Sexually transmitted diseases and other risk factors for cervical dysplasia among southwestern Hispanic and non-Hispanic white women. *JAMA* 1994; **271**: 1181–1188.
8 Olsen AO, Gjøen K, Sauer T *et al.* Human papillomavirus and cervical intraepithelial neoplasia grade II–III: a population-based case-control study. *Int J Cancer* 1995; **61**: 312–315.
9 Liaw K-L, Hsing AW, Chen C-J *et al.* Human papillomavirus and cervical neoplasia: a case-control study in Taiwan. *Int J Cancer* 1995; **62**: 565–571.
10 Guerrero E, Daniel RW, Bosch FX *et al.* Comparison of Virapap, southern hybridization and polymerase chain reaction methods for human papillomavirus identification in an epidemiological investigation of cervical cancer. *J Clin Microbiol* 1992; **30**: 2951–2959.
11 Muñoz N, Bosch FX, de Sanjosé S *et al.* The causal link between human papillomavirus and invasive cervical cancer: a population-based case-control study in Colombia and Spain. *Int J Cancer* 1992; **52**: 743–749.
12 Eluf-Neto J, Booth M, Muñoz N, Bosch FX, Meijer CJLM, Walboomers JMM. Human papillomavirus and invasive cervical cancer in Brazil. *Br J Cancer* 1994; **69**: 114–119.
13 Peng H, Liu S, Mann V, Rohan T, Rawls W. Human papillomavirus types 16 and 33, herpes simplex virus type 2 and other risk factors for cervical cancer in Sichuan province, China. *Int J Cancer* 1991; **47**: 711–716.
14 Koutsky LA, Holmes KK, Critchlow CW *et al.* A cohort study of the risk of cervical intraepithelial neoplasia grade 2 or 3 in relation to papillomavirus infection. *N Engl J Med* 1992; **327**: 1272–1278.
15 Liu T, Soong S-J, Alvarez RD, Butterworth CE. A longitudinal analysis of human papillomavirus 16 infection, nutritional status, and cervical dysplasia progression. *Cancer Epidemiol Biomarkers Prevent* 1995; **4**: 373–380.
16 Ho GYF, Burk RD, Klein S *et al.* Persistent genital human papillomavirus infection as risk factors for persistent cervical dysplasia. *J Nat Cancer Inst* 1995; **87**: 1365–1371.
17 Remmink AJ, Walboomers JMM, Helmerhorst TJM *et al.* The presence of persistent

high-risk HPV genotypes in dysplastic cervical lesions is associated with progressive disease: natural history up to 36 months. *Int J Cancer* 1995; **61**: 306–311.

18 Woodman CBJ, Rollason T, Ellis J, Tierney R, Wilson S, Young L. Human papilloma-virus infection and risk of progression of epithelial abnormalities of the cervix. *Br J Cancer* 1996; **73**: 553–556.

19 Chua K-L, Hjerpe A. Persistence of human papillomavirus (HPV) infections preceding cervical carcinoma. *Cancer* 1996; **77**: 121–127.

20 Muñoz N, Bosch FX, de Sanjosé S *et al*. Risk factors for cervical intraepithelial neoplasia grade III/carcinoma *in situ* in Spain and Colombia. *Cancer Epidemiol Biomarkers Prevent* 1993; **2**: 423–431.

21 Boch FX, Muñoz N, de Sanjosé S *et al*. Risk factors for cervical cancer in Colombia and Spain. *Int J Cancer* 1992; **52**: 750–758.

22 Moreno V, Muñoz N, Bosch FX *et al*. Risk factors for progression of cervical intraepithe-lial neoplasm grade III to invasive cervical cancer. *Cancer Epidemiol Biomarkers Prevent* 1995; **4**: 459–467.

23 Muñoz N, Crawford L, Coursaget P. HPV vaccines for cervical neoplasia. *Lancet* 1995; **345**: 249.

24 Cuzick J, Szarewski A, Terry G *et al*. Human papillomavirus testing in primary cervical screening. *Lancet* 1995; **345**: 1533–1536.

# 2: Epidemiology of Cervical Human Papillomavirus Infection

E. L. Franco,[1] L. L. Villa,[2] H. Richardson,[1] T. E. Rohan[3] & A. Ferenczy[4]

## Summary

The epithelial lining of the anogenital tract is the target for infection by a group of mucosotropic viruses, the human papillomaviruses (HPV). There are more than 70 HPV types, of which nearly 30 infect the anogenital tract. Sexual behaviour and age are the most important determinants of cervical HPV infection and seem to be the most consistent findings in cross-sectional studies. A role for other variables, such as smoking, use of oral contraceptives and reproductive factors has emerged in some studies but less consistently.

Recent evidence suggests that the sexual transmissibility of cervical HPV infection may vary by type. Infection with HPV types of high oncogenicity is strongly associated with sexual activity whereas low-oncogenic-risk types exhibit a weaker association with the same indicators of sexual behaviour. The age-dependence of HPV prevalence seems also to vary on the basis of oncogenicity of viral types. The negative correlation with age seems to be more pronounced for infection with low-oncogenic-risk types.

Over 15% of asymptomatic women who are sexually active can have HPV detected in their cervix using amplified DNA hybridization methods. Most of these infections are transient and are probably of little significance. The concern resides, however, in the small proportion of women who harbour persistent HPV infections. Recent evidence suggests that these women stand a much greater risk of subsequent cervical neoplasia, indicating that persistent, not transient, HPV infections are the actual biological precursor in cervical carcinogenesis. Research on the epidemiology of viral persistence will help in

*Correspondence*: Professor E.L. Franco, Department of Oncology, McGill University, 546 Pine Avenue West, Montreal, QC, Canada H2W 1S6.
[1]Departments of Oncology and [4]Pathology, McGill University, Montreal, Canada, [2]Ludwig Institute for Cancer Research, São Paulo, Brazil, [3]University of Toronto, Toronto, Canada.

the formulation of algorithms and policies for inclusion of some form of HPV testing in cervical cancer prevention.

## Introduction

The epithelial lining of the anogenital tract is the target for infection by a group of mucosotropic viruses, HPV. Subclinical and clinical genital warts, also known as condylomata acuminata, and probably most malignant lesions of the anogenital tract are caused by specific HPV types. There are more than 70 types defined on the basis of DNA homology [1], of which nearly 30 infect the anogenital tract.

## Genital warts

The occurrence of anogenital condylomata can only be measured indirectly, via hospital series or physician consultation statistics. Although we cannot measure the incidence of genital warts directly it seems likely that it has increased substantially in western countries. It is conceivable that clinical and subclinical genital HPV infections may be the most common sexually trans-mitted diseases today. In the USA since 1966 there has been a fivefold increase in the number of initial office visits for diagnosis and treatment of genital warts as monitored by the National Disease and Therapeutic Index (NDTI; IMS America, Ltd), which surveys a stratified random sample of private practitio-ners in the country (see Franco [2] for review).

The true incidence of symptomatic condyloma acuminatum was measured in a study by Mayo Clinic investigators in Rochester, Minnesota, during 1950–1978 [3]. This study found that rates had increased substantially during that period, peaking in 1975 with an average annual incidence of 107 new cases per 100 000. Although a study in a small community in a mid-western state does not reflect national trends, the rate seen in Rochester probably represents a lower bound for present-day rates in most urban centres in North America. Such a level of incidence can be translated into a life-time cumulative risk approaching 10%.

Genital warts are acquired via sexual activity and affect mostly young adults. Low-oncogenic-risk HPVs, particularly of types 6 and 11, the causal agents of condyloma acuminatum, are readily transmitted via breaches in the epithe-lium, which allow the viruses to reach the basal layer cells. Patients with genital warts tend to report more often than controls of the same age a history of multiple sexual partners [4–6]. Autoinoculation is also a likely source of multicentric disease, especially among those who are immunosuppressed. Renal allograft patients have an increased risk of developing condylomata [7,8], as do human immunodeficiency virus-infected individuals [9,10].

Pregnancy exerts a transitory immunosuppression that has been imputed as the cause of condyloma recrudescence [11]. Moreover, long-term use of oral contraceptives also increases the risk of genital warts [5,12], possibly mediated via a lowered immune response to HPVs.

Cigarette smoking is a correlate of risk for condylomata [5] and for subclinical genital HPV infection, although not all studies have uniformly confirmed the association [13]. A recent study found a moderate but significant correlation between the amount of alcoholic beverage consumed and risk of genital warts that persisted after adjustment for potential confounders [14]. A key concern in demonstrating an association between lifestyle and dietary variables and risk of genital HPV infection is that the confounding effect of sexual activity should be appropriately controlled for in the analysis. The difficulty, however, resides in the fact that adjustment in the analysis can only be made by proxy variables, such as age at first intercourse and number of sexual partners, leaving other dimensions of sexual behaviour uncontrolled for.

## Asymptomatic cervical HPV infection

Methods for detecting subclinical HPV infection of the cervix have evolved considerably in the last 15 years. Early molecular epidemiology studies of HPV and cervical cancer that used filter *in situ* hybridization to detect the virus found that cervical HPV infection was not associated with sexual activity variables [15–17] a paradoxical finding resulting from the inadequate specificity and sensitivity of that technique [18]. The advent of polymerase chain reaction (PCR) protocols based on the so-called consensus primers [19,20] has minimized the problem of HPV measurement errors in epidemiological studies.

Cervical HPV infection detected by PCR techniques is found in 5–50% of asymptomatic women of reproductive age presenting for Papanicolaou (Pap) smear screening in different countries [21]. Molecular epidemiology surveys using PCR to detect the virus have unveiled the sexually transmitted profile of cervical HPV infection [22]. However, not all PCR-based studies conducted in different populations have uniformly reproduced these results. Their findings indicate that the association between sexual activity and overall HPV prevalence can be strong [22–24], moderate [25,26] or weak [27]. Since misclassification of HPV infection is less of a concern in these studies it is conceivable that the variability among results might be caused by differences across populations in the relative prevalence of HPV types with greater or lesser transmissibility by the sexual route.

We recently obtained evidence for different degrees of type-specific sexual transmissibility of HPV infection in two cross-sectional studies that we conducted in north-eastern Brazil [28] and in Quebec, Canada [29] – high- and low-incidence areas for cervical cancer, respectively. The Brazilian study included 525 participants in a city-wide cervical cancer screening programme (median age 40 years) in Joao Pessoa, the capital of the state of Paraiba. The Canadian study included 450 female university students (median age 22 years) presenting for routine Pap smear consultation in Montreal. In both studies we tested specimens for the presence of HPV DNA by the so-called MY09/11 L1 PCR, followed by dot blot hybridization of the amplified product with individual oligonucleotide probes specific for HPV types 6, 11, 16, 18, 26, 31, 33, 35, 39, 40, 42, 45, 51–59, 66 and 68 [30]. We analysed predictors of infection with types grouped according to the so-called low- and high-risk HPVs. We used the classification proposed by Bauer *et al.* [23], in which HPV types known to be associated with invasive cervical cancer (HPV 16, 18, 31, 33, 35, 39, 45, 51, 52, 56 and 58) formed the high-risk group, and the remaining types (HPV 6, 11, 26, 40, 42, 53–55, 57, 59, 66, 68 and unknown types) formed the low-risk group.

Table 2.1 shows the association of HPV infection with two indicators of sexual activity as investigated in the Joao Pessoa and in the Montreal studies. The differences in the magnitude of the odds ratios (OR) by oncogenic risk are substantial. In the Brazilian study, infection with low-oncogenic-risk types was only weakly associated with sexual behaviour and only among women younger than 40, whereas sexual activity variables were strong predictors of infection with HPV types classified as of high oncogenic risk, regardless of age. ORs for infection with high-risk HPV types were significantly different than unity for the highest levels of number of sexual partners, in the Joao Pessoa study, and in the highest level of frequency of sexual encounters, in the Montreal study.

**Table 2.1** Odds ratios of infection with low and high oncogenic HPV types according to indicators of sexual activity in two cross-sectional surveys of asymptomatic women conducted by the authors [28,29].

| Study location | Indicator of sexual activity | Categories | Low-oncogenic-risk types | | High-oncogenic-risk types | |
| --- | --- | --- | --- | --- | --- | --- |
| | | | Crude | Age-adjusted | Crude | Age-adjusted |
| Joao Pessoa, Brazil | Lifetime no. of sexual partners | 0–1 | 1.0 | 1.0 | 1.0 | 1.0 |
| | | 2–5 | 1.72 | 1.67 | 1.49 | 1.66 |
| | | 6–10 | 2.17 | 2.05 | 3.84 | 4.09 |
| | | 11 + | 1.63 | 1.63 | 4.49 | 5.06 |
| Montreal, Canada | Monthly frequency of sexual encounters | 0–4 | 1.0 | 1.0 | 1.0 | 1.0 |
| | | 5–13 | 1.18 | 1.20 | 1.96 | 2.17 |
| | | 14 + | 2.19 | 2.24 | 4.49 | 5.22 |

Risk of HPV infection seems also to be independently influenced by other variables, such as parity, oral contraceptive use and current smoking [23]. However, by far the most important determinant of risk of HPV infection is age, with most studies indicating a sharp decrease in prevalence after age 30. The decrease in HPV infection risk with increasing age seems to be independent of sexual activity [23,24].

In the Joao Pessoa study we found that the age-dependence of HPV infection differed by oncogenic risk. Prevalence of low-risk types tended to decrease rapidly until age 20–29 with a slower rate of decline subsequently ($P$ for trend = 0.0503). On the other hand, the prevalence of high-risk types tended to increase slowly with age ($P$ for trend = 0.0430). Since the age-dependence of HPV infection could be due to cumulative exposure via sexual activity we assessed whether the variation in HPV prevalence with age disappeared after controlling for sexual activity. Considering that sexual behaviour contains multiple dimensions, we wanted to capture the entire predictive value of our set of variables with respect to infection by the two HPV groups. The resulting information was embodied in scores computed from two individually fitted logistic regression models containing the same set of covariates (age at first intercourse, number of partners, frequency of sexual encounters, practice of anal intercourse, sexual activity postpartum, vaginal discharge and genital sores). These scores were then divided into tertiles to form strata for analysing the age-specific HPV prevalence.

Table 2.2 shows the results of this analysis. There was no indication that the prevalence of HPV infection varied by age within the individual strata formed the predictive scores, judging from the stratum-specific $P$ values for trend. The opposing trends in combined age-specific prevalence by risk category were marginally significant. However, the score-adjusted test for trend indicated that the crude negative relation between age and prevalence of low-risk types could be accounted for by sexual activity and other characteristics. Likewise, the variation in prevalence of high-risk types with age could also be largely explained by the combined dimensions of sexual activity embodied by the predictor score.

## Persistent HPV infection

Little is known about risk determinants of persistent HPV infection, since cross-sectional surveys can only probe for overall HPV infection, both transient and persistent. Such determinants can only be assessed through prospective cohort investigations with multiple cervical specimens collected over time using sensitive and specific viral assays. Hildesheim *et al.* [30] found that HPV infection is a mostly transient phenomenon. Older age (>30 years), short interval between cervical samplings and presence of an oncogenic type in the

**Table 2.2** Variation in human papillomavirus (HPV) prevalence according to age and tertile of a linear predictor score based on sexual activity variables.

| Tertile of linear score* | HPV prevalence by age group† | | | | | | P value for trend‡ | |
|---|---|---|---|---|---|---|---|---|
| | <20 | 20–29 | 30–39 | 40–49 | 50–59 | 60 + | Crude | Adjusted |
| *Low-risk HPV types* | | | | | | | | |
| 1 | 0/1 | 0/26 | 2/45 | 1/38 | 0/22 | 2/30 | 0.3935 | |
| | (0) | (0) | (4.4) | (2.6) | (0) | (6.7) | | |
| 2 | 1/2 | 1/32 | 4/38 | 8/56 | 3/29 | 1/18 | 0.9332 | |
| | (50.0) | (3.1) | (10.5) | (14.3) | (10.3) | (5.6) | | |
| 3 | 3/9 | 11/44 | 6/56 | 4/34 | 1/15 | 2/10 | 0.0864 | |
| | (33.3) | (25.0) | (10.7) | (11.8) | (6.7) | (20.0) | | |
| Total | 4/12 | 13/105 | 12/142 | 13/132 | 4/68 | 5/66 | 0.0503 | 0.3577 |
| | (33.3) | (12.4) | (8.5) | (9.8) | (5.9) | (7.6) | | |
| *High-risk HPV types* | | | | | | | | |
| 1 | 0/8 | 1/48 | 1/54 | 2/35 | 0/12 | 0/11 | 0.8919 | |
| | (0) | (2.1) | (1.9) | (5.7) | (0) | (0) | | |
| 2 | 1/4 | 3/36 | 3/48 | 6/41 | 3/22 | 2/21 | 0.6941 | |
| | (25.0) | (8.3) | (6.3) | (14.6) | (13.6) | (9.5) | | |
| 3 | 0/0 | 5/18 | 8/37 | 11/52 | 6/32 | 9/26 | 0.6097 | |
| | (—) | (27.8) | (21.6) | (21.2) | (18.8) | (34.6) | | |
| Total | 1/12 | 9/105 | 12/142 | 19/132 | 9/68 | 11/66 | 0.0430 | 0.5481 |
| | (8.3) | (8.6) | (8.5) | (14.4) | (13.2) | (16.7) | | |

* Based on logistic equation predictive for infection with each set of HPV types. See text for details.
† No. of positive/total in each combination. Percentages shown in parentheses.
‡ Crude = tertile-specific or overall unadjusted trends; adjusted = stratified by the linear score.

first specimen were independent predictors of persistence [30]. A high viral burden is also a predictor of persistence of HPV infection in subsequent samplings [31,32].

In 1993 we began an epidemiological study of the natural history of HPV infection and cervical neoplasia in a population of low-income women in São Paulo, Brazil, a high-risk area for cervical cancer. HPV testing by PCR and Pap smear cytology have been performed on multiple visits during follow-up. We have calculated the incidence of HPV infection among the first 680 women admitted, with a total follow-up of 4502 person-months. Table 2.3 shows the incidence by oncogenic risk group and of transient and persistent infections for all women and for only those who were HPV-negative at entry. Infections with high-risk types are more frequent because of the high prevalence of HPV 16 in our population. Most instances of HPV positivity represent transient infections

Among the first 435 subjects enrolled in the cohort, infections by oncogenic HPV types were 2.64 times more likely to persist than those by low-risk

**Table 2.3** Incidence of new cervical human papillomavirus (HPV) infection (per 1000 women per month) among the first 677 women enrolled in the Brazilian cohort study of the natural history of HPV infection and cervical neoplasia (4502 women-months of follow-up, mean follow-up of 6.7 months).

| Cervical HPV infection | Overall (all subjects) | Among those HPV-negative at entry |
| --- | --- | --- |
| Types of low oncogenic risk | 16.0 | 7.9 |
| Types of high oncogenic risk | 20.2 | 9.2 |
| Transient infections | 25.1 | 13.1 |
| Persistent infections with same type | 11.1 | 4.1 |

types (95% confidence interval (CI) 1.23–5.65). Viral burden assayed by quantitative PCR [33] in the first specimen seemed to predict the likelihood of 8-month persistence. The average number of viral copies per cell was 3.8 in transient infections and 111.5 in persistent infections ($P = 0.053$). Transient and persistent infections were associated with markers of sexual activity. The most important risk factor for persistence was the number of sexual partners in the last 5 years (OR = 4.1, 95% CI = 1.7–10.2, for 2 + partners versus ≤1).

## Conclusions and directions

Different HPV types causing cervical infection may vary in terms of their sexual transmissibility. Besides misclassification of HPV infection status, differences in the degree of sexual transmissibility among types may explain why some prevalence surveys have failed to demonstrate a strong association between measures of sexual activity and overall HPV infection, despite using reliable viral detection procedures.

Although there is currently great enthusiasm concerning the possible application of HPV testing as an adjunct to Pap cytology screening for cervical cancer, little is known about epidemiological determinants of cervical HPV infection besides a role for sexual activity. Over 15% of asymptomatic women who are sexually active can have HPV detected in their cervix using current PCR methods. Most of these infections are transient and are probably of little significance. The concern resides, however, in the small proportion of women who harbour persistent HPV infections. These women stand at a much greater risk of subsequent cervical neoplasia, indicating that persistent, not transient, HPV infections are the actual biological precursor in cervical carcinogenesis. Research on the epidemiology of viral persistence and on its determinants will help in the future formulation of algorithms and policies for inclusion of some form of HPV testing in cervical cancer prevention.

## References

1 Zurhausen H, Devilliers EM. Human papillomaviruses. *Ann Rev Microbiol* 1994; **48**: 427–447.

2 Franco EL. Epidemiology of anogenital warts and cancer. In: Reid R, Lorincz A (eds) *Human Papillomaviruses. Obstetrics and Gynecology Clinics of North America*. Philadelphia: W.B. Saunders, 1996, pp 597–623.

3 Chuang TY, Perry HO, Kurland LT *et al*. Condyloma acuminatum in Rochester, Minn, 1950–1978. *Arch Dermatol* 1984; **120**: 469–475.

4 Brisson J, Roy M, Fortier M *et al*. Condyloma and intraepithelial neoplasia of the uterine cervix: a case-control study. *Am J Epidemiol* 1987; **128**: 337–342.

5 Daling JR, Sherman KJ, Weiss NS. Risk factors for condyloma acuminatum in women. *Sex Transm Dis* 1986; **13**: 16–18.

6 Syrjanen K, Vayrynen M, Castren O *et al*. Sexual behaviour of women with human papillomavirus (HPV) lesions of the uterine cervix. *Br J Vener Dis* 1984; **60**: 243–248.

7 Alloub MI, Barr BB, McLaren KM *et al*. Human papillomavirus infection and cervical intraepithelial neoplasia in women with renal allografts. *BMJ* 1989; **298**: 153–156.

8 Halpert R, Fruchter RG, Sedlis A *et al*. Human papillomavirus and lower genital neoplasia in renal transplant patients. *Obstet Gynecol* 1986; **68**: 251–258.

9 Ferenczy A. External genital human papillomavirus infections. *Curr Obstet Gynaecol* 1995; **5**: 98–106.

10 Schneider A. Natural history of genital papillomavirus infections. *Intervirology* 1994; **37**: 201–214.

11 Koutsky LA, Galloway DA, Holmes KK. Epidemiology of genital human papillomavirus infection. *Epidemiol Rev* 1988; **10**: 122–163.

12 Franceschi S, Doll R, Gallwey J *et al*. Genital warts and cervical neoplasia: an epidemiological study. *Br J Cancer* 1983; **48**: 621–628.

13 Schneider A, Koutsky L. Natural history and epidemiological features of genital HPV infection. In: Muñoz N, Bosch FX, Shah KV *et al*. (eds) *The Epidemiology of Cervical Cancer and Human Papillomavirus*. Oxford: Oxford University Press, 1992, pp 25–52.

14 Bairati I, Sherman KJ, McKnight B *et al*. Diet and genital warts: a case-control study. *Sex Transm Dis* 1994; **21**: 149–154.

15 Villa LL, Franco EL. Epidemiologic correlates of cervical neoplasia and risk of human papillomavirus infection in asymptomatic women in Brazil. *J Natl Cancer Inst* 1989; **81**: 332–340.

16 Reeves WC, Brinton LA, Garcia M *et al*. Human papillomavirus infection and cervical cancer in Latin America. *N Engl J Med* 1989; **320**: 1437–1441.

17 Kjær SK, Engholm G, Teisen C *et al*. Risk factors for cervical human papillomavirus and herpes simplex virus infections in Greenland and Denmark: a population-based study. *Am J Epidemiol* 1990; **131**: 669–682.

18 Franco EL. The sexually transmitted disease model for cervical cancer: incoherent epidemiologic findings and the role of misclassificaton of human papillomavirus infection. *Epidemiology* 1991; **2**: 98–106.

19 Manos MM, Ting Y, Wright DK, Lewis AJ, Broker TR, Wolinski SM. Use of polymerase chain reaction amplification for the detection of genital human papillomaviruses. *Cancer Cells* 1989; **7**: 209–214.

20 VanDenBrule AJC, Snijders PJF, Gordijn RLJ, Bleker OP, Meijer CJLM, Walboomers JMM. General primer-mediated polymerase chain reaction permits the detection of sequenced and still unsequenced human papillomavirus genotypes in cervical scrapes and carcinomas. *Int J Cancer* 1990; **45**: 644–649.

21 IARC Working Group. *Human Papillomaviruses. IARC Monograghs on the Evaluation of*

*Carcinogenic Risks to Humans*, vol. 64, Lyon: International Agency for Research on Cancer, 1995.

22  Ley C, Bauer HM, Reingold A *et al.* Determinants of genital human papillomavirus infection in young women. *J Natl Cancer Inst* 1991; **83**: 997–1003.

23  Bauer HM, Hildesheim A, Schiffman MH *et al.* Determinants of genital human papillomavirus infection in low-risk women in Portland, Oregon. *Sex Transm Dis* 1993; **20**: 274–278.

24  Wheeler CM, Parmenter CA, Hunt WC *et al.* Determinants of genital human papillomavirus infection among cytologically normal women attending the University of New Mexico student health center. *Sex Transm Dis* 1993; **20**: 286–289.

25  Rohan T, Mann V, McLaughlin J *et al.* PCR-detected genital papillomavirus infection: prevalence and association with risk factors for cervical cancer. *Int J Cancer* 1991; **49**: 1–5.

26  Hildesheim A, Gravitt P, Schiffman MH *et al.* Determinants of genital human papillomavirus infection in low-income women in Washington, DC. *Sex Transm Dis* 1993; **20**: 279–285.

27  Kjaer SK, Devilliers EM, Caglayan H *et al.* Human papillomavirus, herpes-simplex virus and other potential risk factors for cervical cancer in a high-risk area (Greenland) and a low-risk area (Denmark): a second look. *Br J Cancer* 1993; **67**: 830–837.

28  Franco EL, Villa LL, Ruiz A, Costa MC. Transmission of cervical human papillomavirus infection by sexual activity: differences between low and high risk types. *J Infect Dis* 1995; **172**: 756–763.

29  Richardson H. *Risk factors for cervical HPV infection in female university students in Montreal.* MSc thesis, University of Quebec, 1996.

30  Hildesheim A, Schiffman MH, Gravitt PE *et al.* Persistence of type-specific human papillomavirus infection among cytologically normal women. *J Infect Dis* 1994; **169**: 235–240.

31  Ho GYF, Burk RD, Klein S *et al.* Persistent genital human papillomavirus infection as a risk factor for persistent cervical dysplasia. *J Natl Cancer Inst* 1995; **87**: 1365–1371.

32  Brisson J, Bairati I, Morin C *et al.* Determinants of persistent detection of human papillomavirus DNA in the uterine cervix. *J Infect Dis* 1976; **173**: 794–799.

33  Caballero OL, Villa LL, Simpson AJG. Low stringency-PCR (LS-PCR) allows entirely internally standardized DNA quantitation *Nucleic Acid Res* 1995; **23**: 193–203.

# 3: Geographical and Social Patterns of Cervical Cancer Incidence

## F. X. Bosch,[1] S. de Sanjosé,[1] X. Castellsagué[1] & N. Muñoz[2]

## The burden of cervical cancer in the world

Cancer of the cervix is the second most common cancer in women worldwide after cancer of the breast (excluding non-melanocytic skin cancers) and the most common in developing countries both in women and in both sexes together [1]. Each year, there are approximately 437 000 new cases of invasive cancer of the cervix diagnosed (about 12% of new cases of cancer in women) and in excess of 200 000 deaths from the disease [2]. When males and females are considered together, cancer of the cervix is the fifth most common cancer worldwide, after cancers of the lung, stomach, breast and large bowel, accounting for an estimated 5.7% of all cases of the disease.

For each death from cancer of the cervix, it has been estimated that between 14 and 20 potential years of life before 70 years of age are lost. Assuming, therefore, an average of about 17 years of life lost per death, this gives an estimate of more than 3.4 million woman-years of life before 70 years of age lost due to cancer of the cervix each year worldwide.

## Geographical distribution of cancer of the cervix

The variation in estimated crude incidence rates of invasive cancer of the cervix in the 24 United Nations areas of the world was described by Parkin *et al.* [1]. The highest rates of cancer of the cervix, with corresponding relative frequencies of between 20% and 30%, were observed to occur in the developing areas of the world, particularly parts of Asia, South America and Africa. Intermediate

[1]Servei d'Epidemiologia i Registre del Càncer, Institut Català d'Oncologia, Av. Gran Via s/n km 2.7, E-08907 Hospitalet Llobregat, Barcelona, Spain; [2]International Agency for Research on Cancer, Lyon, France.

rates were particularly evident in areas of eastern, northern and western Europe, while the lowest rates were seen in Australia and New Zealand, southern Europe, North America and western Asia (the Middle East).

Tables 3.1–3.5 show the age-adjusted incidence rates of cancer of the cervix as presented in the publication *Cancer Incidence in Five Continents*, vol. VI [3]. Finland has an anomalous low incidence of invasive cancer of the cervix, presumably because of the extensive population-wide screening carried out in that country. The association of low incidence rates of cancer of the cervix with conservative sexual behaviour in several countries at widely different levels of economic development (like Spain, Ireland, Kuwait and Israel) suggests that

**Table 3.1** Cervical cancer registration in Europe (1982–1988).

| | Cervical cancer | |
|---|---|---|
| Registry/country | AAIR | CR (%) |
| Finland | 4.4 | 0.5 |
| Netherlands* | 6.6 | 0.7 |
| Spain† | 6.7 | 0.7 |
| Italy‡ | 8.4 | 0.9 |
| Switzerland§ | 8.6 | 0.9 |
| Ireland (Eire) | 8.7 | 0.9 |
| Russia, St Petersburg | 9.8 | 1.2 |
| France‖ | 10.9 | 1.2 |
| Hungary¶ | 11.3 | 1.2 |
| Latvia | 11.3 | 1.3 |
| Belarus | 11.9 | 1.4 |
| UK, England and Wales | 11.9 | 1.2 |
| Norway | 12.7 | 1.3 |
| Slovenia | 12.7 | 1.4 |
| Scotland | 13.2 | 1.3 |
| Iceland | 13.5 | 1.3 |
| Estonia | 14.2 | 1.6 |
| Denmark | 15.9 | 1.6 |
| Romania | 16.0 | 1.7 |
| Czechoslovakia** | 17.1 | 1.7 |
| Portugal | 17.8 | 1.8 |
| Poland†† | 18.1 | 1.9 |
| Germany‡‡ | 21.8 | 2.2 |

AAIR = Age-adjusted incidence rates; CR = cumulative rate to age 74.
* Eindhoven, Maastricht.
† Basque country, Tarragona, Granada, Murcia, Navarra, Zaragoza.
‡ Florence, Genoa, Latina, Varese, Parma, Ragusa, Romagna, Torino, Trieste.
§ Basel, Geneva, Neuchâtel, St Gall, Vaud, Zurich.
‖ Bas-Rhin, Calvados, Doubs, Isère, Somme, Tarn.
¶ Szabolcs, Vas.
** Bohemia, Moravia, Slovakia.
†† Cracow city, Lower Silesia, Nowy Sacz, Opole, Warsaw city, Warsaw rural.
‡‡ GDR, Saarland.

**Table 3.2** Cervical cancer registration in Central and South America (1982–1988).

| Registry/country | Cervical cancer | |
| --- | --- | --- |
| | AAIR | CR (%) |
| USA, Puerto Rico | 11.5 | 1.2 |
| Cuba | 20.0 | 2.0 |
| France, Martinique | 24.3 | 2.6 |
| Costa Rica | 26.1 | 2.7 |
| Ecuador, Quito | 34.0 | 3.8 |
| Brazil* | 38.24 | 4.01 |
| Colombia, Cali | 42.2 | 4.7 |
| Paraguay, Asunción | 47.1 | 4.9 |
| Peru, Trujillo | 54.6 | 5.8 |

AAIR = Age-adjusted incidence rates; CR = cumulative rate to age 74.
* Goiania, Porto Alegre.

**Table 3.3** Cervical cancer registration in Africa (1986–1989).

| Registry/country | Cervical cancer | |
| --- | --- | --- |
| | AAIR | CR (%) |
| Algeria, Setif | 10.3 | |
| The Gambia | 10.5 | |
| Mali, Bamako | 23.4 | 2.4 |

AAIR = Age-adjusted incidence rates; CR = cumulative rate to age 74.

**Table 3.4** Cervical cancer registration in North America (1986–1989).

| Registry/country | Cervical cancer | |
| --- | --- | --- |
| | AAIR | CR (%) |
| USA, Japanese* | 4.0 | 0.4 |
| USA, White† | 7.3 | 0.7 |
| USA, Filipino* | 8.8 | 0.9 |
| USA, New York state‡ | 8.8 | 0.9 |
| USA, Chinese* | 9.1 | 0.9 |
| USA, Hawaii* | 10.1 | 1.0 |
| Canada | 10.2 | 1.0 |
| Bermuda§ | 10.9 | 0.9 |
| USA, Black† | 11.7 | 1.2 |
| USA, Los Angeles‖ | 17.4 | 2.2 |
| USA, Los Angeles¶ | 18.4 | 1.9 |

AAIR = Age-adjusted incidence rates; CR = cumulative rate to age 74.
* Los Angeles, Hawaii.
† Surveillance, Epidemiology, and End Results (SEER) program.
‡ New York city and state.
§ Black, white and others.
‖ Spanish surname, white.
¶ Korean.

**Table 3.5** Cervical cancer registration in Asia (1983–1987) and Oceania (1986–1989).

| Registry/country | Cervical cancer | |
| --- | --- | --- |
| | AAIR | CR (%) |
| Israel* | 4.0 | 0.4 |
| China† | 5.4 | 0.7 |
| Kuwait‡ | 7.3 | 0.8 |
| Australia§ | 10.8 | 1.1 |
| Japan‖ | 11.9 | 1.3 |
| New Zealand¶ | 12.8 | 1.3 |
| Kyrgystan | 15.6 | 1.8 |
| Singapore** | 16.3 | 1.7 |
| Hong Kong | 19.2 | 2.2 |
| Philippines†† | 23.3 | 2.6 |
| India‡‡ | 27.7 | 3.0 |
| Thailand§§ | 27.8 | 2.9 |

AAIR = Age-adjusted incidence rates; CR = cumulative rate to age 74.
* All Jews, non-Jews.
† Qidog, Shanghai, Tianjin.
‡ Kuwaitis, non-Kuwaitis.
§ Capital territory, New South Wales, South, Tasmania, Victoria, Western.
‖ Hiroshima, Myyagi, Nagasaki, Osaka, Saga, Yamagata.
¶ Maoris, non-Maoris.
** Chinese, Malay, Indian.
†† Manila, Rizal.
‡‡ Ahmedabad, Bangalore, Bombay, Madras.
§§ Chiang Mai, Khon Kaen.

economic development is not the only factor in determining the geographical variation of this disease.

## Correlation of cervical cancer incidence with the incidence rates of other cancers

The incidence of cervical cancer has been related to the incidence of cancer of the penis and other cancers of the urogenital tract of men and women [4–6]. Using the most recent standardized international incidence data [3]. Figure 3.1 shows the correlation between the age-adjusted incidence rates of cervical cancer with the incidence of other cancers in women. It shows that cervical cancer is significantly correlated (negatively) in affluent countries with the most common cancers such as colorectum, breast, lung and endometrium. Correlation values are however not very high. Positive correlations that reached statistical significance were observed between cervical cancer and placenta and other female genitalia. Consistently, significant (positive) correlations are observed with other cancers of the female genital tract and the

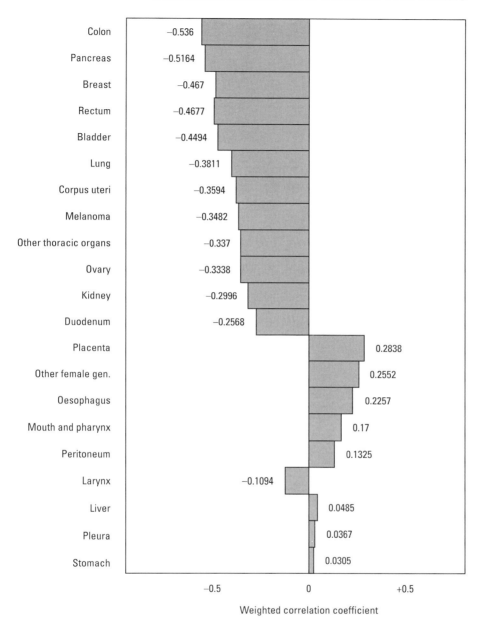

**Fig. 3.1** Correlation of the age-adjusted incidence rates of cervical cancer and other female cancers. Correlation coefficients >0.25 have a P value <0.01.

placenta. Some correlations are also observed with cancers of the oesophagus and mouth and pharynx, all of them relatively more frequent in the poorest areas of the world.

The direction of the correlation coefficients is consistent with the socioeconomic gradient described in the incidence of cervical cancer. In addition, correlations in the incidence of different cancers suggest common aetiological factors. Human papillomavirus (HPV) has now been demonstrated to be the common link for the other genital tract cases. Other hypotheses on common aetiological factors derived from correlation studies (viral, nutritional, tobacco and others) remain to be confirmed.

## Variation of cervical cancer incidence within developed countries

Figure 3.2 shows the range of age-adjusted incidence rates of cervical cancer reported by registries within a selection of developed countries. Given the difficulties in adjusting incidence rates by screening practices in most populations, intracountry comparisons may be the most reliable means of describing minor fluctuations in incidence (assuming egalitarian distribution of services and quality of the registries).

In some countries like Canada, France or Italy, 1.5 to twofold variation in incidence rates can be observed between registries. This suggests, that, in addition to the between-country variability due to differences in socioeconomic level, incidence rates can be modulated by other factors. Some of them are well known, such as within-country social class variation, and some are still poorly described, such as the differences in prevalence of HPV DNA in defined

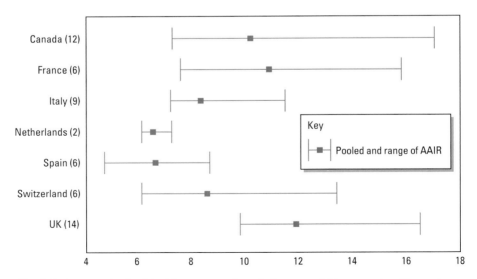

**Fig. 3.2** Age-standardized incidence rates of cervical cancer within countries. Figures in brackets are the number of registries; squares and bars show pooled data and range of age-standardized incidence rates.

subgroups, the predominant sexual behaviour patterns or the efficacy of the local screening strategies.

## Social class and cervical cancer within developed countries

The striking differences in the incidence of cervical cancer observed in developed and developing countries is also reflected by social class within developed countries. In the USA, black populations show a twofold increased incidence rate as compared to whites. In the US population, strong gradients have been reported between cervical cancer incidence, education and income [7]. A gradient by social class has also been found in some developing countries [4,8].

## The central role of human papillomavirus in the aetiology of cervical cancer

It is now established that HPV is the central aetiological factor of cervical neoplasia [9]. Studies using advanced polymerase chain reaction (PCR) technology have reported that over 95% of invasive cervical cancer cases worldwide have HPV markers. These are mostly HPV DNA (>95%) but also antibodies to HPV in the absence of viral DNA (Shah KV, personal communication; [10]).

The International Agency for Research on Cancer's (IARC's) international biological study on cervical cancer [10] suggested that the HPV-type distribution in cases is not geographically uniform. This suggestion is now being confirmed by other studies. However, if it can be assumed that the HPV-type distribution among cases reflects the distribution in the general population, it could be speculated that the geographical variability in the type-specific HPV distribution may be a contributor to the geographical variability in cervical cancer incidence. The study has also shown that the incidence of cervical cancer correlates with the prevalence among cases of the established risk factors for HPV infection, namely sexual and reproductive behaviour variables (unpublished information). Unfortunately, few population-based studies are available describing the correlations of cervical cancer incidence with the prevalence of its relevant risk factors in the population. These studies are likely to be useful to explain the striking geographical variation.

## Correlation of sexual behaviour with the incidence of cervical cancer

To explore the determinants of the geographical variation in the incidence of cervical cancer, a series of ecological analyses using routine population-based surveys [11] is being conducted. In the preliminary results there were no obvious correlations of the age-adjusted incidence rates of cervical cancer and variables such as estimates of the gross national product, fertility rates, oral contraceptive use or use of condoms (results not shown).

More relevant results are provided by some population-based studies on sexual practices recently conducted in the context of the acquired immuno-deficiency syndrome (AIDS) epidemic.

Ecological analyses of number of sexual partners of men and women support the hypothesis that sexual behaviour of men and women is associated with the risk of cervical cancer and may well be one of the main determinants of the geographical variation in incidence. Table 3.6 and Fig. 3.3 summarize a series of reports in which estimates of the average number of life-time sexual partners of men and women are related to the incidence rates of cervical cancer in their countries or in the nearest cancer registry. All the studies included in the table are based on population surveys and the incidence data are based on population-based cancer registries [3,12–17]. The correlation between the average number of sexual partners of men (range 3–40) and the incidence of cervical cancer is statistically significant. In contrast, the variability in the average number of partners reported by women (range 1.6–6.1) is insufficient to show a significant correlation with the incidence of cervical cancer. The apparently negative evidence for female sexual behaviour does not really detract from the firmly established association between the number of partners of the

**Table 3.6** Estimated average number of life-time sexual partners and age-adjusted incidence rates of cervical cancer in selected population surveys.

| Survey | Average number of sexual partners | | | Cervical cancer incidence rates |
| | Men | Women | Men/women ratio | |
|---|---|---|---|---|
| Colombia [12] | 39.5 | 5.1 | 7.7 | 42.21* |
| Denmark [15] | 13.5 | 6.1 | 2.2 | 15.93† |
| France [14] | 11.0 | 3.3 | 3.3 | 10.94‡ |
| Britain [13] | 9.9 | 3.4 | 2.9 | 11.93† |
| USA [17] | 6.3 | 2.8 | 2.3 | 7.76§ |
| Spain [12] | 12.2 | 1.6 | 7.6 | 6.68‡ |
| Utah [16] | 3.3 | 3.7 | 0.9 | 5.92† |
| Finland [17] | 7.2 | 2.9 | 2.5 | 4.40† |
| R-square‖ | 0.94 | 0.38 | 0.34 | |
| (P value) | (0.0001) | (0.11) | (0.13) | |

\* Cancer registry in the city of Cali.
† National/state cancer registries.
‡ Estimated from pooled data of available population-based cancer registries.
§ Estimated from pooled data of the US Surveillance, Epidemiology, and End Results (SEER) cancer registries.
‖ For the correlation between the corresponding variable and age-adjusted incidence rates of cervical cancer.

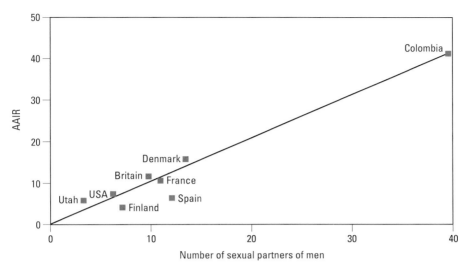

**Fig. 3.3** Correlation between the estimated average number of life-time sexual partners of men and the estimated national age-adjusted rates (AAIR) of cervical cancer. $r^2 = 0.94$ ($P = 0.0001$); $r^2$ excluding Colombia = 0.46 ($P = 0.09$).

women and cervical cancer repeatedly observed in case-control studies. It rather underlines the fact that the greatest proportion of the variability in cervical cancer incidence is attributable to differences in men's sexual behaviour.

## Cervical cancer, social class and participation in screening programmes

Mortality rates to all causes and to cancer are increased among the lower socioeconomic groups in affluent societies [18,19]. Specific studies in relation to cervical cancer have confirmed the finding. Studies in Spain and Colombia have also shown that normal women in the lower social strata have higher rates of HPV DNA and use screening services less frequently than women in the upper social levels [20,21]. Reduced participation in screening programmes in developed countries and limited or absence of screening in developing countries are likely to be major determinants of the observed geographical variation in the incidence of cervical cancer.

## Conclusion

Several studies have convincingly shown that cervical cancer is a long-term sequela of certain unresolved HPV infections of the uterine cervix. As observed for other sexually transmitted diseases, HPV infections and cervical cancer are most common in the poorest countries and among the most deprived social groups in affluent societies. The strongest known determinants of the geographical and social variations in the incidence of cervical cancer are related to the sexual behaviour patterns of the population, to lack of screening or to reduced participation of the population to the available screening programmes.

## Acknowledgements

This study was partially supported by grants from IARC, the European Community (CI 1-0371-F (CD)) and the Fondo de Investigaciones Sanitarias (FIS) of the Spanish Government (FIS 86/753, 87/1513, 88/2049, 90/0901).

## References

1 Parkin DM, Pisani P, Ferlay J. Estimates of the worldwide incidence of 18 major cancers in 1985. *Int J Cancer* 1993; **54**: 594–606.

2 Pisani P, Parkin DM, Ferlay J. Estimates of the worldwide mortality from 18 major cancers in 1985. Implications for prevention and projection of future burden. *Int J Cancer* 1993; **55**: 891–903.

3 Parkin DM, Muir CS, Whelan SL, Gao Y-T, Ferlay J, Powell J. (eds) *Cancer Incidence in Five Continents*, vol. VI. Lyon: IARC, 1992.

4 Franco EL, Campos Filho N, Villa LL, Torloni H. Correlation patterns of cancer relative frequencies with some socioeconomic and demographic indicators in Brazil: an ecologic study. *Int J Cancer* 1988; **41**: 24–29.

5 Bosch FX, Cardis E. Cancer incidence correlations. Genital, urinary and some tobacco-related cancers. *Int J Cancer* 1990; **46**: 178–184.

6 Li Y-L, Li FP, Blot WJ *et al.* Correlation between cancers of the uterine cervix and penis in China. *J Natl Cancer Inst* 1982; **69**: 1063–1065.

7 Baquet CR, Horm JW, Gybbs T, Greenwald P. Socioeconomic factors and cancer incidence among blacks and whites. *J Natl Cancer Inst* 1991; **83**: 551–557.

8 Bouchardy C, Parkin DM, Khlat M. *et al.* Education and mortality from cancer in São Paulo, Brazil. *Am Epidemiol* 1993; **3**: 64–70.

9 *IARC Monographs on the Evaluation of Carcinogenic Risks to Humans*, vol. 64. *Human Papillomaviruses*. Lyon: International Agency for Research on Cancer, 1995.

10 Bosch FX, Manos M, Muñoz N *et al.* Prevalence of human papillomavirus in cervical cancer: a worldwide perspective. *J Natl Cancer Inst* 1995; **87**: 796–802.

11 *World Health Statistics Annual*. Geneva: World Health Organization, 1994.

12 Bosch FX, Muñoz N, de Sanjosé S *et al.* Importance of the human papillomavirus endemicity in the incidence of cervical cancer: an extension of the hypothesis on sexual behavior. *Cancer Epidemiol, Biomarkers Prevent* 1994; **3**: 375–379.

13 Johnson AM, Wadsworth J, Wellings K *et al.* Sexual attitudes, lifestyles and HIV risk. *Nature* 1992; **360**: 410–412.

14 ACSF (Analyse des Comportements Sexuels en France) investigators. AIDS and sexual behaviour in France. *Nature* 1992; **360**: 407–409.

15 Melbye M, Biggar RJ. Interactions between persons at risk for AIDS and the general population in Denmark. *Am J Epidemiol* 1992; **135**: 593–602.

16 Slattery ML, Overall JC, Abbot TM *et al.* Sexual activity, contraception, genital infections, and cervical cancer: support for a sexually transmitted disease hypothesis. *Am J Epidemiol* 1989; **130**: 248–258.

17  Laumann EO, Gagnon JH, Michael RS *et al.* (eds) *The Social Organization of Sexuality.* Chicago: University of Chicago Press, 1994.

18  Pappas G, Queen S, Hadden W, Fisher G. The increasing disparity in mortality between socioeconomic groups in the United States, 1960 and 1986. *N Engl J Med* 1993; **329**: 103–109.

19  Tomatis L. Poverty and cancer. *Cancer Epidemiol, Biomarkers Prevent* 1992; **1**: 167–175.

20  de Sanjosé S, Bosch FX, Muñoz N *et al.* Socioeconomic differences in cervical cancer: two case-control studies in Colombia and Spain. *Am J Public Health* 1996; **86**: 1532–1538.

21  Cuello C, Correa P, Haenszel W. Socio-economic class differences in cancer incidence in Cali, Colombia. *Int J Cancer* 1982; **29**: 637–643.

# 4: The Male Role in Cervical Carcinogenesis: Lessons from the Studies in Colombia and Spain and a Challenge for the Future

F. X. Bosch,[1] N. Muñoz,[2] X. Castellsagué,[1]
S. de Sanjosé[1] & K. V. Shah[3]

## Summary

The studies in Spain and Colombia conducted by the International Agency for Research on Cancer (IARC) have shown a strong relationship between human papillomavirus (HPV) DNA in the penis and the risk of cervical cancer in their wives. The risk is mediated by a reported high number of sexual partners and by sexual contacts with prostitutes. The component of the study in Colombia also suggests that HPV DNA infections in the high-risk populations in Colombia may be extremely common. This indication needs confirmation.

## Introduction

In 1982, a model was proposed whereby the high rates of cervical cancer in Latin America could be explained by a large number of sexual partners among males, including frequent contacts with prostitutes. This sexual behaviour pattern was paralleled by monogamy or few sexual partners among the female population [1]. Studies assessing the contribution of males' sexual behaviour and genital HPV DNA to the risk of developing cervical neoplasia have yielded inconsistent results.

Buckley and coworkers [2] reported that among self-reported monogamous women the risk of cervical cancer increased to eightfold in relation to the number of sexual partners of their husbands. Most subsequent studies [3–5]

[1]Servei d'Epidemiologia i Registre del Càncer, Institut Català d'Oncologia. Av. Gran Via s/n, Km 2.7, 08907 L'Hospitalet de Llobregat (Barcelona), Spain; [2]FIS Unit, International Agency for Research on Cancer (IARC), Lyon, France; [3]Department of Immunology and Infectious Diseases, The Johns Hopkins University, School of Medicine, Baltimore, MD USA.

confirmed the association but other studies did not [6]. The role of contacts with prostitutes was not statistically significant in any of the relevant studies [2,4–6]. Finally, two reports using the early HPV detection assays, filter-*in-situ* [4] and Virapap (Virapap®, Digene Diagnostics Inc., Silver Spring, MD, USA) [6], failed to demonstrate any association between the presence of HPV DNA in the penis and cervical cancer.

One of the aims of the IARC's studies in Spain and Colombia was to evaluate the role of men's sexual behaviour and penile HPV DNA detection in the development of cervical cancer. The studies were conducted concurrently in Spain, a low-risk area for cervical neoplasia and in a high-incidence area in Colombia (where age-adjusted incidence rates of cervical cancer are 6.7 per 100 000 women in Spain and 42.2 per 100 000 women). The results of the studies referring to women's sexual behaviour and HPV DNA have been extensively published [7–11].

## Methods

Husbands of women participating in four case-control studies of cervical neoplasia were recruited in Spain and Colombia. The numbers were 633 in Spain, and 472 in Cali, Colombia, corresponding to 516 husbands of cases and 589 husbands of controls. Participants were interviewed to obtain information on lifestyle habits, including sexual practices. Cytological samples were taken from the distal urethra and the surface of the glans analysed by a polymerase chain reaction (PCR)-based system using a generic probe and 25 type-specific probes [12,13].

Unconditional linear logistic regression models were used to estimate odds ratios (ORs) and 95% confidence interval (CI) after controlling for the effects of potential confounders [14]. The two types of study (cervical intraepithelial neoplasia (CIN) III and invasive cervical cancer) showed very similar risk patterns and were combined in the presentation of results after adding study type as a regressor variable.

## Results

In Spain, the prevalence of HPV DNA in the penis was 17.5% among husbands of cervical cancer cases and 4% among husbands of controls. HPV DNA detection conveyed a fivefold risk of cervical cancer to their wives. The risk was ninefold for carriers of HPV 16. Risk of cervical cancer among women was strongly related to the husband's number of extramarital partners and to the number of extramarital prostitutes as sexual partners.

Presence of antibodies to *Chlamydia trachomatis* and an early age at first sexual intercourse of the husband were also associated with a threefold increase in risk of cervical neoplasia in their wives. After adjusting for these variables and the wife's pack-years of smoking, the husband's smoking was moderately associated with cervical cancer.

In Colombia, limited education and presence of antibodies to *C. trachomatis* were the only identified male risk factors for cervical neoplasia. The prevalence of HPV DNA in the penis was 25.7% among husbands of case women and 18.9% among husbands of control women, and no increased risk was detected. Neither the life-time number of sexual partners nor the life-time number of prostitutes as sexual partners was associated with the risk of cervical cancer. The same results were obtained in both countries when the analyses were restricted to monogamous women.

The key results of these studies have been published [15–17].

## Discussion

In Spain, the study supports the role of men as vectors of the HPV types that are related to cervical cancer. Life-time number of sexual partners, number of prostitutes as sexual partners and detection of HPV DNA in the penis are interpreted as surrogate markers of exposure to HPV during marriage. Our results in Colombia are compatible with the hypothesis that, in the high-risk population of Cali, exposure to HPV among young men is common (perhaps universal) and mediated by contacts with a high number of sexual partners and prostitutes. These widespread sexual practices limit the power of case-control studies to detect significant associations between men's sexual behaviour and cervical cancer risk. HPV DNA detection in the penis of adult men is a poor reflection of life-time exposure to HPV. The role of *C. trachomatis* in cervical carcinogenesis deserves further investigation.

## Conclusions and implications

Men who report multiple sexual partners or who are carriers of HPV DNA may be vectors of high-risk HPV types and place their wives at high risk of cervical cancer. Prostitutes are likely to be important reservoirs of high-risk HPVs.

In more general terms, these results strongly confirm that the HPV types related to cervical cancer are a widespread sexually transmitted disease. Furthermore, they suggest that men can operate as HPV vectors in the epidemiological chain.

Detection of HPV carriers currently requires testing for HPV DNA in exfoliated cells from the penis and a number of problems subsist.

First, sampling from the external genitalia of men is not straightforward in terms of DNA yield and in terms of the areas to be scraped. Colposcopic inspection using acetic acid painting has been recommended and minute

HPV-related lesions are often unveiled among partners of women with CIN or HPV infections. Second, there are at present no reliable treatments for HPV [18]. It has not been shown that condoms would prevent HPV transmission. Therefore there is no obvious advantage at this stage in establishing the diagnosis. Finally, cell scraping from the external genitalia is not within the established screening procedures and may be unacceptable to professionals and populations at large.

It is difficult to issue guidelines as to the clinical management of HPV-infected men and to advise on the appropriate means of interrupting HPV transmission within populations. However, any comprehensive approach to HPV control should include research to further elucidate the male role in cervical carcinogenesis, particularly in populations at high risk for cervical cancer. HPV DNA prevalence surveys and HPV natural history studies in young men will be of great value.

## Acknowledgements

This study was partially supported by grants from the IARC, the European Community (CI 1-0371-F (CD)) and the Fondo de Investigaciones Sanitarias (FIS) of the Spanish government (FIS 86/753, 87/1513, 88/2049, 90/0901).

## References

1 Skegg DCG, Corwin PA, Paul C, Doll R. Importance of the male factor in cancer of the cervix. *Lancet* 1982; **2**: 581–583.
2 Buckley JD, Harris RWC, Doll R, Vessey MP, Williams PT. Case-control study of the husbands of women with dysplasia or carcinoma of the cervix uteri. *Lancet* 1981; **II**: 1010–1015.
3 Slattery ML, Overall JC, Abbott TM, French TK, Robinson LM, Gardner J. Sexual activity, contraception, genital infections and cervical cancer: support for a sexually transmitted disease hypothesis. *Am J Epidemiol* 1989; **130**: 248–258.
4 Brinton LA, Reeves WC, Brenes MM *et al*. The male factor in the etiology of cervical cancer among sexually monogamous women. *Int J Cancer* 1989; **44**: 199–293.
5 Zunzunegui MV, King MC, Coria CF, Charlet J. Male influences on cervical cancer risk. *Am J Epidemiol* 1986; **123**: 302–307.
6 Kjaer SK, De Villiers EM, Dahl C *et al*. Case-control study of risk factors for cervical neoplasia in Denmark. I: Role of the 'male factor' in women with one lifetime sexual partner. *Int J Cancer* 1991; **48**: 39–44.
7 Muñoz N, Bosch FX, de Sanjosé S *et al*. The causal link between human papillomavirus and invasive cervical cancer: a population-based case-control study in Colombia and Spain. *Int J Cancer* 1992; **52**: 743–749.
8 Bosch FX, Muñoz N, De Sanjosé S *et al*. Human papillomavirus and cervical intraepithelial neoplasia grade III/carcinoma *in situ*: a case-control study in Spain and Colombia. *Cancer Epidemiol Biomarkers Prevent* 1993; **2**: 415–422.

9  De Sanjosé S, Muñoz N, Bosch FX *et al*. Sexually transmitted agents and cervical neoplasia in Colombia and Spain. *Int J Cancer* 1994; **56**: 358–363.

10 Bosch FX, Muñoz N, de Sanjosé S *et al*. Risk factors for cervical cancer in Colombia and Spain. *Int J Cancer* 1992; **52**: 750–758.

11 Muñoz N, Bosch FX, de Sanjosé S *et al*. Risk factors for cervical intraepithelial neoplasia grade III/carcinoma *in situ* in Spain and Colombia. *Cancer Epidemiol Biomarkers Prevent* 1993; **2**: 423–431.

12 Manos MM, Wright DK, Lewis AJ, Broker TR, Wolinsky SM. The use of polymerase chain reaction amplification for the detection of genital human papillomaviruses. In: Furth M, Greaves M (eds) *Molecular Diagnostics of Human Cancer*. Cold Spring Harbor, NY: Cold Spring Harbor Press, 1989; pp 209–214.

13 Gravitt PE, Manos MM. Polymerase chain reaction-based methods for the detection of human papillomavirus DNA. In: Muñoz N, Bosch FX, Shah KV, Meheus A (eds) *The Epidemiology of Human Papillomavirus and Cervical Cancer*. Lyon: International Agency for Research on Cancer, 1992, pp 121–133.

14 Breslow NE, Day NE. *Statistical Methods in Cancer Research*, vol. I. *The Analysis of Case-Control Studies*. Lyon: International Agency for Research on Cancer, 1980.

15 Bosch FX, Muñoz N, De Sanjosé S *et al*. Importance of human papillomavirus endemicity in the incidence of cervical cancer: an extension of the hypothesis on sexual behavior. *Cancer Epidemiol Biomarkers Prevent* 1994; **3**: 375–379.

16 Bosch FX, Castellsagué X, Muñoz N *et al*. Male sexual behavior and HPV DNA, key risk factors for cervical cancer in Spain. *J Natl Cancer Inst* 1996; **88**: 1060–1067.

17 Muñoz N, Castellsagué X, Bosch FX *et al*. Difficulty in elucidating the male role in Colombia, a high risk area for cervical cancer. *J Natl Cancer Inst* 1996; **88**: 1068–1075.

18 Barrasso R, de Brux J, Croissant O, Orth G. High prevalence of papillomavirus-associated penile intraepithelial neoplasia in sexual partners of women with cervical intraepithelial neoplasia. *N Engl J Med* 1987; **317**: 916–923.

# 5: Statistical Issues in Studies of Human Papillomavirus Infection and Cervical Cancer

## E. L. Franco

## Summary

Important statistical issues must be considered when interpreting the association of human papillomavirus (HPV) infection with cervical cancer and its cofactors, as seen in epidemiological studies. Perhaps the most serious problem hampering the validity of much epidemiological research on risk factors for cancer and other chronic diseases is the effect of measurement error in study variables. Use of amplified viral DNA detection methods has helped solve the incoherence in results caused by the more severe misclassification of HPV positivity of early molecular epidemiology studies. However, measurement error in exposures, HPV and lesion end-points will always be present to some extent in any epidemiological study and we should be prepared to recognize its effects.

The present report also describes some of the statistical issues arising in experimental trials assessing screening effectiveness when combining HPV testing with conventional Papanicolaou (Pap) smear cytology. In addition, prospective cohort studies of HPV infection and cervical intraepithelial neoplasia (CIN) recently initiated in different countries also pose new statistical analysis challenges because of the multiple and repeated measurements that are performed over time on the same women.

## Introduction

Research on the natural history of HPV infection and CIN, the cytological precursor of invasive cervical cancer, has relied on a number of epidemiological

*Correspondence*: Professor E. L. Franco, Department of Oncology, McGill University, 546 Pine Avenue West, Montreal, QC, Canada H2W 1S6.

study designs, such as case-control, cross-sectional and cohort studies. More recently, with the impetus for using HPV testing as a tool for the secondary prevention of cervical cancer, intervention trials of screening efficacy have begun in different populations.

In all of these studies there are important statistical issues to be considered when interpreting the association of HPV infection (and its determinants) with cervical cancer and on how screening effectiveness should be gauged when combining HPV testing with conventional Pap smear cytology. Prospective cohort studies of HPV infection and CIN recently initiated in different countries also pose new statistical analysis challenges because of the multiple and repeated measurements that are performed over time on the same women. The present report describes some of these statistical challenges.

## Measurement error

To a great extent, epidemiologists have been successful in designing studies that avoid biased population sampling and in developing statistical methods that allow controlling for confounding factors. On the other hand, although measurement errors are recognized as more than a simple methodological nuisance, their biasing effects can seldom be corrected in epidemiological studies. In fact, perhaps the most serious problem hampering the validity of much of the epidemiological research on risk factors for cancer and other chronic diseases is the effect of measurement error in study variables. Those attempting to assess the effects of dietary factors on cancer risk are well aware of the difficulties involved. Epidemiological common sense has it that improper ascertainment of nutritional or any other exposures will bias estimates of relative risk (RR) generally towards the null hypothesis, if the misclassification is random and non-differential with respect to the outcome (being a case of the disease or not). If the measurement error is not random or non-differential with respect to the outcome, the direction and degree of bias are difficult to predict.

In interpreting the epidemiological profile of cervical cancer we assume that the sexual activity correlates of the disease are in reality determinants of risk for acquiring HPV infection, the earliest biological end-point in the natural history of the cervical neoplasia. Interestingly, some inconsistencies emerged in early molecular epidemiology studies of HPV and cervical cancer that used first-generation DNA hybridization methods to detect the virus. Contrary to expectations, these studies found that cervical HPV infection was not associated with sexual activity variables [1–3]–a paradoxical finding considering that cervical cancer risk is strongly associated with sexual behaviour. As shown subsequently [4,5], measurement errors of HPV infection status were the cause for these incoherent findings. Techniques to detect the presence of HPV in cervical cells have evolved considerably, from simply scoring of cytological signs of HPV to immunocytochemical staining, nucleic acid hybridization methods and the polymerase chain reaction (PCR). Modern PCR protocols based on the so-called consensus primers have become the preferred methods in recent years because of their high sensitivity and specificity for epidemiological studies [6,7]. Use of PCR has minimized the problem of misclassification of viral status in epidemiological studies.

The impact of measurement error in natural history studies of HPV and CIN can best be understood by examining simple statistical analysis scenarios in a hypothetical cohort study in which the baseline prevalence of HPV infection and cumulative risk of CIN are comparable to those of actual studies. In a previous report I analysed more complex measurement error scenarios and presented methods for correcting for differential and non-differential misclassification of HPV and CIN [8].

## Misclassification of HPV and CIN status

Figure 5.1 shows the effects of misclassification either of HPV status (Fig. 5.1a) or of cytologically determined CIN as outcome (Fig. 5.1b) on the RR gauging the magnitude of the association between HPV infection and subsequent CIN. Two hypothetical underlying associations are depicted in each graph: one with a RR of 10 and another with a RR of 100. Baseline HPV infection is specified at 20% and cumulative risk of CIN at 2.5%, levels that are comparable to the situation in many natural history investigations in the western populations studied thus far. Under conditions of perfect measurement of cytological outcome (CIN and non-CIN), it is possible to observe that increasing misclassification of baseline HPV status lead to biased estimates of RRs towards unity (Fig. 5.1a). At 10% misclassification, akin to viral testing with 90% sensitivity and 90% specificity, RRs of 10 and 100 are mistakenly estimated as being 5.8 and 18.9, respectively.

Although the biasing effects of HPV misclassification may seem appreciable, they are not as damaging to the validity of a study as misclassification of the cytological outcome, as can be seen in Fig. 5.1b. Under hypothetical conditions of perfect ascertainment of baseline HPV positivity, even moderate levels of cytological misclassification blur the statistical distinction between the strengths of the two underlying associations. At 10% misclassification, equivalent to an impressive cytological performance of 90% sensitivity and 90% specificity to detect CIN, the RRs of 10 and 100 are mismeasured as 1.7 and 1.8—estimates that are statistically indistinguishable in most studies.

## Misclassification of HPV as a covariate

Under the sexually transmitted disease model, certain sexual activity markers (e.g. life-time number of sexual partners) are predictors of risk for acquiring

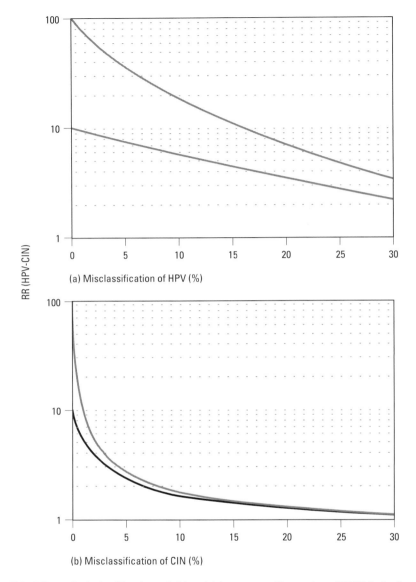

**Fig. 5.1** Effect of misclassification of either (a) human papillomavirus (HPV) infection or of (b) cervical intraepithelial neoplasia (CIN) on the relative risk (RR) estimate for the association between HPV and CIN in a hypothetical cohort study. Baseline prevalence of HPV infection is 20% and the cumulative risk of CIN is approximately 2.5%. Two independent scenarios are assumed: a RR of 10 and one of 100.

HPV infection, an intermediate variable which then influences the risk of cervical neoplasia. In this model the statistical association between sexual activity and cervical neoplasia is only present in analyses that do not control for HPV status. Adjustment of the sexual activity–cancer association for HPV infection status should make it disappear, i.e. its HPV-adjusted RR estimate should be reduced to unity.

Figure 5.2 illustrates the deleterious effect of mismeasurement of HPV status when the purpose of the analysis is to address the role of viral infection as an intermediate variable in the causal pathway between sexual activity and cervical neoplasia. The hypothetical statistical analysis scenario assumes binary variables (S for sexual activity, V for HPV infection and C for CIN) and requires the specification of conditional probabilities of being HPV-positive (V+) given a 'high' sexual activity (S+, e.g. multiple life-time sex partners versus only one) and of becoming CIN-positive (C+) given HPV infection. With the parameters specified as shown in Fig. 5.2, the underlying 'true' RRs for the S–V and V–C associations are 10 and 50, respectively. The RR for the remote association S–C is estimated as 7.4. By varying the specificity of the HPV detection test it is possible to assess the resulting bias in the adjusted RR for the S–C relation. Each curve represents a different sensitivity level for viral

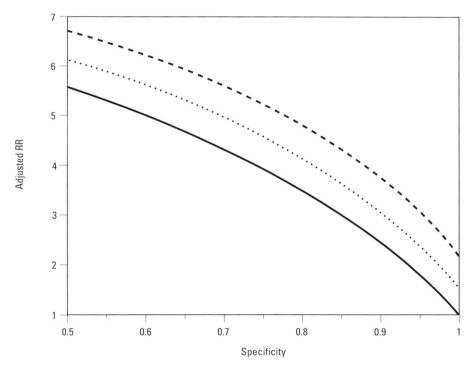

**Fig. 5.2** Relative risk (RR) for the association between sexual activity (S) and cervical cancer (C) after adjustment for misclassified HPV infection (V) when V is assumed as an intermediate variable in the causal pathway between S and C. The following conditions are assumed: prevalence of S+ = 50%; probabilities of being C+ given S+ = 50% and of being C+ given V+ = 5%; $RR_{sv}$ = 10; $RR_{vc}$ = 50. Sensitivity for detecting HPV: solid line = 99%; dotted line = 90%; broken line = 80%.

detection. Misclassification of HPV status as a covariate severely affects the ability to 'adjust away' the indirect S–C association. Even with 99% sensitivity the adjusted RR remains appreciably greater than unity for specificity levels greater than 90%. At 95% sensitivity and specificity the adjusted RR is 2.04, erroneously suggesting an independent effect for S on C.

### Can HPV infection be shown to be a necessary cause of cervical cancer?

Recent evidence from an international collaborative study indicates that meticulous testing of non-fixed cervical carcinomas by PCR results in positivity rates greater than 95% [9]. Combined testing by more than one PCR protocol and systematic testing of multiple specimens of the same primary tumour tend to increase HPV positivity to nearly 100%. Considering that the few HPV-negative tumours may represent instances of decreased detectability, one must entertain the possibility that HPV infection may turn out to be the first cause of a human cancer shown to be a necessary one [10]. In theory, it can be expected that with perfect exposure ascertainment, the RR would tend to infinity if cervical cancer could not arise from routes other than HPV infection. However, demonstration of whether or not HPV infection is necessary for cervical cancer to occur is not an easy task from an epidemiological standpoint because of measurement error in HPV detection. As above, it is possible to examine plausible statistical scenarios for the association between HPV and cervical cancer that illustrate the difficulty in gauging the magnitude of an association when misclassification is present.

Figure 5.3 shows the variation in RRs for the HPV–cervical cancer association under two scenarios: one assuming that HPV is a necessary cause and the other assuming that it is not. Variations as a function of HPV misclassification are examined in two distinct specificity levels, 90% and 99%. Although RRs between these two scenarios can be readily distinguished at low false-negative rates of at most 2%, the curves begin to converge as sensitivity becomes lower than 97%, regardless of the specificity level. This shows that the magnitude of RRs obtained in epidemiological studies of HPV and cervical cancer cannot be used to infer whether or not the exposure to HPV infection is a necessary cause of this neoplastic disease.

## HPV Testing as an adjunct to cytology screening

Frequently, when screening for a disease with a presumptive test with known sensitivity and specificity it is possible to observe that the addition of a second screening test for a separate trait of the same disease will result in increased sensitivity in detecting it. Much of the current enthusiasm about HPV testing

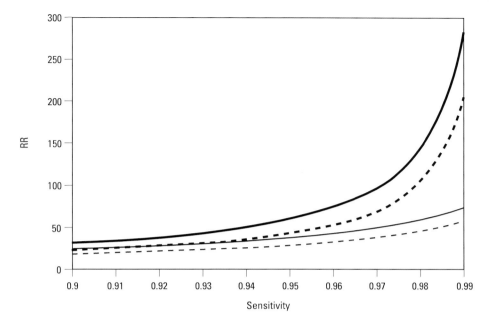

**Fig. 5.3** Effect of misclassification of human papillomavirus (HPV) infection on the relative risk (RR) for the association between HPV and cervical intraepithelial neoplasia (CIN) in a hypothetical cohort study. Two separate possibilities for a causal association are assumed: HPV is a necessary cause (thick lines) or not necessary cause (thin lines) of CIN. The following conditions are assumed: baseline prevalence of HPV infection = 25%; risk of developing CIN given HPV infection = 50%; and risks of developing CIN in the absence of HPV infection = 0% (necessary cause) or 5% (not necessary cause). Specificity for detecting HPV: solid line = 99%; broken line = 90%.

for the intermediate triage of equivocal or low-grade cervical lesions results from this perception of improved sensitivity when adding HPV testing in series to a repeat cytology. Invariably, by referring for colposcopy all women who have either a positive repeat cytology or positive HPV test result, the diagnostic yield of clinically important lesions will increase, giving the clear impression that the combined testing has greater sensitivity than cytology alone.

It can be argued, however, that the real gain is in specificity and not in sensitivity. This is because one must correct for the expected gain in sensitivity by chance alone whenever a new test is added to a previous one, even if the new test brought no new information and were totally random with respect to the attribute or disease being evaluated. In the simplest form, one could conceive of flipping a coin in tandem with Pap cytology testing. Choosing, for instance, heads to indicate positivity and combining this information with the cytology result, interpreting the combination as implying positivity if either of them is positive will invariably increase sensitivity and may give the experimenter a false sense of gain in diagnostic yield. Flipping a coin multiple times tends to produce a 50% prevalence, which is not the ideal randomization scheme to derive expected results. It is better to use a randomization scheme mimicking a hypothetical test that produces the same frequency of positive results as that given by HPV testing in the same patient population. This procedure allows us to use the proper expectation for diagnostic yield in conditions of test combinations.

In a recent study of the diagnostic performance of the Hybrid Capture HPV test combined with cytology for detecting clinically important cervical lesions, we tested women referred to colposcopy because of an abnormal Pap smear [11]. A positive repeat cytology for squamous intraepithelial lesions (SIL) was seen in 53% and a positive HPV test result was obtained in 45% of the women. Figure 5.4 shows the sensitivity and specificity of cytology alone, HPV testing alone, and of the combination of cytology and HPV in detecting

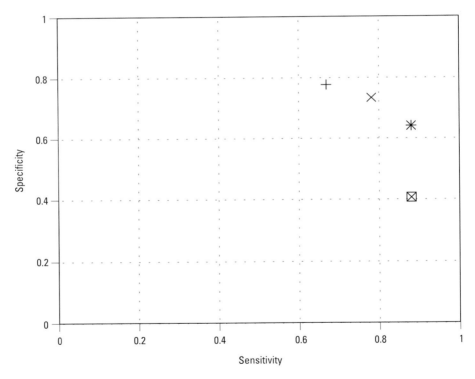

**Fig. 5.4** Sensitivity and specificity of repeat Papanicolaou (Pap) cytology alone (×), of human papillomavirus (HPV) testing alone ( + ), and of a combination of repeat cytology and HPV testing (*) to detect biopsy-confirmed squamous intraepithelial lesions (SIL) or worse lesions among women referred for colposcopy because of an initial abnormal smear. The expected diagnostic performance of a hypothetical combination of the actual repeat cytology results with an adjunct random test (⊠) is shown for comparison. Adapted from Ferenczy *et al.* [11]. See text for details.

SIL or worse lesions verified by histology. Also shown for comparison are the expected sensitivity and specificity of the combination of the two tests if the adjunct test (HPV) were totally random and unrelated to the cytological result and to the outcome (SIL present in the biopsy). Although the sensitivity of the true combination of cytology and HPV testing (87.7%; 95% confidence interval (CI) = 82.2–91.7) seems to indicate a significant gain with respect to the sensitivity of either cytology (78%) or HPV (66.3%), in isolation this interpretation is fallacious because the combination of cytology with the random chance HPV test also produces a significantly greater sensitivity of 87.8% (95% CI = 82.4–91.8). What is relevant in the actual test combination is the fact that the overall specificity (64.6%, 95% CI = 57.3–71.3) was significantly greater than that expected by chance (40.6%) using the combination of the true cytology with a random adjunct test producing the same positivity as the HPV test in this patient population. This translates in substantially improved negative predictive values for the combination of cytology and HPV over that which can be obtained by cytology or HPV testing alone.

## Repeated measurements

Most epidemiological research on the natural history of HPV infection and cervical cancer has been based on designs that require the data to be collected only once on exposure to the virus and its determinants or cofactors, and on cervical lesion end-points. Cross-sectional, case-control and cohort investigations have served a useful role in the current causal paradigm of cervical cancer using the approach of determining the baseline status for key risk factors and the putatively correlated outcomes simultaneously, retrospectively or prospectively. The statistical analysis framework for all of these designs is based on the interpretation of the direction and strength of the correlation present in $2 \times 2$ tables showing the joint frequency distributions of binary risk factor and outcome. Statistical modelling by logistic and proportional hazards regression methods enhanced enormously the ability to probe such correlations in epidemiological datasets, by allowing control of confounding, assessment of interaction among variables, and stratification by design and matching variables and by time between onset of exposure and outcome. However, behind the complexity screen that multivariate modelling brings to epidemiological data analysis, the basic $2 \times 2$ table correlating exposure and outcome remains the fundamental unit of information to generate the evidence for or against causality in an epidemiological study.

What epidemiologists have observed in recent years is that the above paradigm in study design and statistical analysis is overly simplistic to address issues of changes in risk factor status over time (e.g. acquisition of new sexual partners), viral persistence versus transience, onset of anti-HPV antibody response, and progression versus regression of cervical lesions. To understand the role and mechanism of such dynamic changes in the natural history of the disease one must conduct studies that collect data repeatedly on risk factors, HPV and cervical lesions on multiple opportunities during follow-up. The longitudinal structure of the individual resulting datasets on each group of variables can be enormously complex. Such studies pose new challenges in data management and analysis [12,13].

The goal of the statistical analysis in these longitudinal studies is the characterization of the effects of time-dependent, dynamic changes of status for outcome variables with respect to similar changes in status for predictor variables. The most important paradigm change is the elimination of the study subject as the unit of observation. A single individual may contribute observations for distinct risk factor and outcome patterns and be counted multiple times depending on the dynamic changes in study variables. This approach defies the most basic assumption of classical inferential statistics, namely, the assumption of independence of observations. In these analyses, one has to entertain the fact that the overall variation is no longer accounted for by interindividual variability only, but also by the variation among intraindividual observations. Additional assumptions have to be made because of this intra-individual correlation.

Statistical modelling methods now exist for longitudinal studies with repeated measurements over time [14,15]. For instance, they allow us to assess models in which the dependent variable can be a cytological end-point at a visit at a time $t$ and predictor variables can be both time-independent, e.g. race, age at entry, age at first intercouse, etc. and time-dependent, e.g. prior HPV results at times $t$, $t-1$, $t-2$, etc. that can be defined as states representing different definitions of persistent HPV infection. Additional time-dependent covariates, such as number of new partners in recent time intervals, e.g. $t-1-t, t-2-t-1$, etc. can be jointly specified in these models. These techniques are only now becoming part of the computational arsenal of epidemiologists working on HPV and cancer.

A number of natural history studies using repeated measurements for risk factors, HPV variables and cervical lesion end-points have begun in recent years in different populations. These studies are investigating a number of old and new laboratory markers of HPV infection, such as HPV typing, serological response, determination of viral load [13] and the analysis of molecular variants to define viral persistence better [16,17]. Monitoring of cervical lesions is done by Pap cytology augmented with cervicography in some studies. With such a powerful array of virological, immunological and cytomorphological markers we can expect that as the results from these studies are unveiled we will begin a new chapter in the epidemiology of HPV infection and cervical cancer. As epidemiologist, in addition to the challenge of making the best use of a new set of statistical tools, we will have to learn to communicate effectively to clinicians and laboratory scientists the statistical evidence originated from the increased complexity of these studies.

## Acknowledgements

E. Franco is recipient of a senior scholar award from the Fonds de la recherche en santé du Québec.

## References

1 Villa LL, Franco EL. Epidemiologic correlates of cervical neoplasia and risk of human papillomavirus infection in asymptomatic women in Brazil. *J Natl Cancer Inst* 1989; **81**: 332–340.

2 Reeves WC, Brinton LA, Garcia M *et al.* Human papillomavirus infection and cervical cancer in Latin America. *N Engl J Med* 1989; **320**: 1437–1441.

3 Kjær SK, Engholm G, Teisen C *et al.* Risk factors for cervical human papillomavirus and herpes simplex virus infections in Greenland and Denmark: a population-based study. *Am J Epidemiol* 1990; **131**: 669–682.

4 Franco EL. The sexually transmitted disease model for cervical cancer: incoherent epidemiologic findings and the role of misclassification of human papillomavirus infection. *Epidemiology* 1991; **2**: 98–106.

5 Schiffman MH, Schatzkin A. Test reliability is critically important to molecular epidemiology: an example from studies of human papillomavirus infection and cervical neoplasia. *Cancer Res* 1994; **54**: S1944–S1947.

6 Manos MM, Ting Y, Wright DK, Lewis AJ, Broker TR, Wolinski SM. Use of polymerase chain reaction amplification for the detection of genital human papillomaviruses. *Cancer Cells* 1989; **7**: 209–214.

7 VanDenBrule AJC, Snijders PJF, Gordijn RLJ, Bleker OP, Meijer CJLM, Walboomers JMM. General primer-mediated polymerase chain reaction permits the detection of sequenced and still unsequenced human papillomavirus genotypes in cervical scrapes and carcinomas. *Int J Cancer* 1990; **45**: 644–649.

8 Franco EL. Measurement errors in epidemiological studies of human papillomavirus and cervical cancer. In: Muñoz N, Bosch FX, Shah KV, Meheus A (eds). *The Epidemiology of Human Papillomavirus and Cervical Cancer*. Oxford: Oxford University Press, 1992; pp 181–197.

9 Bosch FX, Manos MM, Muñoz N *et al.* Prevalence of human papillomavirus in cervical cancer: a worldwide perspective. *J Natl Cancer Inst* 1995; **87**: 796–802.

10 Franco EL. Cancer causes revisited: human papillomavirus and cervical neoplasia. *J Natl Cancer Inst* 1995; **87**: 779–780.

11 Ferenczy A, Franco E, Arseneau J, Wright T, Richart R. Diagnostic performance of hybrid capture HPV DNA assay combined with liquid-based cytology. *Am J Obstet Gynecol* 1996; **175**: 651–656.

12 Schiffman MH. New epidemiology of human papillomavirus infection and cervical neoplasia. *J Natl Cancer Inst* 1995; **87**: 1345–1347.

13 Ho GYF, Burk RD, Klein S *et al.* Persistent genital human papillomavirus infection as a risk factor for persistent cervical dysplasia. *J Natl Cancer Inst* 1995; **87**: 1365–1371.

14 Zeger SL, Liang KY. Longitudinal data analysis for discrete and continuous outcomes. *Biometrics* 1986; **42**: 121–130.

15 Duffy SW, Rohan TE, McLaughlin JR. Design and analysis considerations in a cohort study involving repeated measurement of both exposure and outcome: the association between genital papillomavirus infection and risk of cervical intraepithelial neoplasia. *Stat Med* 1994; **13**: 379–390.

16 Franco EL, Villa LL, Rahal P, Ruiz A. Molecular variant analysis as an epidemiological tool to study persistence of cervical human papillomavirus infection. *J Natl Cancer Inst* 1994; **86**: 1558–1559.

17 Xi LF, Demers GW, Koutsky LA *et al*. Analysis of human papillomavirus type 16 variants indicates establishment of persistent infection. *J Infect Dis* 1995; **172**: 747–755.

# 6: The Epidemiological Basis for Evaluating Screening Policies

## D. M. Parkin

## The natural history of cervix cancer and screening policy

Reviewing the criteria which should be fulfilled in order that screening for disease can be considered justified, Cole and Morrison [1] identified three characteristics of the disease itself:

1   It should have serious consequences.

2   The preclinical phase which is detected by the screening test should have a high prevalence among the persons screened.

3   There should be a treatment which, when applied to screen-detected disease, is more effective than treatment applied when symptoms have led to diagnosis.

Cervical cancer, in common with all malignant diseases, is certainly a serious disease. It is difficult to be certain of outcome in the absence of treatment, but 5-year survival was no more than 20% in cases seen at the Radiumhemmet in Stockholm prior to 1920 [2]. The natural history of the precursor lesions of carcinoma of the cervix has, in contrast, been the subject of intense study.

### Precursors of invasive cancer

The fact that invasive squamous cell carcinoma of the cervix (accounting for 80–90% of cancers) is preceded by recognizable precursor lesions has been known for some time. Broders [3] was probably the first to recognize carcinoma-*in-situ* as a precursor of invasive disease and Papanicolaou and Traut [4] that the condition could be diagnosed by exfoliative cytology. Later, the existence of dysplasias as precursors of carcinoma-*in-situ* was recognized [5].

*Correspondence*: D.M. Parkin, Unit of Descriptive Epidemiology, International Agency for Research on Cancer, 150 cours Albert Thomas, 69372 Lyon Cedex 08, France.

Since that time, successive nomenclatures for the sequence of pathological conditions which are considered premalignant, or preinvasive, have been introduced, ostensibly for purposes of clarity or simplification. Microscopically, this sequence is characterized by progressive dedifferentiation or atypia of epithelial cells, and progressive involvement of the full thickness of the epithelium, from the basal layer in milder lesions, to the increasingly mature squamous cells as the mucosal surface is approached. Initially, this progression was described in terms of increasing degree of dysplasia (mild, moderate, severe) and carcinoma-*in-situ*, where the full thickness of the epithelium is involved by undifferentiated cells. Of course (and not surprisingly), different degrees of dysplasia may coexist at different sites within the same cervix. But, probably because it was felt that clinicians or scientists would not understand that the two terms implied part of the same continuous process, the terminology cervical intraepithelial neoplasia (CIN) (Fig. 6.1) was introduced [6] and came progressively into use in the early 1980s.

The cytological diagnosis of these lesions was reported in terms of the grading of the smear, with grades I–IV representing increasing degrees of atypia of cells, broadly in line with the severity of the underlying histological lesion. Alternatively, the histological terms themselves were used, to imply cytological features compatible with a particular underlying histology. Recently, cytological appearance has been classified by the Bethesda system [7], and this is sometimes used to describe the histological changes in terms of high-grade or low-grade squamous intraepithelial lesions (SIL).

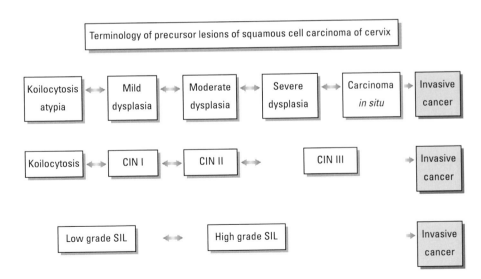

**Fig. 6.1** Natural history of cervical cancer: terminology of precursor lesions of squamous cell carcinoma of cervix.

The category 'low-grade SIL' also includes the cytological diagnosis of koilocytotic atypia, which corresponds to histological changes characteristic of infection with human papillomavirus (HPV) – koilocytosis or frank condylomatous change. Prospective studies have shown that cytologically normal women infected with HPV have a high risk of progressing to SIL/CIN, and that infections with the so-called oncogenic subtypes (16, 18, 31, 33, 35 etc.) predict an elevated risk of progression to high-grade SIL/CIN II–III [8–11].

The prevalence and incidence of preinvasive lesions in different populations must be estimated from the results of screening programmes (bearing in mind that women tested in such programmes may not be entirely representative). Prevalence is determined from tests in women screened for the first time; incidence is estimated from cases detected in previously screened women (assumed to be negative), and relating these to person-years of follow-up [12]. Most studies are cross-sectional in nature, but some [13] do provide estimates of incidence and prevalence in specific birth cohorts.

Figure 6.2 [14] illustrates results of seven studies of age-specific prevalence of carcinoma-*in-situ* in different populations. The actual values have been scaled to the same peak value, but the shape of the curves and age of maximum prevalence (35–40 years) are remarkably similar in all populations.

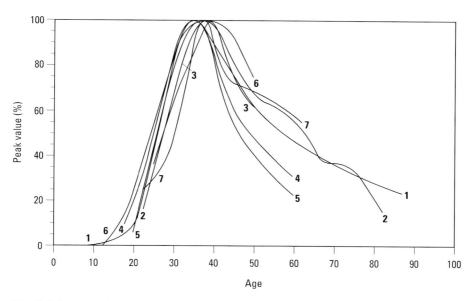

**Fig. 6.2** Age-specific prevalence rates of cancer-*in-situ* as percentage of peak value. Results from: (1) Sweden [88]; (2 and 3) British Columbia [13,52]; (4) Chicago [20]; (5) Leeds/ Wakefield in the UK [89]; (6) USA [90] and (7) Barbados [91]. (Figures smoothed by splines.) From Gustafsson and Adami [14] with permission.

## Progression and regression of precursor lesions: premalignant potential

From the point of view of formulating screening policies, it is important to know the malignant potential of the various precursor lesions. However, since they have long been recognized as posing an enhanced risk of cancer, there has been no opportunity to conduct coherent follow-up studies of the uninterrupted natural history. Observations of untreated carcinoma-*in-situ* [15,16] suggest that a relatively high proportion – 10–15% – will progress to invasive cancer within 3–5 years. Even women who have had carcinoma-*in-situ* treated by excision remained at a threefold risk of cancer in a follow-up study in Sweden [17].

Studies of lower grades of cellular abnormality are very numerous. They involve follow-up of women diagnosed histologically or cytologically by a variety of methods, with estimation of rates of progression to higher-grade, or regression to lower-grade lesions. A review of such studies has been provided by Mitchell *et al.* [18]. They are very difficult to interpret quantitatively. First, studies where lesions are diagnosed and/or followed by cytology suffer from the inevitable problem of lack of sensitivity or specificity of the cytological diagnosis. Studies which use biopsy, however, are complicated by the fact that biopsy of lesions may be curative in many cases. Finally, almost all of these studies, conducted by enthusiastic clinicians, disregard subjects lost to follow-up, and ignore duration of observation, so that *rates* of progression and regression, in relation to severity/age of subject, are almost impossible to calculate. In general terms, it is clear that the majority of low-grade lesions will regress to normal, while as the degree of cellular abnormality increases, the higher is the likelihood that such lesions will progress to *in-situ* or invasive cancer [19–22]. As a consequence, the observed cross-sectional age-specific prevalence of low-grade dysplasia greatly exceeds that of carcinoma-*in-situ* in the same population [12,13,23], and the cumulative incidence of carcinoma-*in-situ* greatly exceeds that of invasive disease [13,24].

A somewhat variant approach to defining natural history of disease has been taken by Gustafsson and Adami [25] using observed incidence of invasive and carcinoma-*in-situ* in periods pre- and post-screening in Sweden and fitting a model which was able to mimic the disturbance in the steady state of these observed parameters with the onset of screening. With some simplifying assumptions (for example, ignoring precursor lesions of a lesser grade than carcinoma-*in-situ* or severe dysplasia) parameters such as age-specific prevalence of carcinoma-*in-situ*, its mean duration (13.3 years) and the proportion progressing to invasive cancer (12.2% of incident *in-situ* cases) could be deduced.

## Design of screening programmes

The importance of these attempts to define and quantify the epidemiology of precursor lesions of invasive squamous cell carcinoma lies in the need for such data in designing optimal screening programmes which aim to interrupt this natural history. Typically, one wishes to know how to optimize a screening programme (in terms of numbers of tests, at what ages, given characteristics such as test sensitivity, specificity and attendance patterns), in order to reduce the numbers of invasive cancers, numbers of deaths from cancer, or person-years of life lost due to cancer. The large number of factors which must be simultaneously considered have prompted the use of simulation models. Initially, these were simple Markov models, in which a transition between defined states is specified in very simple terms of a fixed annual probability [24,26,27]. Unfortunately, such models, while instructive, cannot readily reproduce the observed features of the natural history of cervical cancer, and so tend to be somewhat unconvincing. An alternative approach, using micro-simulation, permits a much more flexible specification of natural history, so that observed data can be reproduced as accurately as possible (e.g. [28,29]). A different approach was adopted by Gustafsson and Adami [14,25] who developed a differential equation model describing natural history based on the use of a computerized identification technique.

Despite these disparate approaches, the findings are generally somewhat similar. Thus, with increasing numbers of tests, the marginal gains become smaller with each additional test (or unit cost). With few tests, the optimal age for screening is around the age of maximum prevalence of CIN (age 35 or so), and that as more tests are added to the schedule, the optimum age at start diminishes, but less than the addition of years for examination at older ages. The efficiency of screening, in terms of attendance for screening, test sensitivity and effectiveness of follow-up, is more important at moderate levels of screening intensity than increasing numbers of tests [14,30].

## The evaluation of established screening programmes

As described above, the basis for screening for cancer of the cervix (recognition of precursor lesions, and their identification by cytology) was recognized in the 1940s, and this approach to prevention of invasive cancer became generally accepted, and introduced, without any formal evaluation of its effectiveness by means of a randomized trial. As a result, evaluation has been based upon observational studies of established programmes. These studies do not distinguish between the relative contributions of the various components of screening – the ability of the tests to detect preclinical disease, the efficacy of treatment in preclinical compared with clinical disease and operational factors such as compliance with screening and follow-up. They do, however, indicate their combined effects in reducing the incidence of invasive cancer, and mortality from it.

**Trends in incidence, or mortality**

Because most cancer registries have been created fairly recently, those able to provide an accurate picture of the age-specific incidence of cervical cancer before the introduction of screening are relatively few. However, although the overall incidence rates (age-standardized rates, for example) vary between different countries, there are considerable similarities in the shape of the curves. Thus, incidence begins to increase at ages 20–29, and rises steeply to a peak. This is at ages 40–50 in some European countries, but a decade later in others, as well as in North America, Latin America, Asia and Africa (Fig. 6.3a). Incidence rates then decline, although the slope is less marked than that of the increase in young women.

For cancer registries providing long-term series of data, it is possible to follow the evolution of the curve of age-specific incidence rates after the introduction of screening programmes. Gustafsson *et al.* [31] have analysed the temporal changes for 17 populations. For 11 of these, there was a 25% or greater reduction in age-standardized incidence. In these registries, age-specific rates showed no change before age 30, a reduction in incidence mainly affecting ages around the peak incidence (with a resulting flattening of the curve), and progressively lesser changes in rates with age after the peak (Fig. 6.3b–e). In regions with no screening (e.g. Bombay; Fig. 6.3f), there has been no change in the curve over time. The lack of effect at young ages (when much opportunistic screening takes place in relation to pregnancy, genital infections, family planning, etc.) seems surprising. It might reflect the short natural history of cervical cancer cases appearing in young women (for which screening will be less effective). In addition, screening activity will result in earlier detection of asymptomatic invasive cancers (with diagnosis at younger ages than before). In post-menopausal women, the lack of large changes in incidence probably reflects the lower intensity of screening in older women [32], as well as the lower test sensitivity [33].

Analyses of time trends in incidence and mortality of cervical cancer in relation to the introduction of screening programmes have been published from the USA [34–36], Canada [37,38], Netherlands [39] and East Germany [40].

Several studies have related the intensity of screening in different areas to the changes in incidence or mortality from cervix cancer. Cramer [41] found a positive correlation between the decline in mortality rates and intensity of screening in different US states. Miller *et al.* [42] related an index of screening

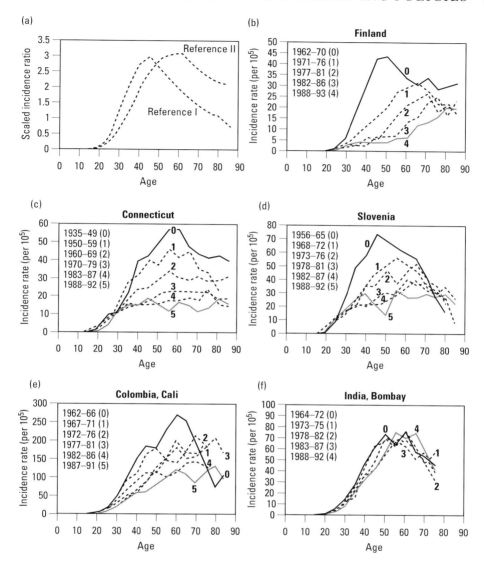

**Fig. 6.3** (a) Scaled age-specific incidence ratios for cervical cancer for time periods prior to screening. Reference I: weighted average from Denmark, Germany (Federal Republic and Democratic Republic), Netherlands, Norway, Slovenia and Sweden. Reference II: weighted average from Finland, Estonia, Latvia, Lithuania, Poland, Connecticut, Brazil, Colombia, Jamaica, Puerto Rico, Hong Kong, India, Israel, Japan, New Zealand, Singapore, Thailand and Africa. Scaling is by dividing each value by the world-standardized rate for the same population. From Gustafsson *et al.* [92]. (b–e) Age-specific incidence curves in successive time periods before (0) and after (1–5) introduction of screening. (f) Age-specific incidence curves in Bombay in five successive time periods during which minimal screening was performed.

intensity in 1966 (smears/1000 women per year) with changes in mortality from cancer of the uterus in Canadian provinces between 1960–1962 and 1970–1972, as well as for smaller geographic areas, and found that mortality declines were related to screening intensity even after adjustment for various sociodemographic variables. Lynge [43] examined data on incidence in women aged 30–59 in different counties of Denmark in relation to intensity of screening, and observed the greatest falls in incidence in those with most screening (particularly in organized programmes). In 24 counties of Sweden, Mahlck *et al*. [44] found that the declines in death rates from cervical cancer since the early 1960s were related to the intensity of screening. In common with all ecological analyses, population-level measures of exposure (here, to screening) may not give good information about the exposure of individuals within the population. Thus, the same average number of tests per woman can result from repeated screening of a small subset of the population, or from few tests in a larger proportion. It is easy to demonstrate that the expected outcome, in terms of incidence or mortality, is quite different.

The most celebrated descriptive studies are probably those comparing incidence trends in the five Nordic countries [45,46]. The extent of the decline in cumulative mortality rates was related to the coverage and extent of the organized screening programmes in the respective countries (Fig. 6.4). In Finland, Iceland and Sweden organized mass screenings have been conducted countrywide since the mid-1960s. In Finland, women between the ages of 30 and 55 years have been invited, women aged 30–49 in Sweden, while in Iceland the age range has been wider. In Denmark, about 40% of the population has been subject to organized mass screening; in Norway, fewer than 5%. It should be noted, however, that in all of the Nordic countries (except Iceland) opportunistic screening outside of the organized programme is extensive, and comprises the great majority of screening tests. In Sweden, there was no difference in the ability of organized and spontaneous screening tests to detect carcinoma-*in-situ* [47], the advantage of the former lying solely in the more appropriate age groups targeted by the organized programme, and more appropriately spaced tests (average of 3.3 years compared with 1.9 years for spontaneous smears). This observation reinforces the message of simulation modelling: that the most cost-effective programmes are those which ensure regular attendance (3–5-yearly) of a high proportion of women in the age groups at greatest risk [48].

An inevitable problem in interpreting time series data is the absence of an appropriate control group, by means of which an expected incidence (or mortality) can be calculated, for comparison with results in the screened population. Nor is any allowance usually made for changing patterns of hysterectomy – a rising prevalence of hysterectomized women would be associated with a decline in incidence in the total female population [49,50]. It is thus possible to interpret declining rates as no more than a continuation of

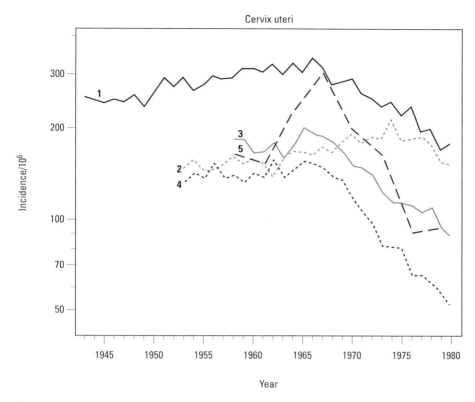

**Fig. 6.4** Trends in the age-standardized incidence of cervix cancer in the Nordic countries. 1, Denmark; 2, Finland; 3, Iceland; 4, Norway; 5, Sweden. From Hakulinen *et al.* [93] with permission.

pre-existing time trends, or a lack of change as evidence of failure of screening. Thus, the lack of a clear decline in incidence and mortality in England and Wales was widely interpreted as a failure of the programme. However, using registration data on *in situ* cancers (and on hysterectomy rates), Parkin *et al.* [32] estimated the 1978 incidence rates in England and Wales in the absence of screening (using a simple model assuming the distribution of lead-times of detected *in situ* cases). The observed increase in incidence in younger women (under age 35) between 1963 and 1978 was the result of cohort-specific increases in risk for generations born since 1931; it would have been considerably greater (50% more) in the absence of screening, and an increased incidence at older ages had been largely prevented (Fig. 6.5).

### Invasive cancer according to past history of screening

There have been rather few attempts to calculate incidence rates of invasive cervical cancer in screened and unscreened women in a prospective approach;

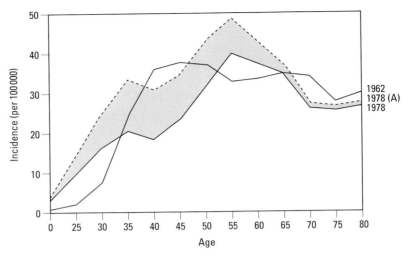

**Fig. 6.5** Annual age-specific incidence rates (per 100 000 uteri) of carcinoma of the cervix uteri in England and Wales in 1962 and 1978. For 1978, the estimated incidence in the absence of screening (A) is also shown. The shaded area represents the reduction in incidence due to screening. Data from Parkin *et al.* [32].

such studies require population registers linked to screening records, so that appropriate denominators can be calculated.

In Iceland [51] it was found that the mortality rate and incidence of advanced tumours were low among women who had had at least one negative smear and were almost zero after two negative tests; rates in the unscreened group were slightly higher than before the introduction of screening, so that the relative risk compared to the screened group was around 10. Fidler *et al.* [52] estimated the ever-screened and never-screened populations in British Columbia and calculated an age-adjusted relative risk for clinical carcinoma of 6.8 in the unscreened compared to the screened group. The screened group excluded women who developed cancer within 10 months of entering the programme (in order to exclude those cases in which the smear was taken as part of an investigation of a symptomatic tumour). Some differences may derive from the lack of comparability of the two groups. It is known, for instance, that certain risk factors for cervical cancer are associated with prior attendance at screening programmes, e.g. social class, marital status [53]. A 10-fold difference in risk, however, cannot plausibly be ascribed to confounding [54]. Furthermore, in Iceland, the unscreened group constituted about 10% of the adult female population and had a mortality rate only marginally higher than that of the general population before screening started. Self-selection for screening would have had at most a minor effect. In British Columbia, Fraser and Boyes [55] suggested that the screened group contains an excess of women of lower social class and a deficit of the sexually inactive.

Furthermore, since the proportion of the population in the screened group increased from 25% to 85% between 1961 and 1973, and assuming that women at higher risk of cancer entered later, the constant rate of invasive cancer in the screened population would not have been observed in the absence of a screening effect [56].

In Sweden, Sparen *et al.* [57] linked the population register and screening register for two counties, in order to calculate incidence rates between 1968 and 1992 in relation to screening history. Age-specific incidence rates pre-screening (1958–1967) were similar to those in the never-screened, arguing for an absence of marked selection bias – except that never-screened women under age 30 had markedly higher rates (perhaps due to increasing exposure to risk factors in recent birth cohorts). Overall, the relative risk in ever- versus never-screened was 0.55, but with much lower risks at ages 40–59 (0.27–0.38). Following a normal smear, the risk of cervical cancer remained significantly reduced for up to 10 years for women of age 50 and above, but for only 2 years for women below 50 years of age. This finding is consistent with the low incidence of precursor lesions above 50 years of age, and implies that, in women who have screened negative up to this age, there is little point in continuing to be screened. It seems that detection of carcinoma-*in-situ* in screening programmes after age 50 is correspondingly rare [33,58].

Case-control studies of screening efficacy have been very popular since the initial pioneering study of Clarke and Anderson in 1979 [59]. However, the design and interpretation of such studies are complex (this has been the subject of several methodological papers [60–63]), and many of them have serious flaws. Ideally, the cases should represent the disease that screening is trying to prevent (invasive cancer of the cervix), with controls drawn from the same population, i.e. having the same opportunity for screening. The 'exposure' evaluated in cases and controls are the screening tests received.

A complication with respect to cervical cancer screening is that, although it aims mainly at detection and treatment of preinvasive precursor lesions (CIN, etc.), and hence to prevent invasive cancer, some of the benefit derives from detection and treatment of early, asymptomatic, invasive disease. Studying this latter component would require the cases to be confined to symptomatic cancers, advanced cancers, or even deaths from cervix cancer. However, the case group in most studies comprises all cases of cervical cancer, including cases found by screening (indeed, confining the case group to screen-detected cancers is one way of controlling for selection bias, see below). In these circumstances, screening tests at which the cancer was diagnosed should not be counted as exposure, which should include all previous tests during an interval corresponding to the preclinical detectable phase of cervical cancer. As described earlier, the natural history of cervical cancer includes a period of variable, but rather long (10 years or more) duration, during which CIN

**Table 6.1** Case control studies of the efficacy of cervical cancer screening.

| Study | Cases/controls | Source of information | Exclusions in exposure tests (cases and controls) | Result (screened) | Estimated relative risk |
|---|---|---|---|---|---|
| Clarke and Anderson (1979) [59] Toronto | 212 Hospital / 212 Neighbourhood | Interview | Symptomatic tests. Tests same year as diagnosis | 32% cases, 56% controls } within 5 years | Screened within 5 years: 0.37 |
| Raymond et al. (1984) [75] Geneva | 186 Registry / 186 Population | Records | Tests following a positive test or a sequence of two tests within 6 months | 18% cases, 38% controls } within 10 years | Screened within 10 years: 0.31 |
| Aristizabal et al. (1984) [76] Cali, Colombia | 204 Incident + 73 Prevalent / 277 Neighbourhood 277 Health centre | Interview | Tests <12 months from diagnosis | 4.3% cases, 31.0% neighbourhood, 52.0% health centre | Screened within 5 years: 0.10, 0.04 |
| La Vecchia et al. (1984) [77] Milan | 191 Hospital / 191 Hospital | Interview | Diagnostic tests | 31% cases, 64% controls | Ever/never: 0.26 |
| Macgregor et al. (1985) [78] Aberdeen | 35 Symptomatic / 175, 80 Screen-detected / 400 | Screening records | Test at diagnosis of case, and matched controls | *Symptomatic:* 66% cases, 81% controls; *Screen detected:* 48% cases, 84% controls had previous test | 0.43 (within 10 years), 0.18 |
| Berrino et al. (1986) [79] Milan | 121 Hospital / 350 Hospital | Records of cytology laboratories | Cases: test after onset of symptoms. Controls: tests after 'midpoint of study minus 4 months' | 17% cases, 25% controls | Ever/never: 0.61 |
| Wangsuphachart et al. (1987) [80] Thailand | 189 Hospital / 1023 | Interview | Tests within 6 months | 30% cases, 37% controls | Ever/never: 0.72 |

| Reference / Location | Cases | Controls | Method | Exposure | Percentage | Odds ratio |
|---|---|---|---|---|---|---|
| Celentano et al. (1988) [81] Maryland | 153 Hospital | 153 'Nominated' by cases/neighbourhood | Interview | Tests within 1 year of diagnosis | 72% cases 93% controls | Ever/never: 0.2 |
| Van der Graaf et al. (1988) [82] Nijmegen | 36 Cancer registry | 120 Community | Questionnaire | Tests < 1 year before diagnosis | 47% cases 68% controls | Ever/never: 0.32 |
| Olesen (1988) [83] Denmark | 428 Cancer registry | 428 General practitioner lists | From general practitioners (records) | Tests for symptoms Tests < 6 months pre-diagnosis | 45% cases 67% cases | Ever/never: 0.29 |
| Sobue et al. (1988) [84] Nose, Japan | 15 Deaths | 150 Population | Records | None | 7% cases 20% controls } within 10 years | 0.22 } within 10 years |
|  | 28 Cases (registry) | 272 Population | Records | Diagnostic tests. Positive tests | 25% cases 38% controls } within 10 years | 0.41 |
| Zhang et al. (1989) [85] Jing-An, China | 119 From a cohort study | 545 | Records | Tests at diagnosis of case | 94% cases 99% controls } within 6 years | 0.13 within 6 years |
| Shy et al. (1989) [86] West Washington State | 92 Symptomatic cases at stage 1b or more Cancer registry | 178 RDD | Interview | Tests at diagnosis of case | 85% cases 93% controls } within 10 years | 0.44 within 10 years |
| Herrero et al. (1992) [68] Bogota, Mexico City, Costa Rica, Panama | 759 Hospital | 1430 Hospital (mainly) and community | Interview | Tests within 1 year of interview | 51% cases 71% controls | 0.40 ever/never |
| Sasieni et al. (1996) [87] 24 British districts | 258 Cases (invasive) | 677 Population matched by general practitioner or district | Screening records | Tests within 6 months of diagnosis | 51% cases 71% controls | 0.51 ever/never (0.42 at age <65) |

RDD, random digit dialling.

lesions are present. It is conventional to exclude tests after the first one found to be positive, since a positive test is often followed by one or more confirmatory tests, prior to definitive diagnostic procedures, and these cannot be considered as screening tests. It is important to exclude Papanicolaou (Pap) smears performed for diagnostic purposes — because of symptoms — since if they are included the cases will have an apparent excess of screening tests. However, because it is very often difficult to decide the motivation for a Pap test (on the part of the subject and/or the examiner), exclusion of symptomatic or diagnostic tests is difficult, and many investigators choose instead to exclude all tests within 6 months or 1 year of diagnosis in the cases, and for an equivalent period in matched controls. This will, of course, exclude some screening tests which proved to be positive, mainly in the cases, and lead to an underestimate of screening in cases and hence an overestimate of its protective efficacy. Screening history is more objectively obtained from records than from verbal reports [64], although clearly this may be difficult where there is no centralized cytology register, so that the majority of studies have relied upon interview data.

Table 6.1 summarizes case-control studies of cervical cancer screening. All of these studies show a lower risk of cervical cancer in screened compared to unscreened women. A major concern, as in all observational studies of screening, is the selection bias involved, that is, women who *choose* to be screened are at lower (or higher) risk of disease, irrespective of receiving the test. One approach to this problem has been to adjust for obvious confounders — factors related to the risk of cervical cancer which are also related to probability of being screened — usually (in addition to age) such items as socioeconomic status/education, parity, sexual history. In general, adjustment makes little difference, and in no study was the conclusion concerning the protective effect of screening changed. Weiss *et al.* [65] propose a different approach to adjusting for 'healthy screenee' bias; to confine analysis to a comparison of tests in a defined interval before diagnosis in the cases (and associated controls), and use earlier tests (which could not possibly have found an asymptomatic cancer) to control for selection bias.

Some of the case-control studies have examined the efficacy of screening in different age groups. In an extension to the Maryland study (see Celentano *et al.* Table 6.1), Klassen *et al.* [66] found that the protective efficacy of screening tests was greater in young women (age 45–64) than older (age 65–84), in whom no significant reduction in risk was seen, even for recent tests. This observation appears consistent with the descriptive data, suggesting that falls in incidence of cervical cancer post-screening are small in older women. However, the case-control studies in Toronto [59], Milan [67] and Latin America [68] did not observe any decline in the efficacy of screening in older women.

The results of observational studies may be analysed with respect to the

**Table 6.2** Geometric mean relative protection against cervical cancer in women with two or more previously negative smears (IARC, 1986).

| Months since last negative smear | Relative protection (95% CI) |
| --- | --- |
| 0–11 | 15.3 (10.0–22.6) |
| 12–23 | 11.9 (7.5–18.3) |
| 24–35 | 8.0 (5.2–11.8) |
| 36–47 | 5.3 (3.6–7.6) |
| 48–59 | 2.8 (1.9–4.0) |
| 60–71 | 3.6 (2.1–5.9) |
| 72–119 | 1.6 (0.6–3.5) |
| 120 $^+$ | 0.8 (0.3–1.6) |
| Never screened | 1.0 |

CI, Confidence interval.

level of risk at different intervals following a negative screening test, relative to an unscreened population. This is itself related to the distribution of the duration of the preclinical detectable phase [69,70]. Using the results from eight screening programmes, the International Agency for Research on Cancer (IARC) Working Group [71] calculated relative protection at different intervals following two negative tests (to exclude false-negative examinations). The results are shown in Table 6.2. The results have been used to estimate the possible outcome of screening programmes involving tests at different frequencies and ages ([72] and see Chapter 7).

It is very unlikely that cytological screening has any effect in reducing the risk of adenocarcinoma of the cervix. Adenocarcinomas occur within the cervical canal (from the glandular epithelium) and do not share the same risk factors or natural history as squamous cell tumours. Many studies show rising incidence rates of adenocarcinoma, in populations where screening has reduced the incidence of cervical cancer [73] and a case-control study [74] has shown that the risk of invasive adenocarcinoma is not reduced by screening.

## References

1 Cole P, Morrison AS. Basic issues in cancer screening. In: Miller AB (ed) *Screening in Cancer*. Geneva: UICC, 1978.
2 Heyman J. (ed) *Annual Report on the Results of Radiotherapy in Cancer of the Uterine Cervix*. Stockholm: International Federation of Gynaecology and Obstetrics, 1937.
3 Broders AC. Carcinoma *in situ* contrasted with benign penetrating epithelium. *JAMA* 1932; **99**: 1670–1674.
4 Papanicolaou GN, Traut HF. *Diagnosis of Uterine Cancer by the Vaginal Smear*. New York: Commonwealth Fund; 1943.
5 Ferenczy A, Winkler B. Cervical intraepithelial neoplasia and condyloma. In: Kurman RJ (ed) *Blausteen's Pathology of the Female Genital Tract*. New York: Springer Verlag, 1989, pp 184–191.

6  Richart RM. Cervical intraepithelial neoplasia: a review. *Pathol Annu* 1973; **8**: 302–328.

7  National Cancer Institute Workshop. The 1988 Bethesda system for reporting cervical/ vaginal cytologic diagnoses. *JAMA* 1989; **262**: 931–934.

8  Stellato G, Nieminen P, Aho H, Vesterinen E, Vaheri A, Paavonen J. Human papillomavirus infection of the female genital tract: correlation of HPV DNA with cytologic, colposcopic, and natural history findings. *Eur J Gynaecol Oncol* 1992; **13**: 262–267.

9  Campion MJ, McCance DJ, Cuzick J, Singer A. Progressive potential of mild cervical atypia: prospective cytological, colposcopic, and virological study. *Lancet* 1986; **2**: 237–240.

10  Schiffman MH, Brinton LA. The epidemiology of cervical carcinogenesis. *Cancer* 1995; **76**: 1888–1901.

11  IARC Monographs on the Evaluation of Carcinogenic Risks to Humans. *Human Papillomaviruses*. Vol. 64. Lyon: IARC, 1995.

12  Parkin DM, Hodgson P, Clayden AD. Incidence and prevalence of preclinical carinoma of cervix in a British population. *Br J Obstet Gynaecol* 1982; **89**: 564–570.

13  Boyes DA, Morrison B, Knox EG, Draper GJ, Miller AB. A cohort study of cervical cancer screening in British Columbia. *Clin Invest Med* 1982; **5**: 1–29.

14  Gustafsson L, Adami HO. Optimisation of cervical cancer screening. *Cancer Causes Control* 1992; **3**: 125–136.

15  Peterson O. Spontaneous course of cervical precancerous conditions. *Am J Obstet Gynecol* 1956; **72**: 1063–1071.

16  Kottmeier HL. Evolution and treatment of epitheliomas. *Rev Fr Gynécol Obstét* 1961; **56**: 821–825.

17  Pettersson F, Silfversward C. Diagnosis and management of cervical abnormalities. In: Hakama M, Miller AB, Day NE (eds) *Screening for Cancer of the Uterine Cervix*. Lyon, France: IARC, 1986, pp 221–237.

18  Mitchell MF, Hittelman WN, Hong WK, Lotan R, Schottenfeld D. The natural history of cervical intraepithelial neoplasia: an argument for intermediate endpoint biomarkers. *Cancer Epidemiol Biomarkers Prev* 1994; **3**: 619–626.

19  Richart RM, Barron BA. A follow-up study of patients with cervical dysplasia. *Am J Obstet Gynecol* 1969; **105**: 386–393.

20  Bibbo M, Keebler CM, Wied GL. Prevalence and incidence rates of cervical atypia. A computerized file analysis of 148 735 patients. *J Reprod Med* 1971; **6**: 184–188.

21  Nasiell K, Nasiell M, Vaclavinkova V. Behavior of moderate cervical dysplasia during long-term follow-up. *Obstet Gynecol* 1983; **61**: 609–614.

22  Nasiell K, Roger V, Nasiell M. Behavior of mild cervical dysplasia during long-term follow-up. *Obstet Gynecol* 1986; **67**: 665–669.

23  Koutsky LA, Holmes KK, Critchlow CW *et al.* A cohort study of the risk of cervical intraepithelial neoplasia grade 2 or 3 in relation to papillomavirus infection. *N Engl J Med* 1992; **327**: 1272–1278.

24  Knox EG. Ages and frequencies for cervical cancer screening. *Br J Cancer* 1976; **34**: 444–452.

25  Gustafsson L, Adami HO. Natural history of cervical neoplasia: consistent results obtained by an identification technique. *Br J Cancer* 1989; **60**: 132–141.

26  Coppleson LW, Brown B. Observations on a model of the biology of carcinoma of the cervix: a poor fit between observation and theory. *Am J Obstet Gynecol* 1975; **122**: 127–136.

27  Eddy D. *Screening for Cancer: Theory, Analysis and Design*. Englewood Cliffs, New Jersey: Prentice Hall, 1980.

28  Parkin DM. A computer simulation model for the practical planning of cervical cancer screening programmes. *Br J Cancer* 1985; **51**: 551–568.

29  van Oortmarssen GJ, Habbama JGF, Lubbe JTN, Jong GA, van der Maas PJ. Predicting the effects of mass screening for disease – a simulation approach. *Eur J Oper Res* 1981; **6**: 399–409.

30  Parkin DM, Moss SM. An evaluation of screening policies for cervical cancer in England and Wales using a computer simulation model. *J Epidemiol Commun Hlth* 1986; **40**: 143–153.

31  Gustafsson L, Ponten J, Zack M, Adami HO. *International Comparison of Screening Effects on Cancer of the Cervix Uteri*. [Personal communication, 1996.]

32  Parkin DM, Nguyen Dinh X, Day NE. The impact of screening on the incidence of cervical cancer in England and Wales. *Br J Obstet Gynaecol* 1985; **92**: 150–157.

33  Gustafsson L, Sparen P, Gustafsson M *et al*. Low efficiency of cytologic screening for cancer *in situ* of the cervix in older women. *Int J Cancer* 1995; **63**: 804–809.

34  Dickinson L, Mussey ME, Soule EH, Kurland LT. Evaluation of the effectiveness of cytologic screening for cervical cancer. I. Incidence and mortality trends in relation to screening. *Mayo Clin Proc* 1972; **47**: 534–544.

35  Christopherson WM, Lundin FE Jr, Mendez WM, Parker JE. Cervical cancer control: a study of morbidity and mortality trends over a 21-year period. *Cancer* 1976; **38**: 1357–1366.

36  Gardner JW, Lyon JL. Efficacy of cervical cytologic screening in the control of cervical cancer. *Prev Med* 1977; **6**: 487–499.

37  Boyes DA, Worth AJ, Anderson GH. Experience with cervical screening in British Columbia. *Gynecol Oncol* 1981; **12**: S143–S155.

38  Anderson GH, Boyes DA, Benedet JL *et al*. Organisation and results of the cervical cytology screening programme in British Columbia, 1955–85. *Br Med J Clin Res Ed* 1988; **296**: 975–978.

39  van der Graaf Y, Zielhuis GA, Vooijs GP. Cervical cancer mortality in the Netherlands. *Int J Epidemiol* 1988; **17**: 270–276.

40  Ebeling K, Nischan P. Organization and results of cervical cancer screening in the German Democratic Republic. *IARC Sci Publ* 1986; **76**: 251–266.

41  Cramer DW. The role of cervical cytology in the declining morbidity and mortality of cervical cancer. *Cancer* 1974; **34**: 2018–2027.

42  Miller AB, Lindsay J, Hill GB. Mortality from cancer of the uterus in Canada and its relationship to screening for cancer of the cervix. *Int J Cancer* 1976; **17**: 602–612.

43  Lynge E. Regional trends in incidence of cervical cancer in Denmark in relation to local smear-taking activity. *Int J Epidemiol* 1983; **12**: 405–413.

44  Mahlck CG, Jonsson H, Lenner P. Pap smear screening and changes in cervical cancer mortality in Sweden. *Int J Gynaecol Obstet* 1994; **44**: 267–272.

45  Hakama M. Trends in the incidence of cervical cancer in the Nordic countries. In: Magnus K (ed) *Trends in Cancer Incidence*. New York: Hemisphere Press, 1982, pp 279–292.

46  Laara E, Day NE, Hakama M. Trends in mortality from cervical cancer in the Nordic countries: association with organised screening programmes. *Lancet* 1987; **1**: 1247–1249.

47  Gustafsson L, Sparen P, Gustafsson M, Wilander E, Bergstrom R, Adami HO. Efficiency of organised and opportunistic cytological screening for cancer *in situ* of the cervix. *Br J Cancer* 1995; **72**: 498–505.

48  Hakama M, Chamberlain J, Day NE, Miller AB, Prorok PC. Evaluation of screening programmes for gynaecological cancer. *Br J Cancer* 1985; **55**: 669–673.

49  Lyon JL, Gardner JW. The rising frequency of hysterectomy: its effect on uterine cancer rates. *Am J Epidemiol* 1977; **105**: 439–443.

50  Marrett LD. Estimates of the true population at risk of uterine disease and an application

to incidence data for cancer of the uterine corpus in Connecticut. *Am J Epidemiol* 1980; **111**: 373–379.

51 Johannesson G, Geirsson G, Day N, Tulinius H. Screening for cancer of the uterine cervix in Iceland 1965–1978. *Acta Obstet Gynecol Scand* 1982; **61**: 199–203.

52 Fidler HK, Boyes DA, Worth AJ. Cervical cancer detection in British Columbia. A progress report. *J Obstet Gynaecol Br Commonw* 1968; **75**: 392–404.

53 Parkin DM, Collins W, Clayden AD. Cervical cytology screening in two Yorkshire areas: pattern of service. *Public Health* 1981; **95**: 311–321.

54 Breslow NE, Day NE. *Statistical Methods in Cancer Research. The Analysis of Case-control Studies*. Lyon: IARC, 1980.

55 Fraser BJ, Boyes DA. The benefit of screening for cancer of the cervix in British Columbia. In: Bostrom H, Larsson T, Ljungstedt N (eds) *Health Control in Detection of Cancer (Skandia International Symposia)*. Stockholm: Almqvist & Wiksell, 1976, pp 215–229.

56 Guzick DS. Efficacy of screening for cervical cancer: a review. *Am J Public Hlth* 1978; **68**: 125–134.

57 Sparen P, Gustafsson L, Hsieh CC, Yuen J, Adami HO. Pap smear screening and the risk of squamous cell cancer of the cervix: a prospective study in Sweden. 1996.

58 Van Wijingaarden WJ, Duncan ID. Rationale for stopping cervical screening in women over 50. *BMJ* 1993; **306**: 967–971.

59 Clarke EA, Anderson TW. Does screening by 'Pap' smears help prevent cervical cancer? A case-control study. *Lancet* 1979; **2**: 1–4.

60 Morrison AS. Case definition in case-control studies of the efficacy of screening. *Am J Epidemiol* 1982; **115**: 6–8.

61 Weiss NS. Control definition in case-control studies of the efficacy of screening and diagnostic testing. *Am J Epidemiol* 1983; **118**: 457–460.

62 Sasco AJ, Day NE, Walter SD. Case-control studies for the evaluation of screening. *J Chronic Dis* 1986; **39**: 399–405.

63 Weiss NS. Application of the case-control method in the evaluation of screening. *Epidemiol Rev* 1994; **16**: 102–108.

64 Gordon NP, Hiatt RA, Lampert DI. Concordance of self-reported data and medical record audit for six cancer screening procedures. *J Natl Cancer Inst* 1993; **85**: 566–570.

65 Weiss NS, McKnight B, Stevens NG. Approaches to the analysis of case-control studies of the efficacy of screening for cancer. *Am J Epidemiol* 1992; **135**: 817–823.

66 Klassen AC, Celentano DD, Brookmeyer R. Variation in the duration of protection given by screening using the Pap test for cervical cancer. *J Clin Epidemiol* 1989; **42**: 1003–1011.

67 Parazzini F, Negri E, La Vecchia C, Bocciolone L. Screening practices and invasive cervical cancer risk in different age strata. *Gynecol Oncol* 1990; **38**: 76–80.

68 Herrero R, Brinton LA, Reeves WC *et al*. Screening for cervical cancer in Latin America: a case-control study. *Int J Epidemiol* 1992; **21**: 1050–1056.

69 Walter SD, Day NE. Estimation of the duration of a pre-clinical disease state using screening data. *Am J Epidemiol* 1983; **118**: 865–886.

70 Brookmeyer R, Day NE, Moss S. Case-control studies for estimation of the natural history of preclinical disease from screening data. *Stat Med* 1986; **5**: 127–138.

71 IARC Working Group on evaluation of cervical cancer screening programmes. Screening for squamous cervical cancer: duration of low risk after negative results of cervical cytology and its implication for screening policies. *BMJ* 1986; **293**: 659–664.

72 Parkin DM. Screening for cervix cancer in developing countries. In: Miller AB, Chamberlain J, Day NE, Hakama M, Prorok PC (eds) *Cancer Screening*. Cambridge: UICC Cambridge University Press, 1991.

73 Kjaer SK, Brinton LA. Adenocarcinomas of the uterine cervix: the epidemiology of an increasing problem. *Epidemiol Rev* 1993; **15**: 486–498.

74 Mitchell H, Medley G, Gordon I, Giles G. Cervical cytology reported as negative, and risk of adenocarcinoma of the cervix: no strong evidence of benefit. *Br J Cancer* 1995; **71**: 894–897.

75 Raymond L, Obradovic M, Riotton G. [A case control study for the evaluation of the cytological detection of cancer of the cervix]. *Rev Epidemiol Sante Publ* 1984; **32**: 10–15.

76 Aristizabal N, Cuello C, Correa P, Collazos T, Haenszel W. The impact of vaginal cytology on cervical cancer risks in Cali, Colombia. *Int J Cancer* 1984; **34**: 5–9.

77 La Vecchia C, Franceschi S, Decarli A, Fasoli M, Gentile A, Tognoni G. 'Pap' smear and the risk of cervical neoplasia: quantitative estimates from a case-control study. *Lancet* 1984; **2**: 779–782.

78 Macgregor JE, Moss SM, Parkin DM, Day NE. A case-control study of cervical cancer screening in north east Scotland. *Br Med J Clin Res Ed* 1985; **290**: 1543–1546.

79 Berrino F, Gatta G, d'Alto M, Crosignani P, Riboli E. Efficacy of screening in preventing invasive cervical cancer: a case-control study in Milan, Italy. *IARC Sci Publ* 1986; **76**: 111–123.

80 Wangsuphachart V, Thomas DB, Koetsawang A, Riotton G. Risk factors for invasive cervical cancer and reduction of risk by 'Pap' smears in Thai women. *Int J Epidemiol* 1987; **16**: 362–366.

81 Celentano DD, Klassen AC, Weisman CS, Rosenshein NB. Cervical cancer screening practices among older women: results from the Maryland Cervical Cancer Case-Control Study [see comments]. *J Clin Epidemiol* 1988; **41**: 531–541.

82 van der Graaf Y, Zielhuis GA, Peer PG, Vooijs PG. The effectiveness of cervical screening: a population-based case-control study. *J Clin Epidemiol* 1988; **41**: 21–26.

83 Olesen F. A case-control study of cervical cytology before diagnosis of cervical cancer in Denmark. *Int J Epidemiol* 1988; **17**: 501–508.

84 Sobue T, Suzuki T, Hashimoto S, Yokoi N, Fujimoto I. A case-control study of the effectiveness of cervical cancer screening in Osaka, Japan. *Jpn J Cancer Res* 1988; **79**: 1269–1275.

85 Zhang ZF, Parkin DM, Yu SZ, Esteve J, Yang XZ, Day NE. Cervical screening attendance and its effectiveness in a rural population in China. *Cancer Detect Prev* 1989; **13**: 337–342.

86 Shy K, Chu J, Mandelson M, Greer B, Figge D. Papanicolaou smear screening interval and risk of cervical cancer. *Obstet Gynecol* 1989; **74**: 838–843.

87 Sasieni PD, Cuzick J, Lynch-Farmery E *et al.* Estimating the efficacy of screening by auditing smear histories of women with and without cervical cancer. *Br J Cancer* 1996; **73**: 1001–1005.

88 Gustafsson L, Adami HO. Cytology screening for the uterine cervix in Sweden evaluated by identification and simulation. *Br J Cancer* 1990; **61**: 903–908.

89 Parkin DM, Hodgson P, Clayden AD. Incidence and prevalence of preclinical carcinoma of cervix in a British population. *Br J Obstet Gynaecol* 1982; **89**: 564–570.

90 Sadeghi SB, Sadeghi FA, Robboy SJ. Prevalence of dysplasia and cancer of the cervix in a nationwide, planned parenthood population. *Cancer* 1988; **61**: 2359–2361.

91 Barron BA, Cahill MC, Richart RM. A statistical model of the natural history of cervical neoplastic disease: the duration of carcinoma *in situ*. *Gynecol Oncol* 1978; **61**: 196–205.

92 Gustafsson L, Ponten J, Bergstrom R, Adami HO. International incidence rates of invasive cervical cancer before cytological screening. *Int J Cancer* 1977 (in press).

93 Hakulinen T, Andersen A, Malker B, Pukkala E, Schou G, Tulinius H. Trends in cancer incidence in the Nordic countries. A collaborative study of the five Nordic Cancer Registries. *Acta Pathol Microbiol Immunol Scand Suppl* 1986; **288**: 1–151.

# 7: Prevention Measures in the Third World: Are they Practical?

R. Sankaranarayanan & P. Pisani

## Summary

Cancer prevention measures aim at reducing the burden of cancer which is expressed in terms of mortality, incidence, prevention, person-years of life lost and, more recently, years of life lost adjusted for disability. It has been estimated that cervical cancer is responsible for 2.8 million years of life lost in developing countries. Though cervical cancer is amenable to prevention by a variety of measures, whether or not these are practical depends upon a number of factors related to competing priorities, public health policy perceptions, sociopolitical issues, health service organization as well as infrastructure and the attitudes of the population. A general improvement in socioeconomic status and educational level of women reduces the risk of cervical cancer by altering some of the known risk factors such as age at marriage and parity. The potential use of human papillomaviral vaccines may provide a long-term approach to prevent cervical cancer, though currently it is experimental. Health education to improve the awareness of the population and professional reorientation measures may facilitate early detection, but this has to be supported by the availability of adequate treatment facilities.

Organized cytology programmes based on western models are not practical in many developing countries. Attempts to introduce such models in some developing regions have not always resulted in comparable reductions in the burden and essentially remained as low-volume, low-coverage programmes. Alternative cytology-based strategies such as low-intensity cytology (screening women aged 35+ once every 10 years or once in a life-time) and visual inspection-based strategies need to be evaluated for their efficacy and cost-

*Correspondence*: Dr R. Sankaranarayanan, Unit of Descriptive Epidemiology, International Agency for Research on Cancer, 150 cours Albert Thomas, 69372 Lyon Cedex 08, France.

effectiveness to allow prudent public health policies. In many developing countries, balanced investments in preventive and therapeutic services, as well as health education to improve the awareness of the general public, will clearly be required if the preventive measures are to be practical.

## Introduction

Cancer prevention aims at reducing the burden of cancer. The impact of preventive measures is evaluated by their effect on burden which is expressed in terms of mortality, incidence, prevalence, person-years of life lost (PYLL) and, more recently, years of life lost adjusted for disability (DALY). The world burden of cancer has been estimated in terms of incidence and mortality [1,2]. The potential for cancer prevention in general is reflected in the remarkable international differences in cancer rates [3]. Cervical cancer rates are higher in South America, Africa and Asia compared to other regions of the world (Table 7.1).

Reduction of mortality is the major objective of interventions. This can be achieved by reducing incidence through primary and secondary prevention or through effective therapy. In the case of cancer, the second option has little potential, particularly in developing countries as they require expensive, advanced technology and highly qualified expertise. Cancer care in the Third World mostly ends up as palliative therapy and pain relief indicating the inability to intervene with effective curative therapies, in view of the advanced disease presentations. Moreover, cancer therapy, even when effective, increases the prevalence of individuals requiring long-term monitoring and carrying disabilities, the cost of which to the individual is often high. When devices to modify the natural occurrence of the disease are known, prevention offers higher potential to reduce the number of deaths and to increase years of life lived in full possession of one's capacities.

Whether prevention measures are practical or not depends upon a number of factors related to the disease, public health policy perceptions and the attitudes of the population (consumers). The incidence of the disease, knowledge of causative factors, the availability of cheap and effective preventive/early detection tests, and effective treatment are the disease-related factors. Cervical cancer is one of the few cancers that satisfies all these requirements. The effectiveness of cervical cancer-preventive measures is well established in developed countries with organized screening where a dramatic decline in incidence and mortality has been observed over the last three decades [4–7].

Cancer is known as a disease of old age, but a substantial number of cases of cervical cancer occur before the age of 55, increasing the number of years of life lost, particularly in developing countries. It has been estimated that 437 000 years of life are lost in developed countries due to premature death from

**Table 7.1** Age-adjusted incidence rates of cervical cancer (per 100 000) in different regions.

| *Africa* | | *South America* | |
|---|---|---|---|
| Setif Wilaya, Algeria | 10.3 | Goiania, Brazil | 48.9 |
| The Gambia | 10.5 | Cali, Colombia | 42.2 |
| Bamako, Mali | 23.4 | Costa Rica | 26.1 |
| | | Cuba | 20.0 |
| *North America* | | Quito, Ecuador | 34.0 |
| Canada | 10.2 | Asunción, Paraguay | 47.1 |
| USA, SEER white | 7.2 | Trujillo, Peru | 54.6 |
| USA, SEER black | 11.7 | | |
| | | *Europe* | |
| *Asia* | | Belarus | 9.0 |
| Shanghai, China | 4.3 | Denmark | 15.9 |
| Hong Kong | 19.2 | Finland | 4.4 |
| Bangalore, India | 31.1 | Bas-Rhin, France | 10.9 |
| Bombay, India | 19.3 | Saarland, Germany | 10.8 |
| Madras, India | 47.2 | Iceland | 13.5 |
| Israel, Jews | 4.2 | Florence, Italy | 7.3 |
| Israel, non-Jews | 2.6 | Norway | 12.7 |
| Osaka, Japan | 13.2 | Warsaw, Poland | 16.3 |
| Kuwait, Kuwaitis | 4.1 | Slovenia | 12.7 |
| Kuwait, non-Kuwaitis | 11.7 | Basque, Spain | 5.9 |
| Manila, Philippines | 25.8 | Sweden | 8.7 |
| Singapore, Chinese | 17.5 | Basel, Switzerland | 6.2 |
| Singapore, Malay | 8.8 | England and Wales | 11.9 |
| Singapore, Indian | 12.7 | Scotland | 13.2 |
| Chiang Mai, Thailand | 29.2 | | |
| | | | |
| *Australia* | | | |
| Victoria | 10.1 | | |

Based on data from Parkin *et al*. [3].
SEER, Surveillance, Epidemiology and End Results programme.

cervical cancer or years spent with disability resulting from the disease [8]. The corresponding figure for the Third World is 2.8 million years or about six times the DALY of western countries.

Public health policy perceptions are determined by a number of factors related to the relative importance of the disease in question among an array of other common ailments (competing priorities), health care resources (fiscal, staffing and organization/infrastructure), and sociopolitical factors. Socio-cultural phenomena, education, economic status and attitudes of the public towards the disease and preventive measures affect the population acceptability and compliance.

We review the existing cervical cancer prevention programmes in the Third World and discuss the limitations which make them ineffective in order to establish practical measures to improve efficacy. However, the nature and intensity of the programmes may justifiably vary in different settings, within and among countries, as dictated by the above-mentioned factors.

## Primary prevention

Though it is well known that sexual behaviour is strongly associated with the risk of cervical cancer, implementing primary prevention by changing sexual practices is a difficult task. However, social changes and political policies aiming to improve the status and educational attainment of women should lead to some success in the primary prevention of cervical cancer.

A general improvement in socioeconomic status and educational attainment of women reduces the task of cervical cancer by altering some of the known risk factors such as age at marriage, and parity. This was partly responsible for the general reduction in incidence and mortality from cervical cancer in developed countries before the introduction of screening programmes [5] and may account for some of the decline in some developing countries. The falling cervical cancer incidence in more recent birth cohorts in Bombay over the last two decades has been attributed to increasing age at marriage and declining fertility [9].

Human papillomaviruses (HPV) have been recognized as responsible for more than 70% of the cervical cancers worldwide [10–12]. HPV DNA was detected in over 93% of cervical cancers worldwide [12]. Four types of (HPV 16, 18, 31 and 45) account for about 80% of HPV infections associated with cervical cancer. The potential use of HPV vaccines in the prevention of cervical cancers, though currently thematic, may provide a long-term approach to prevent cervical cancers in the Third World. Proper characterization of the distribution of the various HPV types in cervical cancer from different geographical areas is essential to the development of vaccination strategies to curb the burden of cervical cancer [12]. The large experience accumulated in this century on immunization programmes against communicable diseases shows that these could be made practical and very successful. Therefore, current investments should bear in mind that this option will be available in the near future for cervical cancer prevention. Efforts to promote the use of condoms, as part of acquired immunodeficiency syndrome (AIDS) control efforts, may have a beneficial impact on the incidence of cervical cancer, considering the causal role of HPV infection.

## Secondary prevention

Secondary prevention aims at reducing death from cervical cancer by early diagnosis, either at preinvasive (dysplasia/carcinoma-*in-situ*) or early invasive stage of the disease and by providing appropriate treatment. The approaches considered in the context of developing countries are health education, improving professional awareness and skills, and screening.

### Health education and professional awareness (information education campaigns)

Health education aims to improve public awareness and accessibility to health services by informing people of the risk factors of the disease, its symptoms, diagnostic and treatment methods and the locally available health facilities. Health education about risk factors should delicately avoid inducing a stigma of promiscuity and multipartner experience. The major thrust should be to counteract tendencies of denial or ignorance. A positive message on the possibility of preventing invasive cancer and the high chance of cure with early detection and treatment is aimed to encourage women to take personal measures to pursue an appropriate health behaviour. Professional orientation measures aim to improve the diagnostic and referral capability of the health-care providers by reinforcing their skills in clinical suspicion, early diagnosis, referral and treatment. This may motivate them to use the routine health care interactions to facilitate prevention and early detection.

The major improvements in survival from cervical cancer in Sweden before the introduction of screening programmes has been partly attributed to the information education measures targeted to the general public and health profession [13]. Early detection accompanied by accessible and effective therapy resulted in the reduction in mortality from cervical cancer in Sweden in the first half of this century.

In Barshi, a rural district in central India, an improved awareness created by the health workers among the predominantly illiterate villagers resulted in significant increase of subjects presenting with early cervical cancers [14]. The proportion of stage I cancers increased from 37% in 1988 to 55% in 1992 among the cases diagnosed from a region subjected to health education as compared to no change in stage distribution from the control area. In Kerala, India, hospital-based data indicated that the combined proportion of stage I and II cancers increased from 15% in 1979 to 45% in 1989 [15]. This has been attributed to improved public awareness (health education facilitated by high female literacy rate ($\sim 90\%$), wide newspaper readership and accessibility to electronic media) and professional orientation measures.

### The outcome of cytology-based programmes in some developing countries

A brief review of existing cytology-based screening and their impact on disease burden in some developing countries is worthwhile while considering the practicality of cervical cancer prevention in the Third World. Most developing country programmes are limited to offering a Papanicolaou (Pap) smear to women attending the primary health care, antenatal, gynaecology and family planning clinics in urban areas, with no organized efforts to ensure that high-risk women attend for screening, follow-up and treatment [16]. In some countries, Pap smear services are widely available, but not necessarily in an organized manner; in most countries, cytology services are less widely provided, either on opportunistic basis or on demand, with little inbuilt quality control mechanisms.

Evaluation of effectiveness was generally by time trends in incidence and mortality (with the assumption that without screening, no change would be observed) or by case-control studies. The latter estimate individual risk (of invasive cancer, or death from cancer) in relation to screening history, but the estimates will, in general, tend to inflate the magnitude of the protective effect, due to the selection bias.

In *Costa Rica*, nationwide cytology services have been available, since 1970, for women aged 15 years and above receiving obstetric and gynaecological care. Mass communication methods were used to encourage women to have annual Pap smears. Invariably, in all pelvic examinations, a smear is included [17]. In 1987, 242 219 smears were taken (287.3/1000 women above 15 years). However, most of the women above 55 years have never had cytology, as they seldom attend family planning and prenatal clinics. A wide regional variation in cervical cancer incidence has been observed [18,19]. The incidence is about twice as high in the rural coastal regions of poor socioeconomic status as in the interior urban areas. Though there is some reduction in mortality in women under 55 years, the overall crude- and age-adjusted mortality rates from cervical cancer have not decreased significantly over the last two decades [7,19]. Case-control studies, conducted in Costa Rica to evaluate cervical cancer screening, have reported that those who had had at least one smear experienced about one-half the risk of invasive cervical cancer, compared to women who had had none [17,18].

A cervical cancer screening programme initiated in *Cuba* in 1967 advised women aged 20 years and above to have Pap smears once in 2 years [20]. Pap smears, taken by a primary care nurse (1 for 800 people) in the family doctor's office, are processed in one of the 36 laboratories. It is claimed that approximately 60% of the women aged 20–60 have been screened at least once; the coverage was reportedly 73.8% among women aged 20–25, but only 20.1% for women 50 years and above. No reduction in incidence and mortality from cervical cancer has been observed so far in Cuba over the last three decades [7,20]. The age-adjusted incidence rates were 16.1, 17.1 and 20.0 during 1968–1972, 1973–1977 and 1986, respectively. The proportion of stage I cancer has steadily increased from 26% in 1982 to 50% in 1988 with a proportional decrease in stage II and III cancers [20]. However, staging information was not available for one-quarter of the cases.

An early detection programme for cervical cancer was established in *Puerto Rico* in the 1960s. This covered only metropolitan areas until 1962, but was expanded at all the health regions of the whole island thereafter and approximately 150 000 cervical smears are taken annually [21]. Pap smears are offered to females aged 15 years and above. The incidence and mortality from cervical cancer have steadily declined over the last three decades [7,22]. The average annual age-adjusted incidence rate dropped from 38 during 1950–1954 to 19.9 in 1990 and the mortality rate from 19.1 to 5.2.

In Cali, *Colombia*, cytology screening is being offered to all sexually active women through the prenatal clinics since the late 1960s and a decrease in the incidence of cervical cancer has been observed [7,23]. The age-adjusted rates were 52.9, 48.2 and 42.2 during 1972–1976, 1977–1981 and 1982–1986, respectively. A case-control study found a relative risk of 9.9 for invasive cancer among women with no history of screening, compared to apparently healthy women with history of screening [23]. In Colombia, cytology services are now widely offered in several regions.

In São Paulo, *Brazil*, though cytology screening was introduced in the 1970s and 981 000 women were examined between 1970 and 1985, no decline in incidence has been observed [7,24]. A case-control study of cervical cancer involving cases and controls from Bogota, Colombia; Costa Rica; Mexico City, Mexico; and Panama reported a relative risk of 2.5 with never having been screened [25].

In *Zimbabwe*, the national cytology service maintains facilities for examining and reporting cervical smears in Harare and Bulawayo [26]. Cytology services are provided on an opportunistic basis. In 1991, some 35 292 smears were examined, most of them coming from low-risk women. Zimbabwe has the potential to provide a Pap smear once in 3 years to all women at risk in the country and the limitations seems to be the lack of an organization rather than the availability of cytoscreeners and facilities.

In *South Africa*, Pap smear services are usually provided on demand in antenatal, postnatal, gynaecology and family planning clinics [27]. A national policy taken in 1989 to screen women once in their life-time at age 40 has not yet been implemented. The South African Institute of Medical Research organized the infrastructure to handle some 90 000 smears annually in order to provide mass screening for the female population of Soweto (Project Screen Soweto) [28]. However, the project failed due to the poor participation of the population. Between 20 000 and 32 500 smears were taken annually by the programme during 1980–1984. The lack of a planned education/awareness programme to motivate eligible women was considered to be the major reason for failure.

The marked decline in cervical cancer incidence in all age groups in Shanghai, *China* and *Hong Kong* is attributed to the cervical cytology programmes initiated in the early 1970s [7,29]. In Jingan, a high-risk rural community in China, some 22 000 women aged over 25 years (95% of the eligible population) attended for screening at least once over a 12-year period between 1974 and 1985 [30]. In a case-control study reported from this region, the relative risk of cervical cancer was found to be 0.33 in women who had had three or more smears. A mass screening programme provided by the cancer society of *Taiwan*, through some 700 gynaecological clinics throughout the country during 1974 to 1984, covered only 5.3% of the eligible women [31].

In general, most developing country programmes are low-volume, institution or commercial laboratory-based (with little inbuilt quality control measures), isolated and opportunistic ones without systematic recruitment, follow-up and treatment of women at risk. They cover a negligible proportion of women, and that too, of women at low risk and screen the low-risk women too often.

## Cytology-based programmes for developing countries

Any strategy based on cervical cytology for the control of cervical cancer in developing countries aiming at a major public health impact should take the following factors into consideration:
1   Experience from organized screening in developed countries.
2   Outcome of screening endeavours in some developing countries.
3   The following ground realities in developing countries:
    (a) low health care resources;
    (b) relatively low priority rating for cervical cancer among the health problems;
    (c) limited capability of existing staffing levels, laboratory and treatment resources in many countries.
    (d) quality control issues;
    (e) low awareness among the risk groups on cervical cancer and the Pap smear;
    (f) the need for appropriate strategies to ensure participation and follow-up attendance by the eligible subjects;
    (g) the natural history of cervical cancer.
Cervical cancer prevention methods require a pelvic examination. In many cultures in developing countries this is often unacceptable for asymptomatic women. This is a major barrier for cervical cancer prevention measures affecting participation of women as evidence shows low compliance in developing country programmes. Illiteracy and ignorance among women are other

**Table 7.2** Relative protection against cervical cancer with two or more positive smears.

| Months since last smear | Relative protection |
| --- | --- |
| 0–11 | 15.3 |
| 12–23 | 11.9 |
| 24–35 | 8.0 |
| 36–47 | 5.3 |
| 48–59 | 2.8 |
| 60–71 | 3.6 |
| 72–119 | 1.6 |
| 120 + | 0.8 |
| Never screened | 1.0 |

From Hakama *et al.* [4] with permission.

impediments. Focused awareness programmes are necessary to overcome these obstacles.

Data from developing countries indicate that more than 80% of cervical cancer occur among women 35 years or older [32,33]. The average age of women with carcinoma-*in-situ* and invasive cancer varies between 35 and 45 years and 45 and 55 years, respectively [25,32–35].

The focus in a developing country programme should be to cover women at high risk at least once and to ensure that those with abnormalities return for follow-up and treatment. Some of the theoretical considerations that emerged from the evaluation of the developed country screening programmes by the International Agency for Research on Cancer (IARC) working group also provide the justification to this [7]. The relative protection by two or more negative smears, in relation to the duration of time elapsed since the last negative smear, based on the data from eight screening programmes in developed countries is shown in Table 7.2. Using these data, the effects of different screening policies on cervical cancer incidence in Cali, Colombia in 1977–1981 have been calculated (Table 7.3) [16]. Even screening women once in a life-time at an appropriate age in low-resource countries may reduce the incidence of cervical cancer by 30% [36–38]. Theoretical benefit (as per Table 7.3) can be deduced from models, but it is not clear whether it can be achieved in reality. Randomized clinical trials would not only demonstrate feasibility and operational aspects, but also the precise preventive impact on a population offered screening.

## Visual inspection-based strategies

There is some interest in screening for cervical cancer by visual inspection of the uterine cervix of women aged 35 and above, either by the naked eye using a speculum (unaided visual inspection) or visualization of the acetic acid-

**Table 7.3** Effects on cervical cancer incidence of different screening policies

| Screening schedule | Cumulative rate per 100 000 | Reduction in incidence (%) | No. of tests |
|---|---|---|---|
| None | 3311.5 | | |
| Every 10 years, 25–64 | 1298 | 61 | 4 |
| Every 10 years, 35–64 | 1476 | 55 | 3 |
| Every 10 years, 45–64 | 1895 | 43 | 2 |
| Every 5 years, 20–64 | 544 | 84 | 9 |
| Every 5 years, 30–64 | 630 | 81 | 7 |
| Every 3 years, 20–64 | 303 | 91 | 15 |
| Every year, 20–64 | 216 | 93 | 45 |

From *Control of Cancer of the Cervix Uteri* [36] with permission, assuming incidence rates from Cali, Colombia.

impregnated cervix with the help of a simple magnifying device called a gynoscope (aided visual inspection) or without magnification (cervicoscopy). This is based on three premises:

1   Many developing countries do not have adequate facilities, even for a limited cytology approach, as described above.
2   Direct inspection of the cervix per speculum in asymptomatic women may allow detection of cancers in an early stage.
3   Treatment of such lesions will reduce morbidity and mortality from cervical cancer.

A review of visual inspection-based strategies suggests that it is still an unproven experimental approach [39] (see Chapter 48). Visual inspection-based strategies should not be considered for implementation unless their efficacy and cost-effectiveness are established in randomized trials.

## Health services, health policy factor

Monetary, staffing and hardware resources as well as the organization of health services are major factors to be considered. Currently in most developing countries the health services are predominantly provided by governments with varying extent of participation by the non-profit voluntary organizations and profit-oriented private agencies. The development and expansion (?shrinkage) of government health services are dictated by several competing priorities, political and policy perceptions of changing (political, civil) administrations and pressures from national and international financial bodies. The major orientation in health services seems to be towards maternal child health activities, general therapeutic services and control of infectious diseases.

In the case of cancer, in most countries the services are often non-equitably developed; limited, centralized establishments are oriented towards therapy.

In sub-Saharan Africa both the preventive as well as therapeutic services for cancer are only sparingly available and leave cervical cancer aside. Even in regions of the developing world with reasonably well-developed cancer health services, the preventive services are rather inadequately developed. As an example, the cancer health services in Kerala can be cited. This province in India has achieved excellent health indices and cancer services are equitably developed. Cytology services are evenly distributed, and available on demand. Though sophisticated facilities to treat invasive cervical cancer are available in six locations, colposcopy and therapeutic facilities for cervical precancers are not widely available there.

The lack of impact of cytology programmes in developing countries may also be explained by lack of or inadequate quality control measures and policies/facilities in the health services to manage the preinvasive lesions detected.

Though setting right priorities and establishing cost-effective strategies should allow rational development of balanced preventive and therapeutic cancer health services even with the limited resources and attention towards cancer care, it is not uncommon to see proportionately large amounts of resources expended for cancer therapy in hospitals serving selected populations with little public health impact. A rational development of health services is even more important in future, in view of the structural readjustment programmes forcing national governments increasingly to withdraw from service sectors. This means even fewer resources will be available to health services in future, which will force health services reorganization based on recommendations from financial institutions to achieve fiscal objectives rather than on the basis of epidemiological data reflecting the real needs of the population. Priority to disease prevention will thus assume even more importance as a public health policy in future, if governments wish to balance the health care costs and the available resources.

Unless rational insurance-based schemes are rapidly implemented, the health care costs must be increasingly met by the consumer. In the long run, empowering the consumer to take preventive action will be one among the measures to avoid overextended health services and to reduce the overall health care expenditure of the consumer.

## Conclusions

We have made an attempt to describe the rationale and the current experience with the various strategies for the control of cervical cancer in developing countries. The information and education programme using printed and electronic media can be implemented in all countries by health services. It does not involve active case-finding, as implied in the case of visual inspection of asymptomatic women, but seeks to encourage those with symptoms to seek medical attention early in the course of their disease. However, considerable care should be taken to avoid tendencies of denial and social stigma. Though it may not achieve an immediate reduction in mortality, the outcome of treatment of early-stage disease is satisfactory with good quality of life. The messages need to be clear, brief and should respect local cultures. Health education programmes could be a forerunner for screening programmes, when this is feasible for the health services to provide.

Organized cytology programmes, based on the western models, are not practical in many developing countries. The fact that smears taken outside the organized programmes account for a major proportion of overall smears in developed countries needs to be highlighted [40]. Attempts to introduce such models in some regions have not always resulted in comparable reductions in burden, as discussed earlier. Strategies based on low-intensity cytology and visual inspection need to be evaluated in trial settings for their efficacy in reducing mortality and for their cost-effectiveness. Implementation of these procedures without sufficient scientific know-how may result in depletion of the limited health care resources in the event of lack of efficacy. Randomized intervention trials, with the above approaches, should be encouraged in settings wherever this is possible. The outcome of such trials could provide valuable information for implementing cervical cancer prevention programmes in developing countries.

Empowering individuals to purchase prevention procedures seems to be another practical approach to cervical cancer prevention. Though an overutilization of low-risk groups and underutilization by high-risk groups is a distinct possibility, resulting in very little impact on disease burden, a recent report from Sweden [40] found no support for the belief that opportunistic screening selectively reaches women at low risk. This study found that the difference in efficiency between organized and opportunistic screening in the detection of carcinoma-*in-situ* was slight. The conclusion by Gustafsson *et al.* [40] that a well-conceived promotion of smear-taking initiated by women or the health-care providers might be an efficient way to stimulate prevention activities seems to have implications in the developing country environment.

## Acknowledgements

The authors gratefully acknowledge the useful comments by Dr D.M. Parkin, Chief, Unit of Descriptive Epidemiology, IARC, Lyons, France on a draft of this paper. We thank Mrs E. Bayle and Ms O. Bouvy for their help in preparing this manuscript.

## References

1 Parkin DM, Pisani P, Ferlay J. Estimates of the world-wide incidence of 18 major cancers in 1985. *Int J Cancer* 1993; **54**: 594–606.

2 Pisani P, Parkin DM, Ferlay J. Estimates of the world-wide mortality from 18 major cancers in 1985; *Int J Cancer* 1993; **55**: 891–903.

3 Parkin DM, Muir CS, Whelan SL *et al*. (eds) *Cancer Incidence in Five Continents*, vol. VI. IARC Scientific Publications no. 120. Lyon: International Agency for Research on Cancer, 1992.

4 Hakama M, Miller AB, Day NE. (eds) *Screening for Cancer of the Uterine Cervix*. IARC Scientific Publication no. 76. Lyon: International Agency for Research on Cancer, 1986.

5 Laara E, Day NE, Hakama M. Trends in mortality from cervical cancer in the Nordic countries: association with organized screening programmes. *Lancet* 1987; **i**: 1247–1249.

6 Coleman MP, Esteve J, Damiecki P, Arsalan A, Renard H. (eds) *Trends in Cancer Incidence and Mortality*. IARC Scientific Publication no. 121. Lyon: International Agency for Research on Cancer, 1993.

7 Anderson GH, Boyes DA, Benedect JL *et al*. Organization and the results of the cervical cytology screening programme in British Columbia, 1955–85. *BMJ* 1988; **296**: 975–978.

8 Murray CJL, Lopez AD. Quantifying disability: data, methods and results. In: Murray CJL, Lopez AD (eds). *Global Comparative Assessments in the Health Sector*. Geneva: World Health Organization, 1994, pp 55–95.

9 Yeole BB, Jayant K, Jussawalla DJ. Declining trend in cervical cancer incidence in Bombay, India (1964–1985). *J Surg Oncol* 1989; **42**: 267–271.

10 Muñoz N, Bosch FX, Shah KV, Meheus A (eds) *The Epidemiology of Human Papilloma Virus and Cervical Cancer*. IARC Scientific Publications no. 119. Lyon: IARC, 1992.

11 Eluf-Neto J, Booth M, Muñoz N, Bosch FX, Meijer CJLM, Walboomers JMM. HPV and invasive cervical cancer in Brazil. *Br J Cancer* 1994; **69**: 114–119.

12 Bosch FX, Manos MM, Muñoz N *et al*. Prevalence of HPV in cervical cancer; a world-wide perspective. *J Natl Cancer Inst* 1995; **87**: 796–802.

13 Ponten J, Adami HO, Bergstrom R *et al*. Strategies for global control of cervical cancer. *Int J Cancer* 1995; **60**: 1–26.

14 Jayant K, Rao RS, Nene BM, Dale PS. Improved stage at diagnosis of cervical cancer with increased awareness in a rural Indian population. *Int J Cancer* 1995; **63**: 161–163.

15 Miller AB. *Cervical Cancer Screening Programmes. Managerial Guidelines*. Geneva: World Health Organization, 1992.

16 Parkin DM. Screening for cervix cancer in developing countries. In: Miller AB, Chamberlain J, Day NE, Hakama M, Prorok PC (eds) *Cancer Screening*. Cambridge: Cambridge University Press, 1991, pp 184–198.

17 Irwin LR, Oberle MW, Rosero-Bixby L. Screening practices for cervical and breast cancer in Costa Rica. *Bull PAHO* 1991; **25**: 16–26.

18 Herrero R, Brinton LA, Hartge P *et al*. Determinants of the geographic variation of invasive cervical cancer in Costa Rica. *Bull PAHO* 1993; **27**: 15–25.

19 Sierra R, Parkin DM, Barrentes R, Bieber CA, Leiva GM, Calero NM. (eds) *Cancer in Costa Rica*. IARC Technical Report no. 1. Lyons: International Agency for Research on Cancer, 1988.

20 Cuban Inform to WHO working group on National Cancer Control Programs. Report presented in Banff, Canada, 1993. Havana: National Institute of Oncology and Radiobiology.

21  Dueno JR, Martinez I, Llauger RT. *Cancer en Puerto Rico*. Estado Libre Asociad de Puerto Rico, Departmento de Salud, Programa Control del Cancer, Registro Central del Cancer, 1980.

22  Zapata JS, Hernandez de Freer A, Castellanos R, Llauger RT, Martinez I. Cancer en Puerto Rico 1990, Departmento de Salud de Puerto Rico, 1992.

23  Aristazabal N, Cuello C, Correa P, Collazos T, Haenzel W. The impact of vaginal cytology on cervical cancer risks in Cali, Colombia. *Int J Cancer* 1984; **34**: 5–9.

24  Goes JS, Lemos LB, Donoso NF *et al*. Practical approaches to screening for cervical cancer. *Cancer Detect Prev* 1987; **10**: 265–277.

25  Herrero R, Brinton LA, Reeves WC *et al*. Screening for cervical cancer in Latin America: a case control study. *Int J Epidemiol* 1992; **21**: 1050–1056.

26  Prevention and early detection of cervical cancer, a pilot study in a district in Zimbabwe. A Government of Zimbabwe, University of Zimbabwe, World Health Organization co-operative investigation. Harare: University of Zimbabwe, 1994.

27  Fonn S, Klugman B, Dehaeck K. *Towards a National Screening Policy for Cancer of the Cervix in South Africa*. Paper no. 31, Johannesburg: The Centre for Health Policy, Department of Community Health, Medical School, University of Witwatersrand, 1993.

28  Leiman G. 'Project Screen Soweto' – a planned cervical cancer screening programme in a high risk population. *S Afr Med J* 1987; **2**: 61–68.

29  Parkin DM. Cancer in developing countries. *Cancer Surv* 1994; **20**: 519–561.

30  Zhang JF, Parkin DM, Yu SZ, Esteve, J, Yang X, Day NE. Cervical screening attendance and its effectiveness in a rural population in China. *Cancer Detect Prev* 1989; **13**: 337–342.

31  Chou P, Chen V. Mass screening for cervical cancer in Taiwan from 1974 to 1984. *Cancer* 1989; **64**: 962–968.

32  Parkin DM. *Cancer Occurrence in Developing Countries*. IARC scientific publications no. 75. Lyon: International Agency for Research on Cancer, 1986.

33  Jain DK. *Biennial Report 1988–1989*. National Cancer Registry Programme. New Delhi: Indian Council of Medical Research, 1990.

34  Sierra R, Barrentes R. Epidemiology of cancer of the uterine cervix in Costa Rica, 1980–83. *Bull PAHO* 1989; **23**: 431–437.

35  Luthra UK, Prabhakar AK, Seth P *et al*. Natural history of pre-cancerous early cancerous lesions of the uterine cervix. *Acta Cytol* 1987; **31**: 226–233.

36  World Health Organization. Control of cancer of the cervix uteri. A WHO meeting. *Bull WHO* 1986; **64**: 607–618.

37  Prabhakar AK. Cervical cancer in India strategy for control. *Ind J Cancer* 1992; **104**: 29–32.

38  Murthy NS, Agarwal SS, Prabhakar AK, Sharma S, Das DK. Estimation of reduction in life time risk of cervical cancer through one life-time screening. *Neoplasma* 1993; **40**: 255–258.

39  Sherris J, Wells ES, Tsu VD, Bishop A. *Cervical Cancer in Developing Countries. A Situation Analysis*. Women's Health and Nutrition working paper. Washington: The World Bank, 1993.

40  Gustafsson L, Sparen P, Gustafsson M, Wilander E, Bergstorm R, Adami HO. Efficiency of organised and opportunistic cytological screening for cancer *in situ* of the cervix. *Br J Cancer* 1995; **72**: 498–505.

# 8: Prevention of Sexually Transmitted Infections through Health Education and Counselling: A General Framework

## A. Meheus

## Background

The spectrum of sexually transmitted diseases (STD) has expanded considerably in the past 25 years and includes now more than 20 different aetiological agents. It is increasingly obvious that much of the STD problem does not result from contact with clinically apparent diseases but rather from unnoticed and frequently subclinical infections. This means that in our prevention and control activities we should aim to prevent sexually transmitted infections (STI) or, at the vary least, to detect and treat STI before transmission occurs and disease or complications develop.

The priorities for STI/STD prevention and control are: the four bacterial infections of gonorrhoea, syphilis, chancroid and *Chlamydia*; the four viral infections of human immunodeficiency virus (HIV), herpes simplex virus (HSV; genital herpes), human papillomavirus (HPV) and hepatitis B virus (HBV); and trichomoniasis/bacterial vaginosis.

One can use a broad definition of behavioural interventions which encompasses any effort that aims to alter one or more behavioural determinants of STI. These behavioural interventions can be categorized into: (i) interventions to reduce risk of infection (sexual behaviour); (ii) interventions to reduce infectiousness and further transmission (health-care-seeking behaviour); (iii) interventions to improve behaviour of health-care providers; and (iv) public laws to reduce transmission of STI.

The objectives of these four broad types of behavioural interventions are given in Table 8.1 [1].

Most of our intervention efforts in industrialized countries have focused on

*Correspondence*: Professor André Meheus, Epidemiology and Community Medicine, University of Antwerp, 2610 Antwerp, Belgium.

**Table 8.1** Objectives of specific behavioural interventions to control sexually transmitted infections.

*Reduce risk of exposure to and acquisition of STI through changes in sexual behaviour*
Postpone coital debut
Reduce number of sexual partners
Select sexual partners by infection status
Reduce use of substances that result in loss of control
Reduce sexual contact with individuals from high-STI prevalence groups
Increase use of condoms and/or spermicides
Reduce frequency of sexual practices associated with high rates of transmission

*Reduce risk of transmission and complications of STI through improvements in health-care-seeking and compliance behaviour*
Increase early recognition of risk and/or symptoms of STI
Increase compliance with extended treatment regimens
Increase compliance with test-of-cure and other follow-up visits
Increase compliance with partner notification

*Increase accessibility, effectiveness and acceptability of STI treatment and prevention services by improving health-care provider behaviour*
Improve STI training in professional schools
Provide STI and HIV prevention training centres
Establish STI specialty training and recognition
Improve private care providers' willingness and ability to detect and care for STI
Improve and expand partner notification
Improve counselling on STI risk reduction
Improve promotion, distribution and instructions for condoms

*Reduce transmission of STI through the use of public laws*
Registration and/or periodic health examinations of prostitutes
Punitive fines and/or restrictive measures
Regulating and/or prohibiting certain establishments such as bathhouses for homosexual men and massage parlours

From Judson and Paalman [1], with permission.
HIV, Human immunodeficiency virus.

reducing an individual's risk of infection through changes in sexual behaviour. This primary prevention effort for STI became more emphasized since the recognition of the public health importance of viral STI, for which primary prevention through a change in sexual behaviour is the major control strategy. Genital herpes in the 1970s and HIV/acquired immunodeficiency syndrome (AIDS) in the 1980s have put behavioural interventions high on the public health agenda. A common assumption was that much of sexual behaviour is under cognitive control, and consequently methods that emphasized information, education and communication (IEC) were stressed. An alternative explanation is that modifying community norms, structural barriers or sexual drive is much more difficult.

Interventions directed at health-care seeking and compliance behaviour are intended to minimize the period of infectiousness of treatable STI and to reduce further transmission of all STI.

In this chapter, we shall restrict the discussion to reduction of risk of infection and health-care-seeking behaviour as they apply to all STI and specifically to HPV infection and transmission.

## Interventions to reduce the risk of acquiring STI

The first line of defence is through avoiding exposure to STI: postponing coital debut, which also is a strategy to prevent teenage pregnancies; sexual abstinence; non-penetrative sexual practices such as masturbation; and by selecting uninfected partners. In this regard, any type of sexual practice with an uninfected partner will be safer than safer sex with a partner known to be infected or whose infection status is unknown, but in practice this type of intervention is difficult.

The second line of defence is through interventions that reduce the risk of exposure: reduction of use of alcohol and other substances that result in loss of control over sexual behaviour; reduction of number of sexual partners; reduction of specific types of sexual relationships, such as anonymous partners, 'one-night stands', partners likely to have high-risk lifestyles, sex with prostitutes. The rationale behind this intervention is that most STI are transmitted in the community within core-group transmitters and only occasionally STI spread from core groups into low-prevalence populations [2].

The third line of defence aims to minimize the chances of infection when exposure to STI occurs: reduction of the frequency of high-risk sexual practices (e.g. receptive anal intercourse); increasing the use of condoms and spermicides. Since the HIV epidemic, condom promotion has become a cornerstone of STI prevention programmes, particularly important for HIV and other viral STI. It would be expected, but firm evidence is lacking, that condom use would give adequate protection from HPV infection.

## Interventions directed at the general public

There are many reasons to direct IEC activities for STI to the public at large [3]: to raise personal and political awareness of the problem; to influence favourably general attitudes toward STI, safer sex and health-care-seeking behaviour; to counteract discrimination against and stigmatization of infected people and risk groups; to reach individuals who cannot be accessed through targeted programmes.

A mass-media approach has the advantage of reaching large numbers of people at a low unit cost, generating free publicity and setting the stage for behavioural change. The disadvantages are that the public nature of the communication often makes it necessary that the messages cannot be explicit, that much of the information goes to people who are already well informed through other sources or who are not at risk at all (creating a pool of worried unrisky).

Behavioural interventions for general public use, separately or in combination, are information brochures, posters, leaflets, hotlines, mass media campaigns, condom promotion and provision.

Sweden and other Scandinavian countries used IEC in the late 1960s and early 1970s to fight the gonorrhoea epidemic. Temporally associated with these health promotion efforts, gonorrhoea incidence declined since 1970; a recent evaluation indicates however that not so much sexual behavioural change caused the decline but shorter duration of gonorrhoea infection through early detection, adequate treatment and counselling of persons with gonorrhoea [4]. With the arrival of HIV/AIDS the number of IEC interventions has increased tremendously (television spots, posters, brochures, advertisements, etc.). There have been great differences in the tone of campaigns: some used fear to induce behavioural change, others took a neutral stance and gave primarily information, while others used humour to get the message across. The dilemma of IEC is to indicate that sex is in itself a healthy, normal, pleasurable activity, and that sexuality as such is not to be controlled, but that risks involved should be minimized.

## Interventions directed at defined groups

Interventions directed at specific groups allow IEC activities to be targeted. It is essential to work through key group members (peer groups) who know the values and habits of other members, the channels to reach them and the authorities they listen to.

To prevent infections in future generations, adolescents and young people are an important target group [5,6]; it is also easier to develop safer sex behaviour from the start than to change established unsafe practices. Therefore school education is a targeted intervention with great potential impact [7]. The best approach might be to integrate education on HIV/AIDS and other STI with contraception into a curriculum on sex education or family health education.

Specific educational materials have been produced and distributed to different target groups such as STI patients, female prostitutes and their clients, homosexual men, ethnic minorities, women, tourists, young people, students, military personnel and health-care workers.

## Interventions directed at the individual

Much of the IEC directed at the individual is not part of a professional service: patients tell their children to be careful, friends talk together about sex, partners ask each other questions.

Behavioural intervention by professional health workers delivered on a one-to-one basis is called counselling. This individual behavioural intervention provides the opportunity to personalize information to fit individual needs, beliefs, levels of knowledge, sexual preference and perceived and true risk of infection. A 19-year-old girl who contracted genital warts from her first sexual partner clearly needs different counselling from an HIV-seropositive man presenting with gonorrhoea.

Top priority for counselling should be given to those with high-risk sexual behaviour: patients with STI, male and female prostitutes, male homosexuals, injecting drug users, poor inner-city ethnic minorities, seafarers, migrant workers.

Counselling is a major component of comprehensive management of patients with STD [8]. Counselling should include the importance of risk reduction so as to avoid contracting STI in the future and should deal with the patient's actual STD. Whether the patient has a curable bacterial infection or a treatable but not curable viral STI, the following should be discussed:

1   the treatment;
2   whether the infection is curable, and if not what the long-term effects will be;
3   the complications, if any;
4   when sex can be resumed;
5   the special issues of fertility, pregnancy and risks to neonates;
6   the fact that the infection was caught from one partner and may already have been transmitted to others;
7   the risk that reinfection can occur if sex is resumed with an untreated partner;
8   the consequences to a partner of failure to receive treatment;
9   the risk of other unsuspected STD, including HIV infection;
10   partner notification.

In STD clinics, there are usually trained health workers who act as counsellors. Outside special STD clinics, the clinician most often has to do the counselling; in settings where many of the STD are seen by private physicians, their role as counsellors should be stressed.

As STD patients very often belong to the core transmitter groups in the population, control and prevention of an STI in them has a far greater impact on STD incidence than prevention in a non-core group member [2].

## Interventions to reduce infectiousness and further transmission

Improvements in health-care-seeking behaviour and compliance behaviour coupled with effective and comprehensive management of persons infected has great potential in decreasing further transmission of STI. Patients with symptoms and signs of an STD should present as early as possible at the health services for diagnosis and treatment. Persons with a promiscuous lifestyle should be aware of their increased risk of infection and be encouraged to seek periodic examinations for STI (men and women with multiple partners, male and female prostitutes, persons with a previous STI, persons from high-prevalence STI groups).

An important component of comprehensive care for STI, be it in a patient with symptomatic disease or in a person proven infected after screening or case-finding, is partner notification [9]. Partner notification encompasses a spectrum of public health activities in which sexual partners of persons with an STI are notified, counselled on their exposure and offered services.

The general objective is to break the chain of infection. There are two approaches to partner notification (also called contact-tracing): provider referral, when a health-care worker notifies the index patient's partner or partners, and patient referral, when the infected patient notifies the partner or partners of their possible infection.

Partner notification undoubtedly is important in STI control and has been successful in the UK and Sweden. Opponents to this intervention voice concerns about cost-effectiveness relative to other behavioural interventions and the potential to invade privacy. Partner notification and treatment of those found to be infected are accepted interventions in patients with symptomatic HPV infection, such as anogenital warts. But it is much more controversial to perform partner notification in asymptomatic women for instance, in whom condylomata have been found through routine cervical cytology or colposcopy.

## Conclusions

There has been an impressive reduction in STI morbidity in industrialized countries in the last 25 years. Precise data are lacking concerning the relative contribution of behavioural interventions and non-behavioural interventions [10]. The fact that viral STI are much less under control than bacterial ones tends to support that improved clinical services linked to public health interventions and adequate health-care-seeking behaviour had the greatest impact. But experience showed that no magic bullet is identifiable when it comes to prevention and control of STI; broadly balanced programmes are needed in which behavioural interventions have an important part.

## References

1 Judson FN, Paalman M. Behavioural interventions in industrialized countries. In: Wasserheit J, Aral S, Holmes K (eds) *Research Issues in Human Behavior and Sexually*

*Transmitted Diseases in the AIDS Era.* Washington DC: American Society for Microbiology, 1991, pp 296–317.

2 Brunham RC, Ronald AR. Epidemiology of sexually transmitted diseases in developing countries. In: Wasserheit J, Aral S, Holmes K (eds) *Research Issues in Human Behavior and Sexually Transmitted Diseases in the AIDS Era.* Washington, DC: American Society for Microbiology, 1991, pp 61–82.

3 Paalman M, Sandfort T. Promoting safer sex among the public at large. In: Paalman M (ed) *Promoting Safer Sex: Prevention of Sexual Transmission of AIDS and other STD.* Proceedings of an international workshop, May 1989. Amsterdam: Swets & Zeitlinger, 1990, pp 199–216.

4 Aavitsland P. Epidemiology and national strategy for prevention of sexually transmitted diseases in Norway. Abstract, 9th Meeting of Scandinavian Society for Genitourinary Medicine, Stockholm, May 31–June 2, 1996.

5 World Health Organization. *Meeting on the Prevention and Control of Sexually Transmitted Diseases/AIDS in Young People.* Unpublished document WHO/VDT/87.441, Geneva, 1987.

6 Meheus A. Sexually transmitted diseases among adolescents: epidemiology and prevention. In: Bennett DL (ed) *The Control of Hepatitis B, The Role of Prevention in Adolescence.* London: Gower Medical, 1992, pp 17–20.

7 World Health Organization. *School Health Education to Prevent AIDS and Sexually Transmitted Disease.* WHO AIDS series no. 10. Geneva: WHO, 1992.

8 World Health Organization. *Management of Patients with Sexually Transmitted Diseases.* WHO Technical Report series no. 810. Geneva: WHO, 1991.

9 Potterat JJ, Meheus A, Gallwey J. Partner notification: operational considerations. *Int J STD AIDS* 1991, **2**: 411–415.

10 Holmes KK, Aral S. Behavioural interventions in developing countries. In: Wasserheit J, Aral S, Holmes K (eds) *Research Issues in Human Behavior and Sexually Transmitted Diseases in the AIDS Era.* Washington, DC: American Society for Microbiology, 1991, pp 318–344.

# Section 2
# Natural History and Management of Cervical Cancer Precursors

# 9: Biological Behaviour of Cervical Intraepithelial Neoplasia

## K. J. Syrjänen

The biological relevance of any novel classifications of cervical precancer lesions can only be established by well-controlled, prospectively followed up cohort studies. While reviewing the reported prospective follow-up studies on cervical intraepithelial neoplasia (CIN), Östör [1] found 3529 cases of CIN I, of which 57% showed regression, 32% were persisting, progression to CIN III was established in 11%, and progression to invasive cancer estimated in 1% of cases. The corresponding figures for CIN II were 43%, 35%, 22%, and 5%, respectively. The association of human papillomavirus (HPV) with CIN has further complicated the natural history studies on these lesions. Results from the early prospective follow-up studies are remarkably consistent, however. Progression from HPV NCIN (koilocytosis without CIN) to CIN I or greater was reported for 8% (18/232) of women followed by Syrjänen *et al.* [2] for an average of 25 months, for 8% (26/314) of those followed by de Brux *et al.* [3] for 15–18 months, and for 13% (113/846) of women followed up for 6 years by Mitchell *et al.* [4] During a 42-month follow-up period, a 10% progression rate was found in 1269 women with HPV CIN I, and in 17% of 762 women with HPV CIN II by de Brux *et al.* [5]. The spontaneous regression rates were 53% and 39% in these cohorts, respectively. This is fully consonant with our experience from a 15-year follow-up (1981–1996) of 530 women in Kuopio, where the spontaneous regression rate seems to increase in parallel with the extent of the follow-up time, currently 66.7% for HPV NCIN and 55.7% for HPV CIN I. The figures for progression are 6.3% and 14.2%, respectively. It is obvious from these data that the risk of a cervical precancer lesion progressing to invasive disease increases in parallel with the severity of the lesion grade.

*Correspondence*: Professor Kari J. Syrjänen, Department of Pathology and Forensic Medicine, Kuopio Cancer Research Centre, University of Kuopio, POB 1627, FIN-70211 Kuopio, Finland.

Another distinct prognostic factor is HPV type; HPV 16 lesions possess a significantly (>fivefold) higher risk for progression than infections due to low-risk HPV types 6 and 11, or lesions remaining HPV DNA-negative with conventional hybridization techniques (i.e. issues of the viral load).

The natural history data of cervical precancer lesions should have important implications in the treatment practice of these lesions, whether to treat or follow-up. CIN I and even CIN II lesions can be safely followed up, provided that patient compliance can be ensured. It is essential to realize, however, that CIN III lesions represent the immediate cancer precursor lesions, advocating prompt ablative treatment with histopathological confirmation of the free margins. The unsolved problem still remains; these natural history data apply neatly to a large series of women but, unfortunately, are of little help in predicting disease outcome in individual women.

## Cancer precursor lesions of the uterine cervix

During the past several decades, the nomenclature for cervical precancer lesions has undergone a series of marked changes, starting from the early 1900s with the classical monograph of Schottländer and Kemauner [6] and continuing to the present. The widely used World Health Organization (WHO) terminology identifies two types of lesions – dysplasia and carcinoma-*in-situ* (CIS) [7]. In the WHO system, dysplasia is regarded as a bivalent lesion that may regress to normal, remain unchanged or progress to an invasive carcinoma, whereas CIS is considered a lesion that frequently develops into an invasive carcinoma, if left untreated [7].

In the late 1960s, a new terminology was presented, introducing the concept of CIN [8]. According to this system, precancer lesions are categorized into three grades (CIN I–III), in which CIN III groups together severe dysplasia and CIS lesions. The CIN nomenclature has gained wide acceptance among both clinicians and cytopathologists during these decades. In 1988, a National Cancer Institute workshop published recommendations and guidelines for reporting the results of cervical cytology, known as the Bethesda system [9]. The Bethesda system proposes to replace the terms dysplasia-CIS or CIN with two terms – low-grade squamous intraepithelial lesion (SIL) and high-grade SIL. The former includes lesions that show cellular changes associated with HPV infection or mild dyplasia (CIN I), whereas the latter includes moderate dysplasia (CIN II) or severe dysplasia/CIS (CIN III) [9].

The biological relevance of any new classification of cervical cancer precursors can only be established by carefully conducted prospective follow-up studies, capable of establishing their natural history. In this communication, the data on the natural history of cervical precancer lesions are reviewed on the basis of available prospective follow-up studies.

## Progressive potential of cervical precursor lesions

### Invasive cancer develops from precancer lesions

General agreement prevails that most, if not all, squamous cell carcinomas of the uterine cervix arise from intraepithelial precursor lesions. The supporting evidence for this presumption includes the following observations, as recently discussed in more detail [1,10]:

1  In most cases, CIN occurs at last 10 years earlier than the invasive cancer, supporting the concept of a temporal evolution of cervical cancer.

2  Women with such epithelial abnormalities develop invasive cancer much more frequently than women without those lesions.

3  Early invasive carcinoma frequently arises from CIN, and areas of CIS almost invariably surround the foci of invasive tumours.

4  Other evidence (e.g. cytogenetics, molecular biology, tissue culture) supports similarities between the dysplastic and frankly malignant epithelia.

5  Epidemiological studies have shown that cervical cancer precursors and invasive cancers share identical risk factors.

6  Prospective cohort studies address the problems of regression, persistence and progression of the precursors, i.e. the natural history of CIN [5].

These studies will be discussed in more detail below.


### Prevalence, incidence and prevention

As evident from the above, cervical cancer is considered an appropriate model disease known to develop through well-defined precursor lesions, called dysplasia/CIS, CIN or SIL. Of key importance in preventing and predicting the development of cervical cancer is the assessment of the biological character of these precancer lesions. The time-honoured means of preventing the development of an invasive cervical cancer are the organized, nationwide mass screening programmes using Papanicolaou (Pap) smears. Such programmes have proven to be effective in strikingly reducing the prevalence of this disease, for example, in Scandinavian countries (except Norway) since the 1960s [2, 11]. Pap smear also provides a means of assessing the prevalence of CIN lesions, which seems to have increased throughout the 1970s and 1980s [12,13]. Based on analysis of almost 800 000 Pap smears in 1981, the prevalence of biopsy-proved CIN lesions (all grades) in a teenage population in the USA was 13.3/1000 [14]. This, of course, is a substantially higher figure than the annual incidence of invasive cervical cancer, for example, in the low-risk countries like Finland, which is currently 2.7/100 000 [15]. Accordingly, it seems clear that the vast majority of cervical precancer lesions never progress to invasive cancer; they are either eradicated after detection or they regress spontaneously without any treatment. Indeed, this has been shown to be the case, when large cohorts of women with cervical precancer lesions have been prospectively followed up for prolonged periods.

## Prospective follow-up studies

### Conceptual problems

The methodological and conceptual problems inherent in the prospective follow-up studies conducted during the past several decades for dysplasia/CIN lesions were pointed out by Koutsky *et al.* [14] and meritoriously discussed by Östör [1]. These same problems are also encountered in prospective HPV cohort studies, as pointed out in the recent summary [10]. Because they are relevant to the proper interpretation of all prospective follow-up studies, these problems are listed here. For detailed discussion, however, the reader is referred to the recent reviews [1,10,14].

   While interpreting the natural history data of cervical precancer lesions, one should carefully consider a number of issues which potentially influence the course of the disease. These include the following:

1   The effect of biopsy [16–20].
2   Criteria of selection [21,22].
3   Diagnostic criteria.
4   Methods of follow-up.
5   End-point of follow-up.
6   Complexity of the transformation zone (TZ).
7   Problems of cytology [9,14,23–28].
8   Resolution of colposcopy [29].
9   Extent of follow-up.
10  Ethical considerations. This has been highlighted recently by the 'unfortunate experiment' in New Zealand, where a significant percentage of women with CIN III progressed to invasive cancer when left untreated [30].
11  Statistical analysis. The statistical modelling of the follow-up data of the precancer lesions can be difficult, especially when HPV is taken into account [31–34]. As recently pointed out, the clinical course of these lesions is a complex one; at least six distinct disease patterns can be differentiated among a large cohort of women examined at regular intervals for prolonged periods [25,34].

### Natural history of low-grade lesions

Recently, long-term follow-up data were published from Sweden, where 328 women with normal colposcopy and histology at the onset were followed up for an average of 10.6 years [35]. During that time, CIN occurred in 72 (22%) cases, including 20 cases of CIN I (6.1%), 17 of CIN II (5.2%) and 35 of CIN III (10.7%). This is one of the few studies where prospective follow-up results are available for women with normal histology. It is to be emphasized, however, that even in this study, the basis for patient recruitment was an initially abnormal Pap smear suggestive of CIN [35]. Similarly, the vast majority of antedating smears collected from 82 biopsy-proven CIN III patients revealed evidence of cervical abnormalities from 24 to 12 months prior to the development of CIN III, thus emphasizing the value of annual cytological follow-up of women at increased risk [36]. In another series of 1454 women with abnormal cytology, triage of even low-grade smears based on histopathological examination is encouraged to disclose the eventual progression [37]. Contradictory experience was recently reported by Bertelsen and Hartveit [38] who examined the previous cervical smears of 850 women with established CIN in 1989, and could not establish any predictive value for the previous smear history. These data were interpreted to suggest that some progressive lesions may be acute in origin [38], not necessarily detectable in the preceding smears.

The natural history studies on cervical precancer lesions were critically reviewed by Östör [1] summarizing all the papers over the past 40 years, with particular emphasis on disease regression, persistence and progression. There are follow-up series including mild dysplasia (or CIN I), mild and moderate dysplasia (CIN I and II) together, moderate dysplasia or CIN II, dysplasia (CIN) unspecified, and severe dysplasia—CIS or CIN III. The studies on low-grade lesions are summarized in Table 9.1 [3,4,16,18,21–23,39–51]. The total number of CIN cases subjected to prospective follow-up was 4504. Of these, 2567 showed regression, giving a regression rate of 57%. When stratified into the various grades of severity, the composite data indicate the likelihood of regression for CIN I to be 57%, persistence 32%, progression to CIN III 11%, and progression to invasive cancer 1% [1].

In a second category of longitudinal studies, the works were included where mild and moderate dysplasia (CIN I and II) were lumped together; the results are also summarized in Table 9.1 [13,17,26,28,43,50–62]. The total

**Table 9.1** Natural history of cervical intraepithelial neoplasia (CIN) lesions.*

| Grade of lesions | No. of cases | Regress | Persist | Progress (to CIS) | Follow-up (years) |
|---|---|---|---|---|---|
| CIN I/mild dysplasia | 4504 | 57% | 32% | 11% | 1–18 |
| CIN I and CIN II | 4155 | 43% | 35% | 22% | 0.5–16 |

* CIS, Carcinoma-*in-situ*.
Table compiled and modified from the data reviewed by Östör [1].

number of lumped (CIN I and CIN II) cases with follow-up was 4155 [13,17,26,28,43,50–62]. Here the composite data indicate the likelihood of regression for CIN II to be 43%, persistence 35%, progression to CIN III 22% and progression to invasive cancer 5% [1].

## HPV-associated precancer lesions

The connection of a viral infection with a spectrum of distinct morphological manifestations (CIN) in itself is hard to assess, and the scene is rendered more complex by the recognition of subclinical and latent HPV infections [14, 24,25,34,63–65]. As with CIN, the natural history of HPV lesions can be reliably evaluated by prospective follow-up studies, a large number of which have been completed during the late 1980s and early 1990s (see detailed reviews [63–65]). The data from these follow-up studies are laborious to interpret, for the reasons discussed recently by Kataja *et al.* [33] including: (i) the different study populations; (ii) different methods of follow-up (i.e. Pap smear or biopsy); (iii) the length of the follow-up period; and (iv) the reproducibility problems of grading the precancer lesions [19,20,22,33,52,66–69].

## Early prospective studies of HPV

Until the mid-1980s, the natural history of cytologically defined cervical HPV infections in relation to the development of CIN has been studied among three cohorts of women (see reviews [70–74]). Results from these three studies are remarkably consistent. Progression from HPV-NCIN (i.e. koilocytosis without CIN) to CIN I or greater was reported for 18 (8%) of 232 women followed by us for an average of 25 months [27,75] for 26 (8%) of 314 women followed by de Brux *et al.* [5] for 15–18 months; and for 113 (13%) of 846 women followed up for 6 years by Mitchell *et al.* [4]. In the last study, 30 cases of CIS were observed – compared to only 1.9 cases expected in the general population – giving a relative risk of 15.6 [4]. Campion *et al.* [21] found that 22 (56%) of 39 women with HPV 16-associated CIN I progressed to CIN III, whereas only 1 (4%) of 26 women with HPV 6 progressed to CIN III. The most extensive of these follow-up studies (albeit retrospective) was reported by de Brux *et al.* [3] based on observations of 2466 women out of 7257 cases diagnosed among 1 036 020 Pap smears between 1979 and 1982. During a 42-month follow-up period, a 10% progression rate was found in 1269 women with HPV CIN I, and in 17% of 762 women with HPV CIN II [3]. On the other hand, the spontaneous regression rates were 53% and 39% in these cohorts, respectively. As evident from these figures, the progression rates in these different studies are remarkably constant, varying from 8% to 17%, depending on the length of the follow-up time. This is fully consonant with our experience from a 15-year follow-up of >530 women in Kuopio [33,34, 39].

## Kuopio follow-up study

To elucidate the natural history of genital HPV infections, a prospective follow-up study of the women infected with this virus was started in our clinic in 1981. During 1981–1985, 530 women were invited to participate in the study, and their genital HPV lesions have been followed up for a mean of almost 10 years (mean ± s.d. 101 ± 42 months) by now, using colposcopy, Pap smears and punch biopsies, but without any kind of therapy [24,25,27,31–33, 75,76]. The results of this extensive study have been reported in a series of previous publications [24,25,27,31–33,75,76].

There are two major trends emerging, when individual women are being followed up for prolonged periods. The rate of spontaneous regression increases in parallel with the extent of the follow-up time, from 28% at 25 months of mean follow-up, to 56% at 57 months, up to 67% after 101 months of observation [33]. In practice, this means that marked difference exists in the regression rates obtained when the follow-up is continued for 2 years, 4 years and up to 7 years. After that, however, the regression rate does not show any further significant increase.

From the clinical point of view, even more important is the progression of HPV lesions towards CIS. As repeatedly emphasized, the main attention should be focused on predicting the lesions eventually progressing among the clinical lesions [24,25,34]. In contrast to the increasing trend of the regression rate as a function of time, no such trend can be observed in the progression rate. In fact, the progression rate remains unchanged (around 14%) after 25 months of mean follow-up time. In practice, this means that the lesions destined to clinical progression do so quite rapidly, almost invariably during the first 2 years from the diagnosis. This should have important clinical implications while planning strategies for diagnosis, treatment and follow-up of genital HPV infections [40].

## Recent follow-up studies

The number of prospective follow-up studies carried out for genital HPV infections (mainly focused on cervical lesions) has increased during the late 1980s and early 1990s. Because of the difficulties discussed above, the results of these studies are difficult to interpret and even more difficult to compare with each other. A summary of the recent follow-up studies is given in Table 9.2.

The major clinical impact of these studies would be to give the definite

**Table 9.2** Natural history of human papillomavirus (HPV)-associated cervical intraepithelial neoplasia (CIN) lesions.

| Reference no. | No. of patients | Follow-up time (months) | Rate of regression (%) | | Rate of progression (%) | |
|---|---|---|---|---|---|---|
| | | | HPV-NCIN | CIN I | HPV-NCIN | CIN I |
| [102] | 51 | 12 | 47.0 | n.d. | 11.8 | n.d. |
| [3] | 30 | 24 | n.d. | 83.0 | n.d. | n.d. |
| [86] | 20 | 28 | n.d. | n.d. | 15.0 | n.d. |
| [103] | 45 | 11 | 40.0 | n.d. | 33.3 | n.d. |
| [104] | 12 | 4 | 50.0 | n.d. | n.d. | n.d. |
| [91] | 50 | 6 | 22.4 | n.d. | n.d. | n.d. |
| [82] | 415 | 36 | n.d. | n.d. | 3.5 | n.d. |
| [77] | 82 | 18 | 21.4 | 3.6 | 9.7 | 22.2 |
| [84] | 38 | 36 | n.d. | 26.6 | n.d. | 73.3* |
| [80] | 146 | 18 | n.d. | 85.3† | n.d. | 14.7* |
| [81] | 2.709‡ | 60 | n.d. | n.d. | n.d. | n.d. |
| [83] | 101 | 73 | n.d. | n.d. | n.d. | 13.0§ |
| [92] | 100 | 120 | 47.0 | 13.3 | 49.0 | n.d. |
| [79] | 525 | 54 | n.d. | 77.3‖ | n.d. | 7.8 |
| [78] | 91 | 9 | 78.3¶ | n.d. | 3.4¶ | n.d. |
| [87] | 24 | 2–65 | n.d. | 37.5 | n.d. | 4.2** |
| [85] | 241 | 25 | n.d. | n.d. | 28.0†† | n.d. |
| [39] | 487 | 70 | 66.7 | 55.7 | 6.3 | 14.2 |
| [105] | 124 | 12 | n.d. | 48.3 | n.d. | 7.2 |
| [106] | 87 | >60 | | 50.6 | n.d. | 4.6 |

n.d., Not defined.
* Includes both persistence and progression.
† Includes CIN 0 and CIN I lesions.
‡ Papanicolaou (Pap) smears only.
** Progression fo CIN III or invasive carcinoma.
¶ Progression defined by Pap smear only.
‖ Includes both CIN I and CIN II cases.
§ Low-grade squamous intraepithelial lesions.
†† Women with positive test for HPV.

answers to two key questions: first, what is the spontaneous regression rate of HPV lesions of different grades? Second, what is the inherent potential of different grades of HPV lesions to progress towards an invasive cancer? As evident from the figures in Table 9.2, no such unanimous answers can be obtained from these extensive studies, unfortunately. Concerning the first issue, fairly unanimous agreement seems to exist in that the regression rate for HPV lesions without CIN (HPV-NCIN) is substantial, i.e. ranging from 21% [77] up to 78% [78]. Highly unfortunately, these figures have not been determined in many of the follow-up studies of longest duration [53,78–87]. According to our experience from the Kuopio study, we would be apt to accept the concept that the vast majority (two-thirds, maybe) of these lesions will eventually regress when controlled long enough [10,39].

Even more controversial are the data on the regression rates of HPV-CIN I lesions, the figures extending from 3.6% [77] to 85.3% [80]. Here again, these data were not recorded in the majority of these studies, and notable differences in the categorizing criteria exist between the different studies. The regression data for HPV-CIN II lesions are even more meagre, being available in only four of these reports [39,80,84,87]. It seems evident, however, that even the CIN II lesions possess a substantial regression tendency, ranging from 25% [87] to 60.8% [80]. Surprisingly few reports are able to give the data on the regression rate of HPV CIN III lesions [39,84]. This is explained by the fact that, for safety reasons, most authors are apt to institute an immediate treatment for CIN III lesions – a policy that cannot be protested against with any reasonable argument. The general impression is obtained, however, that the regression tendency for CIN III lesions is significantly lower than that of the lower-grade lesions, CIN II included.

The transient nature of HPV infections in sexually active young women has been emphasized by a number of recent studies as well [88–90]. Accordingly, of the 173 women with Pap smears demonstrating only koilocytosis, only 16.2% had underlying CIN or progressed to CIN over a 21-month follow-up [88]. This suggests that koilocytosis as such is associated with a low risk of CIN, advocating a conservative attitude to management. Similar data were obtained in a recent polymerase chain reaction (PCR) study, where 93% (25/27) initially HPV-infected women failed to demonstrate any HPV DNA in the smears four menstrual cycles later [89], suggesting a transient character of HPV infection in young women with a normal Pap smear. This accords with another study from Sweden, where regression (disappearance of HPV DNA) was shown in 80% of 276 young women examined by PCR during a 2-year interval [90].

Of even greater clinical significance are the lesions with potential to progress, as discussed before [10,24,25,34,73]. From the above studies, progression data are available even for women assessed as normal at the onset of the follow-up [53,77,81,85,86,91]. As could be expected, the progression rates for such cases (i.e. the development of HPV lesion of any grade) is relatively low, ranging from 0.65% [81] to 21.7% [84], even after a lengthy observation period. As with the regression, the deviation is marked in the figures of progression for HPV lesions without CIN; from 3.4% [78] to 49% [92]. Some of these discrepancies are due to different criteria of categorization, as indicated by the footnotes of Table 9.2. The studies are surprisingly consistent, however, in reporting the progression rates of HPV CIN I. If the extreme of 73.3% (due to different ranking) is ignored, the range is quite narrow, from 4.2% [87] to 22.2% [77] the majority settling around 10%

**Table 9.3** Natural history of cervical intraepithelial neoplasia (CIN) and human papillomavirus (HPV) CIN lesions.*

| Lesion | Regress | Persist | Progress to CIS | Progress to invasion |
|---|---|---|---|---|
| CIN I | 57% | 32% | 11% | 1% |
| CIN II | 43% | 35% | 22% | 5% |
| CIN III | 32% | <56% | | >12% |
| HPV-NCIN | 80% | 15% | 5% | 0% |
| HPV-CIN I | 65% | 21% | 14% | 0% |
| HPV-CIN II | 59% | 19% | 21% | 0% |
| HPV-CIN III | 12% | 9% | 79%† | ? |

* Table compiled from the data reviewed by Östör [1] and from the figures of Kuopio Prospective Follow-up study (1981–1996) Syrjänen [10].
† Progression based on colposcopy (lesion severity and extent) and histology (progress from severe dysplasia to CIS in two subsequent biopsies).
HPV-NCIN, HPV lesion without concomitant CIN (see Syrjänen [10]); CIS, carcinoma-*in-situ*.

[39,79,80,83]. Too few data are available to draw definite conclusions from the progression tendency of HPV CIN II. Because of the ranking differences, the two highest figures, 39.2% and 57.1% [80,84] cannot be compared with those of our study (20.6%) [39]. As pointed out before, it is ethically unjustified to establish the progression rate of CIN III by prospective follow-up of any significant length. In our study, a careful attempt was done to survey the HPV CIN III lesions by colposcopy, Pap smear and punch biopsy repeated at 3–4 month intervals. Even during such short periods and high patient compliance, a substantial proportion of lesions showed a clear progressive tendency, making necessary early eradication to ensure patient safety (see figures in Table 9.3).

## HPV type and clinical course

As part of the Kuopio follow-up study, factors influencing the natural history of cervical precancer lesions have been elucidated [24,25,27,28,31]. As repeatedly emphasized, one of the key factors affecting the disease progression is the lesion grade at the time of diagnosis [31,34,39]. As evidenced by the fact, however, that even a proportion of high-grade lesions may regress, it seems clear that the lesion grade *per se* is not the only determinant of clinical progression [10,31,39,73,93].

Another prognostic factor of considerable importance seems to be the HPV type [32,39]. Using a life-table analysis, HPV 16 infections seem to start progression earlier than those induced by other HPV types, and if follow-up is continued long enough, almost 80% of HPV 16 lesions will eventually make progression [32]. The most benign clinical course was ascribed to HPV lesions induced by HPV 6 and even more so to those which remained HPV DNA-negative with the conventional typing techniques (PCR excluded). When applied to Cox's proportional hazards analysis, HPV types can be clearly divided into low- and high-risk types according to their potential to progress [32,39]. Accordingly, HPV 16 infections show a progression rate more than five times higher than that of the low-risk types HPV 6 and HPV 11 [32,39]. Thus, data are convincing to substantiate the concept that the high-risk-type HPV 16 infection is a distinct risk factor predisposing the cervical precancer lesions to clinical progression significantly more often than infections by other HPV types.

Confirmation of this concept has been provided by evidence from other studies as well [94–97]. Thus, type-specific persistence and high viral load were significant predictors of high-grade cervical dysplasia [98]. The risk seems to be particularly confined to HPV types 16 and 18 [99]. In another series, HPV 33 was included in this category of viruses which, as persisting infections, increased the risk of CIN III and invasive cancer [100]. Indeed, the cumulative risk of progression was shown to be 17% after 36 months in women who were positive for the high-risk types HPV 16 and 18 [101]. In a multivariate analysis adjusting for confounding factors (age, race, smoking, oral contraceptives, plasma retinol), HPV 16 infection proved to be related to disease progression with a relative risk of 1.19 (95% confidence interval 1.03–1.38) [102].

## Conclusions

It is evident from the above discussion that HPV infections and cervical precancer lesions are intimately linked, even when considered on the basis of their natural history. This fact is clearly demonstrated by the figures in Table 9.3. To illustrate the point, this table was constructed by utilizing the summary date reviewed by Östör [1] in his excellent survey of almost 100 prospective follow-up studies, and adding the current natural history data on the clinical course of the genital HPV lesions in 530 women prospectively followed up since 1981 in our clinic [39]. Undoubtedly, genital HPV lesions and CIN are one and the same disease, with its natural history directly related to the severity of the lesion at first diagnosis.

To conclude, it seems to be established that the probability of a cervical precancer lesion progressing into an invasive disease increases with the severity of the atypia. Equally evident is, however, the fact that progression does not occur in every case, and even the high-grade lesions may spontaneously regress in a proportion of cases. The risk for progression seems to be closely linked with the type of HPV involved, i.e. whether it is a low-risk or a high-risk HPV type. The risk for progression is particularly high in HPV 16-induced lesions. Ideally, this kind of information should have implications in the therapy as well. Unfortunately, however, the basic problem still remains; the above natural history observations apply only to a large series of women but are of little or no help in predicting the disease outcome in individual women. In the future, major efforts should be focused on delineating the factors capable of predicting disease progression in individual patients.

## References

1 Östor AG. Natural history of cervical intraepithelial neoplasia – a critical review. *Int J Gynecol Pathol* 1993; **12**: 186–192.
2 Syrjänen K, Yliskoski M, Kataja V, Hippelainen M, Syrjänen SM, Saarikoski S. Prevalence of genital human papillomavirus infections in a mass-screened Finnish female population aged 20–65 years. *Int J STD AIDS* 1990; **1**: 410–415.
3 de Brux J, Cochard IB, Kaeding MH. Epidemiologie morphologie evolution des condylmes cervicaux. *Gynecologie* 1981; **32**: 314–318.
4 Mitchell H, Drake M, Medley G. Prospective evaluation of risk of cervical cancer after cytological evidence of human papillomavirus infection. *Lancet* 1986; **1**: 573–575.
5 de Brux J, Orth G, Croissant O, Cochard B, Ionesco M. Lesions condylomateuses du col uterin evolution chez 2466 patientes. *Bull Cancer* 1983; **70**: 410–422.
6 Schottländer J, Kemauner F. *Zur Kenntnis des Uteruskarzinoms: Monographische Studie über Morphologie, Entwicklung Wachstum. Beiträgen zur Klinik der Erkrankung*. Berlin. S. Karger, 1912.
7 Riotton G, Christopherson WM. *Cytology of the Female Genital Tract*. Geneva: World Health Organization, 1973.
8 Richart RM. Cervical intraepithelial neoplasia. *Pathol Ann* 1973; **8**: 301–328.
9 National Cancer Institute Workshop. The 1988 Bethesda system for reporting cervical/vaginal cytological diagnoses. *JAMA* 1989; **262**: 931–934.
10 Syrjänen KJ. Spontaneous evolution of intraepithelial lesions according to the grade and type of the implicated HPV. *Eur J Obstet Gynecol Reprod Biol* 1996; **65**: 45–53.
11 Syrjänen K, Hakama M, Saarikoski S, Vayrynen M, Yliskoski M, Syrjänen SM. Prevalence, incidence, and estimated life-time risk of cervical human papillomavirus infections in a nonselected Finnish female population. *Sex Transm Dis* 1990; **17**: 15–19.
12 Fredricsson B, Nasiell M, Sennerstam R, Wadås AM. Is there a changing epidemiology of premalignant lesions of the cervix? *Acta Obstet Gynecol Scand* 1977; **56**: 435–439.
13 Sadeghi SB, Hsieh EW, Gunn SW. Prevalence of cervical intraepithelial neoplasia in sexually active teenagers and young adults. *Am J Obstet Gynecol* 1984; **148**: 726–729.
14 Koutsky LA, Galloway DA, Holmes KK. Epidemiology of genital human papillomavirus infection. *Epidemiol Rev* 1988; **10**: 122–163.
15 Finnish Cancer Registry. *Cancer Incidence in Finland 1988*. Helsinki: Cancer Statistics of the National Agency for Welfare and Health, 1991, pp 8–16.
16 Bibbo M, Dytch HE, Alenghat E, Bartels PH, Wied GL. DNA ploidy profiles as prognostic indicators in CIN lesions. *Am J Clin Pathol* 1989; **92**: 261–265.
17 Byrne MA, Parry GC, Morse A, Taylor Robinson D, Malcolm AD, Coleman DV. A prospective study of human papillomavirus infection of the cervix. *Cytopathology* 1990; **1**: 329–337.
18 Nasiell K, Roger V, Nasiell M. Behavior of mild cervical dysplasia during long term follow up. *Obstet Gynecol* 1986; **67**: 665–669.
19 Nasiell K, Nasiell M, Vaclavinkova U. Behavior of moderate cervical dysplasia during

long term follow up. *Obstet Gynecol* 1983; **61**: 609–614.

20 Stern E, Neely PM. Dysplasia of the uterine cervix: incidence of regression recurrence and cancer. *Cancer* 1964; **17**: 508–512.

21 Campion MJ, McCance DJ, Cuzick J, Singer A. Progressive potential of mild cervical atypia: prospective cytological, colposcopic, and virological study. *Lancet* 1986; **2**: 237–240.

22 Richart RM, Barron BA. A follow up study of patients with cervical dysplasia. *Am J Obstet Gynecol* 1969; **105**: 386–393.

23 Sondheimer SJ, Casey MV, Rubin M, Mangan C, Atkinson B, Huggins GR. Mild cervical dysplasia experience in a family planning clinic. *J Reprod Med* 1983; **28**: 489–495.

24 Syrjänen K. Epidemiology of human papillomavirus (HPV) infections and their associations with genital squamous cell cancer. Review article. *APMIS* 1989; **97**: 957–970.

25 Syrjänen KJ. Natural history of genital HPV infections. *Papillomavirus Rep* 1990; **1**: 1–5.

26 Kwikkel HJ, Timmers T, Boon ME, Vanrijswijk MMM, Stolk JG. Relation of quantitative features of visually normal intermediate cells in cervical intraepithelial neoplasia I, II. *Anal Quant Cytol Histol* 1987; **9**: 405–410.

27 Syrjänen K, Vayrynen M, Saarikoski S *et al.* Natural history of cervical human papillomavirus (HPV) infections based on prospective follow-up. *Br J Obstet Gynaecol* 1985; **92**: 1086–1092.

28 Syrjänen K, Saarikoski D, Väyrynen M, Syrjänen S, Saastamoinen J, Castren A. Factors associated with the clinical behaviour of cervical papillomavirus infections during a long term prospective follow up. *Cervix* 1989; **1**: 131–143.

29 Burghardt E, Östör AG. *Colposcopy, Cervical Pathology. Textbook and Atlas*, 2nd edn. New York: Georg Thieme, 1991, p 247.

30 Chang AR. Carcinoma *in situ* of the cervix and its malignant potential. A lesson from New Zealand. *Cytopathology* 1990; **1**: 321–328.

31 Kataja V, Syrjänen K, Mantyjarvi R *et al.* Prospective follow-up of cervical HPV infections: life table analysis of histopathological, cytological and colposcopic data. *Eur J Epidemiol* 1989; **5**: 1–7.

32 Kataja V, Syrjänen K, Syrjänen SM *et al.* Prospective follow-up of genital HPV infections: survival analysis of the HPV typing data. *Eur J Epidemiol* 1990; **6**: 9–14.

33 Kataja V, Syrjänen SM, Mantyjarvi R, Yliskoski M, Saarikoski S, Syrjänen K. Prognostic factors in cervical human papillomavirus infections. *Sex Transm Dis* 1992; **19**: 154–160.

34 Syrjänen KJ. Genital human papillomavirus (HPV) infections and their associations with squamous cell cancer: Reappraisal of the morphologic, epidemiologic and DNA data. In: Fenoglio-Preiser CM, Wolff M, Rilke F (eds) *Progress in Surgical Pathology*, vol XII. New York: Field & Wood, 1992, pp 217–245.

35 Hellberg D, Nilsson S, Valentin J. Positive cervical smear with subsequent normal colposcopy and histology – frequency of CIN in a long-term follow-up. *Gynecol Oncol* 1994; **53**: 148–151.

36 Troncone G, Gupta PK. Cytologic observations preceding high grade squamous intraepithelial lesions. *Acta Cytol* 1995; **39**: 659–662.

37 Lonky NM, Navarre GL, Saunders S, Sadeghi M, Woldetsadik G. Low-grade Papanicolaou smears and the Bethesda system: a prospective cytohistopathologic analysis. *Obstet Gynecol* 1995; **85**: 716–720.

38 Bertelsen B, Hartveit F. The cervical smear record: its relevance to the subsequent development of cervical neoplasia. *Acta Obstet Gynecol Scand* 1995; **74**: 729–733.

39 Syrjänen K, Kataja V, Yliskoski M, Chang F, Syrjänen SM, Saarikoski S. Natural history of cervical human papillomavirus lesions does not substantiate the biologic relevance of the Bethesda system. *Obstet Gynecol* 1992; **79**: 675–682.

40 Raymond CA. For women infected with papillomavirus, close watch counseled. *JAMA* 1987; **257**: 2398–2399.

41 Weaver MG, Abdul-Karim FW, Dale G, Sorensen K, Huang YT. Outcome in mild and moderate cervical dysplasias related to the presence of specific human papillomavirus types. *Mod Pathol* 1990; **3**: 679–683.

42 Robertson JH, Woodend BE, Crozier EH, Hutchinson J. Risk of cervical cancer associated with mild dyskaryosis. *BMJ* 1988; **297**: 18–21.

43 Luthra UK, Prabhakar AK, Seth P *et al*. Natural history of precancerous and early cancerous lesions of the uterine cervix. *Acta Cytol* 1987; **31**: 226–234.

44 Lindgren J, Vesterinen E, Purola E, Wahlström T. Prognostic significance of tissue carcinoembryonic antigen in mild dysplasia of the uterine cervix. *Tumour Biol* 1985; **6**: 465–470.

45 Fu YS, Reagan YW, Richart RM. Definition of precursors. *Gynecol Oncol* 1981; **12**: S220–S231.

46 Srivannaboon S, Bhamarapravati N. Prevalence and outcome of dysplasia of cervix in self-selected population in Thailand. *J Med Assoc Thailand* 1974; **57**: 351–356.

47 Patten SF. Dysplasia of the uterine cervix. In: Lewis GC Jr, Wentz WB, Jaffe RM (eds) *New Concepts in Gynecological Oncology*. Philadelphia: FA Davis, 1966, pp 33–44.

48 Pahl IR, Stein AA, Rome D, Plotz EJ. Basal cell proliferative disease of the cervix. *Obstet Gynecol* 1965; **25**: 201–208.

49 Lambert B, Woodruff DJ. Spinal analysis of the cervix. *Cancer* 1963; **16**: 1141–1150.

50 Nieburgs HE. The significance of tissue cell changes preceding uterine cervix carcinoma. *Cancer* 1963; **16**: 141–159.

51 Galvin GA, Jones HW, Te Linde RW. The significance of basal-cell hyperactivity in cervical biopsies. *Am J Obstet Gynecol* 1955; **70**: 808–817.

52 Fox CH. Biologic behavior of dysplasia and carcinoma *in situ*. *Am J Obstet Gynecol* 1967; **99**: 960–974.

53 Cheetham D, Smith J, Wilson C, Munday PE, Colman DV. Clinical significance of human papillomavirus infection of the uterine cervix in the development of cervical intraepithelial neoplasia. *Br J Vener Dis* 1984; **60**: 182–185.

54 Navone R, Pich A, Margaria E, Ghiringhello B. Immunohistochemical identification of the papillomavirus in uterine cervix: relationship with dysplasia, koilocytosis and evolution of the lesions. *Appl Pathol* 1987; **5**: 136–144.

55 Cotton R, Elwood JM, Jones GM. Results of delayed follow up of abnormal cervical smears. *BMJ* 1986; **292**: 799–800.

56 Heinzl S, Szalmay G, Jochum L, Roemer V. Observations on the development of dysplasia. *Acta Cytol* 1982; **26**: 453–456.

57 Rummel HH, Frick R, Heberling D, Schubert D. Verlaufskontrolle bei Patientinnen mit suspekter Zytologie. *Geburtsh Frauenheilk* 1977; **37**: 521–526.

58 Berget A. Epithelial dysplasia of the cervix uteri. *Dan Med Bull* 1971; **21**: 169–171.

59 Hulka BS. Cytological and histologic outcome following an atypical cervical smear. *Am J Obstet Gynecol* 1968; **101**: 190–199.

60 Ayre JE. Is carcinoma *in situ* reversible? In: Wied GL (ed) *Proceedings of the First International Congress of Exfoliative Cytology*. Vienna: International Academy of Cytology, 1962, pp. 94–102.

61 Simon TR, Sheehan JF. Reversible atypia of cervical epithelium. In: Wied GL (ed) *Proceedings of the First International Congress of Exfoliative Cytology*. Vienna: International Academy of Cytology, 1962, pp 116–120.

62 Peckham B, Greene RR. Follow-up on cervical epithelial abnormalities. *Am J Obstet Gynecol* 1957; **74**: 804–815.

63 Syrjänen KJ. Current concepts of human papillomavirus infections in the genital tract and their relationship to intraepithelial neoplasia and squamous cell carcinoma. *Obstet Gynecol Surv* 1984; **39**: 252–265.

64 Syrjänen K. Human papillomavirus (HPV) infections of the female genital tract and their associations with intraepithelial neoplasia and squamous cell carcinoma. *Pathol Annu* 1986; **21**: 53–89.

65 Syrjänen KJ. Papillomaviruses and cancer. In: Syrjänen KJ, Gissmann L, Koss L (eds) *Papillomaviruses and Human Disease*. Heidelberg: Springer Verlag, 1987, pp 468–503.

66 Hall JE, Walton L. Dysplasia of the cervix: a prospective study of 206 cases. *Am J Obstet Gynecol* 1968; **100**: 662–671.

67 Spriggs AI. Natural history of cervical dysplasia. *Clin Obstet Gynaecol* 1981; **8**: 65–76.

68 Varga A. The relationship of cervical dysplasia to *in situ* and invasive carcinoma of the cervix. *Am J Obstet Gynecol* 1966; **95**: 759–762.

69 Villa Santa U. Diagnosis and prognosis of cervical dysplasia. *Obstet Gynecol* 1971; **38**: 811–816.

70 de Palo G, Rilke F, zur Hausen H (eds) *Herpes and Papilloma Viruses*, vol II, vol 46. Serono Symposia Publications. New York: Raven Press, 1988.

71 Gross G, Jablonska S, Pfister H, Stegner HE (eds) *Genital Papillomavirus Infections: Modern Diagnosis and Treatment*. Heidelberg: Springer Verlag, 1990.

72 Monsonego J (ed) *Papillomaviruses in Human Pathology. Recent Progress in Epidermoid Precancers*, vol 78. Serono Symposia Publications. New York: Raven Press, 1990.

73 Syrjänen K, Gissmann L, Koss LG. *Papillomaviruses and Human Disease*. Heidelberg: Springer Verlag, 1987; pp 1–518.

74 von Krogh G, Rylander E (eds) *Genital Papilloma Virus Infection: A Survey for the Clinician*. Karlstad: Conpharm, 1989.

75 Syrjänen K, Mäntyjärvi R, Väyrynen M *et al*. Human papillomavirus (HPV) infections involved in the neoplastic process of the uterine cervix as established by prospective follow-up of 513 women for two years. *Eur J Gynaecol Oncol* 1987; **8**: 5–16.

76 Syrjänen K, de Villiers E-M, Väyrynen M *et al*. Cervical papillomavirus infection progressing to invasive cancer in less than three years. *Lancet* 1985; **i**: 510–511.

77 Kitchener HC, Neilson L, Burnett RA, Young L, Macnab JC. Prospective serial study of viral change in the cervix and correlation with human papillomavirus genome status. *Br J Obstet Gynaecol* 1991; **98**: 1042–1048.

78 Montz FJ, Monk BJ, Fowler JC, Nguyen L. Natural history of the minimally abnormal Papanicolaou smear. *Obstet Gynecol* 1992; **80**: 385–388.

79 Carmichael JA. The management of minor degrees of cervical dysplasia associated with the human papilloma virus. *Yale J Biol Med* 1991; **64**: 591–597.

80 Courtial I, Bremond A, Aknin D. Regression spontanee des condylomes plan du col uterin. *J Gynecol Obstet Biol Reprod* 1991; **20**: 527–531.

81 de Villiers E, Wagner R, Schneider A, Wesch H, Munz F, zur Hausen H. Human papillomavirus DNA in women without and with cytological abnormalities: results of a 5-year follow-up study. *Gynecol Oncol* 1992; **44**: 33–42.

82 Franceschi S, Doll R, Gallway J, La Vecchia C, Peto R, Spriggs AI. Genital warts and cervical neoplasia: an epidemiological study. *Br J Cancer* 1983; **48**: 621–628.

83 Hirschowitz L, Raffle AE, Mackenzie EFD, Hughes AO. Long term follow up of women with borderline cervical smear test results effects of age and viral infection on progression to high grade dyskaryosis. *BJM* 1992; **304**: 1209–1212.

84 Hörding U, Saugaard S, Bock JE, Sebbelow AM, Norrild B. HPV 11, 16 and 18 DNA sequences in cervical swabs from women with cervical dysplasia prevalence and associated risk of progression. *Eur J Obstet Gynecol Rep Biol* 1991; **40**: 43–48.

85 Koutsky LA, Holmes KK, Critchlow CW *et al*. A cohort study of the risk of cervical intraepithelial neoplasia grade 2 or 3 in relation to papillomavirus infection. *N Engl J Med* 1992; **327**: 1272–1278.

86 Lörincz AT, Schiffman MH, Jaffurs WJ, Marlow J, Quinn AP, Temple GF. Temporal associations of human papillomavirus infection with cervical cytologic abnormalities. *Am J Obstet Gynecol* 1990; **162**: 645–651.

87 Pich A, Margaria E, Ghiringhello B, Navone R. *In situ* hybridization for human papillomavirus as a method of predicting the evolution of cervical intraepithelial neoplasia. *Arch Gynecol Obstet* 1992; **252**: 11–19.

88 Dudding N, Sutton J, Lane S. Koilocytosis; an indication for conservative management. *Cytopathology* 1996; 7: 32–37.

89 Hinchliffe SA, van Velzen D, Korporaal H, Kok PL, Boon ME. Transience of cervical HPV infection in sexually active, young women with normal cervivovaginal cytology. *Br J Cancer* 1995; **72**: 943–945.

90 Evander M, Edlund K, Gustafsson A *et al*. Human papillomavirus infection is transient in young women: a population-based cohort study. *J Infect Dis* 1995; **171**: 1026–1030.

91 Walker PG, Singer A, Dyson JL, Oriel JD. Natural history of cervical epithelial abnormalities in patients with vulval warts. A colposcopic study. *Br J Vener Dis* 1983; **59**: 327–329.

92 Handley J, Lawther H, Horner T, Maw R, Dinsmore W. Ten year follow-up study of women presenting to a genitourinary medicine clinic with anogenital warts. *Int J STD AIDS* 1992; **3**: 28–32.

93 Morrison EAB. Natural history of cervical infection with human papillomaviruses. *Clin Infect Dis* 1994; **18**: 172–180.

94 Downey GP, Bavin PJ, Deery ARS *et al*. Relation between human papillomavirus type 16 and potential for progression of minor-grade cervical disease. *Lancet* 1994; **344**: 432–435.

95 Kenemans P. HPV genotype as a prognostic factor for progression to cervical carcinoma in young women. *Eur J Obstet Gynecol Reprod Biol* 1994; **55**: 24–25.

96 Iwasaka T, Yokohama M, Matsuo N, Fukuda K, Mvula M, Sugimori H. *In situ* hybridization analysis of human papillomavirus DNA in cervical intraepithelial neoplasia. Prospective follow-up. *Cervix & Ifgt* 1994; **12**: 55–60.

97 Terry G, Ho L, Mansell M, Singer A. Relation between human papillomavirus type 16 and potential for progression of minor-grade cervical disease. *Lancet* 1994; **344**: 1096–1097.

98 Ho GYF, Burk RD, Klein S *et al*. Persistent genital human papillomavirus infection as a risk factor for persistent cervical dysplasia. *J Natl Cancer Inst* 1995; **87**: 1365–1371.

99 Saito J, Sumiyoshi M, Nakatani H, Hoshiai MIH, Noda K. Dysplasia and HPV infection initially detected by DNA analysis in cytomorphologically normal cervical smears. *Int J Gynecol Obstet* 1995; **51**: 43–48.

100 Takahashi Y, Yamade I, Nakamura T *et al*. Infection by human papillomavirus types 6, 11, 16, 18, 31, 33 and 35 of the cervix in Japanese women. *Int J Gynecol Cancer* 1995; **5**: 45–48.

101 Remmink AJ, Walboomers JMM, Helmerhorst TJM *et al*. The presence of persistent high-risk HPV genotypes in dysplastic cervical lesions is associated with progressive disease: natural history up to 36 months. *Int J Cancer* 1995; **61**: 306–311.

102 Liu T, Soong SJ, Alvarez RD, Butterworth CE. A longitudinal analysis of human papillomavirus 16 infection, nutritional status, and cervical dysplasia progression. *Cancer Epidemiol Biomarkers Prev* 1995; **4**: 373–380.

# 10: Optimal Management of Cervical Cancer Precursors: Low-Grade Squamous Intraepithelial Lesions

## A. Ferenczy

## Summary

The objective of this study was to review current data on the management options for women with an initial minor-grade cytological atypia (atypical squamous cells of undetermined significance/low-grade squamous intraepithelial lesion – ASCUS/LGSIL) smear, through review of literature and personal experience.

The results showed that only a small proportion of women with ASCUS/LGSIL smears have persistent/progressive-type low-grade lesion or have pre-existent high-grade squamous intraepithelial lesions (HGSIL). Modern management guidelines are thus centred on identifying those at risk for having clinically significant lesions. Low-risk patients (< 25 years, reliable for follow-up, negative history of cervical cytology and/or therapy, monogamous, cytology laboratory with high rates of false-positives) benefit from colposcopy only if minor-grade atypia persists on cytology. Those at high risk (> 25 years, unreliable, suspected/known previous history of positive cytology and/or therapy, promiscuous and cytology laboratory with low false-positives) should have colposcopy at once.

An alternative diagnostic triage to high-risk women uses the combination of cytology and human papillomavirus (HPV) DNA testing. According to several clinical trials, the sensitivity of the HPV DNA triage to detect HGSIL amongst women with an initial ASCUS/LGSIL smear is equal to colposcopy but has the potential to reduce unnecessary colposcopic referrals by 50%. A clinically suspicious cervix mandates immediate colposcopy/biopsy despite minor-grade atypia on cytology.

*Correspondence*: Professor Alex Ferenczy, Department of Pathology, Sir Mortimer B. Davis Jewish General Hospital, 3755 Côte Ste Catherine Road, Montreal, Quebec, Canada H3T 1E2.

The conclusions were that current management of women with minor-grade cytology atypia should focus on identifying those with clinically significant lesions. Persistent LGSILs can be successfully treated by ablative methods, particularly with cryotherapy, whereas loop electroexcision is the preferred technique for treating incidentally found HGSILs. Cytological follow-up must be part of the overall management scheme.

## Introduction

LGSILs have been shown to form a heterogeneous group with respect to their natural history and viral content. In a multicentre study involving 2600 women with LGSIL, 17% had HPV type 6 and 11, 20% had HPV 16 and 18, 11% HPV 31, 33 and 35, 22% other types and in 30% HPV was not detected [1]. While the majority (two-thirds) of LGSIL regress during long-term follow-up [2], between 8% and 25% progress to HGSIL, and occasionally to invasive carcinoma [3–5]. Progression seems to be related to DNA ploidy and HPV type. In one study, the majority (91%) of lesions with polyploid DNA values regressed, whereas those with aneuploidy persisted (81%) and 12% progressed to HGSIL [6]. Regarding progression and viral type, in 22 (85%) of 26 cases of LGSIL that progressed to HGSIL during a follow-up of 19–30 months were positive for HPV 16 [7]. Conversely, in a study on 342 women with LGSIL, no progression was observed in the absence of HPV DNA or with low-oncogenic-risk HPV types 6 or 11, whereas 17 (89%) of the 19 women with progressive disease to HGSIL were positive for high oncogenic HPV types, mainly type 16. Others found that an increased amount of HPV 16 DNA in cervical smears as determined by polymerase chain reaction (PCR) technology predicted the subsequent presence of HGSIL on biopsy specimens in nearly 90% of patients [8].

## Management options

Currently, there are two major options for the management of patients with minor-grade cytological atypia, including ASCUS and LGSIL [9]. One recommends colposcopy for only those women who have persistent low-grade abnormality, e.g. at least two positive smears within a 2-year follow-up period; the other favours colposcopy at once for all patients with a single abnormal cytology suggestive of or consistent with LGSIL. Both options have clinical merits provided they are applied according to whether the patient represents low or high risk for having or developing clinically significant lesions (Table 10.1; Fig. 10.1) [10]. The single most important demographic risk factor seems to be age; those aged 25 years and younger are very unlikely to have either cancer or HGSILs, as most women with an LGSIL revert to normal

**Table 10.1** Risk factors in patients with minor-grade cytological atypia.*

|  | Low-risk patient | High-risk patient |
|---|---|---|
| Age (years) | < 25 | > 25 |
| Reliability for follow-up | High | Low |
| Past history of abnormal cytology or therapy | No | Yes |
| Known to physician | Yes | No |
| Sexual habits | Monogamous | Polygamous |
| Cytology with high rates of false-positive results | Yes | No |
| Clinically suspicious cervix | No | Yes |

* Initial smear.

[11]. Those aged 25 years or older are candidates for immediate colposcopic examination, as the likelihood of lesional tissue is high. Conversely, cytological practices in which the false-positive rates are high (> 10%) lead to too many unnecessary colposcopic examinations. In such situations, it is more economical to follow women with cytology to ascertain persistent cytological abnormality.

## Pretreatment diagnostic work-up

It is important to realize that cervical cytology is not a diagnostic, but rather a screening test. In other words, a negative test has no significance in the face of a clinically suspicious cervix. Such patients should be colposcoped and biopsied at once to rule out invasive cancer. Conversely, a positive test suggestive of a low-grade cytological abnormality only indicates the least severe abnormality the patient may have. For example, HGSIL can be found in nearly 7% and 20% of patients with an initial ASCUS and LGSIL smear, respectively [12] and 30% of patients with invasive cancer of the cervix have had two ASCUS smears.

Traditionally, it was recommended to obtain directed (target) biopsies of the colposcopically 'worse' areas. The drawback of this approach was that it has encouraged taking one or two samples and what seemed to the clinician the worst area was not necessarily the area of occult invasion. In order to enhance recognizing occult invasive disease, it is advisable to be redundant and routinely to perform an endocervical curettage (ECC) in all pregnant patients to establish a disease-free endocervical canal and to take multiple punch biopsies, including the squamocolumnar junction (SCJ) of the atypical transformation zone (ATZ) [13]. The latter area is particularly important, as the

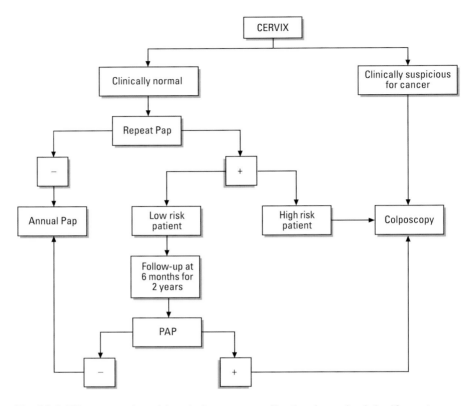

**Fig. 10.1** When an equivocal (atypical squamous cells of undetermined significance) or low-grade squamous intraepithelial lesion smear on cytology is not supported by a repeat Papanicolaou (Pap) test and the cervix is clinically normal, the patient is followed with annual Pap tests. Any patient with a clinically suspicious cervix should be sent to colposcopy. If the repeat Pap smear is positive for minor-grade cytological atypia, the low-risk patient (see text for description) may be followed with Pap tests at 6-month intervals for up to 2 years to determine whether her lesion will remain persistent or regress. High-risk patients (see text for description) should be colposcoped at once and, if appropriate, treated to prevent the development of invasive disease. From: Ferenczy and Jenson [10] with permission.

majority of early invasive lesions are located within a few millimetres from the SCJ of the ATZ. Using a 'redundant' diagnostic work-up, the information obtained is similar to that offered by a diagnostic cone, and virtually ensures that the patient with cancer is not treated as if she had SIL.

## Alternative HPV-based diagnostic triage

The presently available data clearly indicate that the common denominator separating LGSILs with cancer potential from those with benign behaviour is the persistent presence of high values of high-risk HPV types [8,14]. The use of modern HPV DNA testing (Hybrid Capture HPV DNA assay, Digene Corporation, MD, USA) of women with minor-grade cytological atypia has been evaluated as one of the options for managing women with ASCUS and LGSIL smears [12,15,16]. According to the HPV-based triage approach (alternate between colposcopy for all versus cytological follow-up), only women aged 25 years and older, and those at high risk at any age, with minor-grade smears who test positive for high-risk HPV DNA would be referred to colposcopy (Fig. 10.2). The sensitivity of the combination cytology and HPV testing for detecting HGSIL in these women is 95–100%. On the other hand, HPV-negative women with a clinically normal cervix would have colposcopy deferred.

A repeat negative cytology and HPV test on follow-up confer a negative value of close to 100% [12,15,16]. Using the HPV-based triage, unnecessary

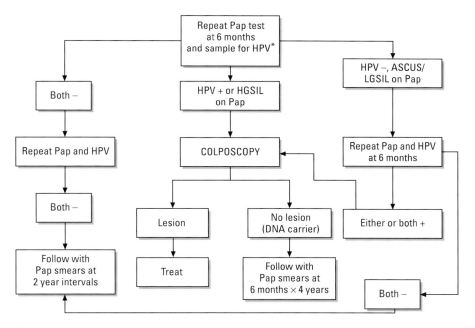

**Fig. 10.2** Human papillomavirus (HPV)-based triage. Flow chart illustrating the intermediate triage approach for the evaluation of women with atypical squamous cells of undetermined significance (ASCUS) or low-grade squamous intraepithelial lesions (LGSIL) on conventional Papanicolaou (Pap) smears. Two negative Pap tests and HPV tests have a very high negative predictive value, hence the 2-year rather than annual follow-up with Pap smears. Colposcopy is mandatory for patients with a positive HPV test or HGSIL on a repeat smear, whereas those with a negative HPV with an ASCUS/LGSIL smear may either be colposcoped or followed with a Pap smear and HPV tests. If either or both tests persist or become positive, colposcopy is indicated. Patients with latent HPV infection (HPV DNA carriers) are followed with Pap tests at 6-month intervals for 4 years, after which they are returned to the routine follow-up pool. From Ferenczy [17] with permission.

colposcopic examinations and overtreatment may be reduced by 30–50%. Measurable reduction in cost is foreseen if the patient with minor-grade cytologic atypia was not required to return to the physician's office for obtaining samples for HPV DNA testing. In this triage protocol, routine cytology is performed with liquid-based cell collection and processing technology and HPV DNA is assayed in the cellular residues of liquid-based collection kits (Preservcyt, Cytyc Corporation, MA, USA) used for preparing thin-layer type slides. HPV DNA testing is done only in those women whose thin-layer slides were read as positive for minor-grade cytologic atypia [18]. Using this scheme, an office visit for HPV DNA sampling and repeat smear could be eliminated, which in turn may result in further cost saving.

There are several ongoing clinical trials, including two Centers for Disease Control and one very large-scale National Cancer Institute-sponsored studies addressing the clinical utility of HPV DNA testing in women with ASCUS/ LGSIL smears.

## Treatment options

Management algorithms based on patient's risk factors are illustrated in Fig. 10.1. Once persistent low-grade SIL have been documented and invasive cancer ruled out by histology, the choice of therapy may be tailored according to the size and position of the endocervical margin of the lesional epithelium. Very large lesions with extension into the external os are best treated with loop electroexcision (central portion of the lesion) under local anaesthesia and electrofulgurating the periphery of the lesional tissue. Fortunately, most LGSILs are exocervical in their presentation and can be easily and successfully ablated using cryotherapy [13]. It is customary to follow patients for 1 year after either ablative or excisional therapy by cytology and colposcopy (first-3–6 months post-treatment visit) and, if the results are negative, the patients are followed regularly with cytology at annual intervals.

## References

1 Lorincz AT, Reid R, Jenson AB et al. Human papillomavirus infection of the cervix: relative risk associations of 15 common anogenital types. *Obstet Gynecol* 1992; **79**: 328.
2 Montz FJ, Monk BJ, Fowler JM et al. Natural history of the minimally abnormal Papanicolaou smear. *Obstet Gynecol* 1992; **80**: 385.
3 Richart RM, Barron BA. A follow-up study of patients with cervical dysplasia. *Am J Obstet Gynecol* 1969; **105**: 386.
4 Syrjänen, K, Mäntyjärvi R, Väyrynan M et al. Assessing the biological potential of human papillomavirus infections in cervical carcinogenesis. In: Steinberg BM, Brandsma JL, Taichman LB (eds) *Papillomavirus*, vol. 5. *Cancer Cells*. Cold Spring Harbor, NY: Cold Spring Harbor Laboratory, 1987; p 281.

5 Campion MJ, McCance DJ, Cuzick J et al. Progression potential of mild cervical atypia: prospective cytological, colposcopic and virological study. *Lancet* 1986; **2**: 237.

6 Fu YS, Reagan JW, Richart RM. Definition of precursor. *Gynecol Oncol* 1981; **12**: S220.

7 Remmink A, Helmerhorst T, Walboomers JM et al. HPV in follow-up of patients with cytomorphologically abnormal cervical smears: a prospective nonintervention study. *Int J Cancer* 1995; **61**: 1.

8 Cuzick J, Terry G, Ho L et al. Human papillomavirus type 16 DNA in cervical smears as predictor of high-grade cervical intraepithelial neoplasia. *Lancet* 1992; **339**: 959.

9 Kurman RJ, Henson DE, Herbst AL et al. Interim guidelines for management of abnormal cervical cytology. The 1992 National Cancer Institute Workshop. *JAMA* 1994; **23**: 1866.

10 Ferenczy A, Jenson AB. The key to rational triage of cervical neoplasia. In: Lorincz A, Reid R (eds) *Obstetrics and Gynecology Clinics of North America.* Philadelphia: WB Saunders, 1996, in press.

11 Schiffman MH. Recent progress in defining the epidemiology of human papillomavirus infection and cervical neoplasia. *J Natl Cancer Inst* 1992; **84**: 394.

12 Wright TC, Sun XW, Koulos J. Comparison of management algorithms for the evaluation of women with low-grade cytologic abnormalities. *Obstet Gynecol* 1995; **85**: 202.

13 Ferenczy A. Management of the patient with an abnormal Papanicolaou test: recent developments. In: Wright VC (ed) *Obstetrics and Gynecology Clinics of North America. Contemporary Colposcopy.* Philadelphia: WB Saunders, 1993; p 189.

14 Ho GYF, Burk RD, Klein S et al. Persistent genital human papillomavirus infection as a risk factor for persistent cervical dysplasia. *J Natl Cancer Inst* 1995; **87**: 1365.

15 Cox JT, Lorincz AT, Schiffman MH et al. HPV testing by hybrid capture is useful in triaging women with a cytologic diagnosis of ASCUS. *Am J Obstet Gynecol* 1995; **172**: 946.

16 Hatch KD, Schneider A, Abdel-Nour MW. An evaluation of human papillomavirus testing for intermediate- and high-risk types as triage before colposcopy. *Am J Obstet Gynecol* 1995; **172**: 1150.

17 Ferenczy A. Viral testing for genital human papillomavirus infections: recent progress and clinical potentials. *Int J Gynecol Cancer* 1995; **5**: 321.

18 Ferenczy A, Franco E, Arseneau J et al. Liquid-based Thin-Prep smear technology can be used for HPV DNA testing. *Am J Obstet Gynecol* 1996; **175**: 651.

# 11: Optimal Management of Cervical Cancer Precursors: High-Grade Lesions

## A. Ferenczy

## Summary

The objective of this study was to review the rationale for choosing one over another modality to treat patients with high-grade squamous intraepithelial lesions (HGSILs), comparing ablative versus excisional methods.

The results showed that ablative therapy such as electrofulguration or cryotherapy for relatively small-size ($\leqslant 2.5$ cm) exocervical HGSILs is appropriate and results in a 90% cure rate after one treatment and 95% after repeat therapy. Large HGSILs respond poorly to ablative therapies, with cure rates not higher than 50% after repeat therapies. Carbon dioxide laser vaporization results in excellent cure rates (90%+) regardless of lesional size: however, the equipment is expensive, thus precluding its universal availability. Excisional techniques using cold knife cone, laser cone or electroexcisional cones for HGSIL of any size and distribution result in over 90% cure rate after a single treatment session. Complications associated with excisional techniques are higher (about 20%) than with ablative methods (about 2%). Among excisional techniques used, the loop electrosurgical excision procedure (LEEP) or large loop excision of the transformation zone (LLETZ) provides for the most cost-effective means to treat HGSILs.

In conclusion, ablative therapy is appropriate for small, exocervical lesions of high-grade histology provided invasive cancer has been ruled out and the patient is reliable to be followed at regular intervals. Of all excisional techniques, LEEP/LLETZ is preferred to treat large HGSILs. Only patients with cytologically and colposcopically unequivocal HGSILs should be managed

*Correspondence*: Professor Alex Ferenczy, Department of Pathology, Sir Mortimer B. Davis Jewish General Hospital, 3755 Côte Ste Catherine Road, Montreal, Quebec, Canada H3T 1E2.

with the 'see-and-treat' electroexcisional approach. Those with borderline lesions should be histologically documented by endocervical curettage and punch biopsies prior to initiating definite treatment.

## Introduction

There is compelling evidence to suggest that a substantial proportion of HGSIL if untreated progress to invasive disease [1]. HGSILs correspond to lesional epithelium of the cervix which, on cytological and histological grounds, contains abnormal morphology traditionally attributed to moderate to severe dysplasia to carcinoma-*in-situ* or cervical intraepithelial neoplasia (CIN grades II and III). The rationale for using the term HGSIL is that the above subsets of names really represent the same disease process and that their morphological distinction is arbitrary at best and impossible to reproduce in any consistent fashion at worst [2].

It has abundantly been documented that successful removal of HGSILs prevents the later development of most invasive squamous cell carcinomas and results in a measurable reduction in incidence and mortality due to cervical cancer [3]. As a result of better understanding of the natural history of HGSIL and advances made in instrumentations, the techniques and algorithms for treating patients with HGSIL have undergone modifications and refinement over the years [4].

Until the late 1960s, the choice of treatment was primarily based on the histological grade of lesions; CIN III were considered best treated by cervical conization or hysterectomy under general anaesthesia, whereas conization or ablation was carried out for CIN II lesions. The rationale for this two-disease/two-treatment approach was that CIN III was more likely to invade endocervical glands and/or associated with early invasion then CIN II.

With the increasing acceptance of colposcopy as a means of diagnostic yield from the 1970s, lesional size and distribution rather than morphological grade became factors that influenced choice of treatment [4]. It was shown that small HGSILs (measuring less than 2.5 cm in greatest diameter) responded favourably to ablative procedures (Table 11.1), whereas large lesions and those with endocervical gland involvement failed ablative therapies using alternating electric current or cryocoagulation. On the other hand, carbon dioxide ($CO_2$) laser photovaporization and radical diathermy yielded excellent results irrespective of the size of HGSIL (Table 11.1). Among all ablative techniques, other than external os stenosis, cryotherapy has proven to have the lowest complication rates (Table 11.2); the equipment is inexpensive, and for small-sized lesions, it seems to be the most cost-effective therapeutic approach. Electrofulguration is associated with very high rate of external os stenosis, particularly in women over 40 years of age; radical diathermy is expensive by

**Table 11.1** Results of treatment for high-grade squamous intraepithelial lesions by ablative techniques.

| Method | Failures (%) | |
|---|---|---|
| | Small (<2.5 cm) | Large* (>2.5 cm) |
| Electrofulguration | 10 | 60 |
| Radical diathermy | 1 | 7 |
| Cryotherapy | 10 | 40 |
| Carbon dioxide laser vaporization | 6 | 8 |

* With endocervical gland involvement.
From Ferenczy [4] with permission.

virtue of requiring general anaesthesia, whereas the $CO_2$ laser is expensive to purchase and maintain, limiting its use in referral centres.

Over the past 25 years, it became clear that a certain number of patients with invasive cancers have been treated with ablative methods as they had intraepithelial lesions [5–7]. The main reasons for missing invasion are failure to sample the cervix adequately and endocervical canal for histology prior to ablative therapy, and lack of abnormal vascular pattern by colposcopy or inexperience for recognizing invasive cancer vessels [5–9]. Because failure to provide adequate therapy for women with invasive cancer within a relatively short time-frame may be associated with loss of lives as well as leading to malpractice suits, many have suggested a return to excisional techniques for treating HGSILs [10–15].

Among these, cold knife conization has the longest history. While the results are excellent, the technique is expensive, as it is performed under general anaesthesia and, because it is essentially a blind procedure, it removes unnecessarily a large portion of normal tissue which in turn may lead to relatively high complication rates [16] (Table 11.3). In some hands, the scalpel has been replaced by the $CO_2$ laser beam [10]. The advantage of this technique is that, because it is guided by colposcopy less normal tissue is removed compared to the cold knife conization technique. The disadvantages of $CO_2$ laser conization are the high cost of the equipment and high rates of charred,

**Table 11.2** Complications of ablation for high-grade squamous intraepithelial lesions.

| Method | Complication | % |
|---|---|---|
| Electrofulguration | Mainly os stenosis >40 years | 60 |
| Radical diathermy | Postoperative bleeding | 1.4 |
| Cryotherapy | Mainly os stenosis >40 years | 20 |
| Carbon dioxide laser | Postoperative bleeding | 10 |

From Ferenczy [4] with permission.

**Table 11.3** Complications of excision for high-grade squamous epithelial lesions.

| Method | Patients with complications % | |
|---|---|---|
|  | Bleeding* | Os stenosis |
| Cold knife cone | 14–22 | 17 |
| LEEP | 8 | 4 |

LEEP, Loop electrosurgical excision procedure.
* Perioperative and postoperative combined.
From Ferenczy [4] with permission.

histologically uninterpretable specimens [17]. In current practice, loop electro-conization is the preferred technique for treating HGSILs [11–15]. The procedure known as LLETZ or LEEP is performed in the office under local anaesthesia with the use of loop-shaped electrodes. Clinical experience with LLETZ/LEEP both in the UK and North America has yielded excellent cure rates and relatively low complications (Table 11.3). In addition, using this technique up to 4% of unexpected findings, including adenocarcinoma-*in-situ* and early invasion, are encountered [15]. In the early phases of the learning curve, thermocoagulation injury to tissue margins may make histological interpretation difficult; however, after half a dozen cases or so, the technique is mastered and thermocoagulation-related diagnostic problems are eliminated.

Because of the relative simplicity of the technique yet its great excisional power, two problems have been noted with loop electroconizations: first, the danger of removing an excessive amount of tissue and second, too frequently removing histologically disease-free tissue. Indeed, LEEP-negative specimen rates range between 5% and 60% [14]. In general, low-grade lesions are associated with the highest rates of histologically negative specimens, whereas the lowest rates are observed with their high-grade counterparts.

The first problem relates to the use of loop electrodes with depth greater than 1.5 cm or performing double excisional procedures or still failure of using colposcopic guidance during electroexcision. When loop electrodes measuring 8 mm in depth are used and the procedure is performed under colposcopic control, the danger of removing an excessive amount of tissue and the inherent complications, including bleeding, stenosis and premature deliveries, associated with such inappropriate instruments and techniques are eliminated [15,18].

The two major factors resulting in overtreatment are first, misclassification of benign (atypia of repair) or normal (squamous metaplastic) conditions and second, multiple punch biopsies of relatively small lesions performed prior to loop electroexcisions. In the latter case, the lesions are often removed entirely or the residual lesion is destroyed during the process of repair of the biopsied areas.

While no technique prevents overtreating some patients, high rates of LEEP-negative specimens can be avoided by applying the traditional diagnostic triage for patients with cytologically and colposcopically equivocal and low-grade-type lesions. Patients with unequivocal lesions, particularly the high-grade variant, may be managed with the 'see-and-treat' protocol in one sitting. In over 90% of these patients (provided the specimen contains no invasion), loop electroexcision results in cure in one office visit. There are additional advantages of 'see-and-treat'. These are improved patient compliance with treatment (patients lost to therapy may be as high as 30% [19]) and reduced patient anxiety by eliminating the wait between biopsy and treatment.

Poor compliance with treatment of cervical cancer precursors is a particularly important issue in developing countries, as nearly 80% of women may be lost to follow-up after either an abnormal cervical cytology or colposcopy and biopsy. In these countries, cervical cancer is the leading malignancy and cause of death among women, and paradoxically the comparatively more expensive cold knife conization or hysterectomy is the choice of therapy. LEEP in these countries seems to be the ideal technique to manage women with cervical cancer precursors, inexpensively and adequately.

## References

1 McIndoe WA, McLean MA, Jones RW *et al.* Treatment of carcinoma *in situ*: evaluation of 1609 cases. *Obstet Gynecol* 1984; **64**: 451.

2 Tabbara S, Saleh ADM, Anderson WA *et al.* The Bethesda classification for squamous intraepithelial lesions: histologic, cytologic and viral correlates. *Obstet Gynecol* 1992; **79**: 338.

3 Miller AB, Anderson G, Brisson J *et al.* Report of a national workshop on screening for cancer of the cervix. *Can Med Assoc J* 1991; **145**: 1301.

4 Ferenczy A. Management of patients with high grade squamous intraepithelial lesions. *Cancer* 1995; **76**: 1928.

5 Townsend DE, Richart RM. Diagnostic errors in colposcopy. *Gynecol Oncol* 1981; **12**: S259.

6 Shumsky AG, Stuart GCE, Nation J. Carcinoma of the cervix following conservative management of cervical intraepithelial neoplasia. *Gynecol Oncol* 1994; **53**: 50.

7 Pearson SE, Whittaker J, Ireland D *et al.* Invasive cancer of the cervix after laser treatment. *Br J Obstet Gynaecol* 1989; **96**: 486.

8 Benedet JL, Anderson GH, Boyes DA. Colposcopic accuracy in the diagnosis of microinvasive and occult invasive carcinoma of the cervix. *Obstet Gynecol* 1985; **65**: 557.

9 Helmerhorst TJM. Clinical significance of endocervical curettage as part of colposcopic evaluation: a review. *Int J Gynecol Cancer* 1992; **2**: 256.

10 McIndoe GA, Robson MS, Tidy JA *et al.* Laser excision rather than vaporization: the treatment of choice for cervical intraepithelial neoplasia. *Obstet Gynecol* 1989; **74**: 165.

11 Keijser KGG, Kenemans P, van der Zanden PHTH *et al.* Diathermy loop excision in the management of cervical intraepithelial neoplasia: diagnosis and treatment in one procedure. *Am J Obstet Gynecol* 1992; **166**: 1281.

12 Wright TC, Richart RM, Ferenczy A. *Electrosurgery for HPV-related Diseases of the Lower*

*Genital Tract: A Practical Handbook for Diagnosis and Treatment by Electroexcision and Fulguration Procedures.* Montreal: Arthur Vision and BioVision, 1992.

13 Houghton SJ, Luesley DM. LLETZ-diathermy loop excision. *Curr Obstet Gynaecol* 1995; **5**: 107.

14 Hodges DJ. Loop excision of the transformation zone (LETZ) for cervical dysplasia – a review. *J SOGC* 1994; **16**: 2017.

15 Ferenczy A, Choukroun D, Arseneau J. Loop electrosurgical excision procedure for squamous intraepithelial lesions of the cervix: advantages and potential pitfalls. *Obstet Gynecol* 1996; **87**: 332.

16 Luesley DM, McCrum A, Terry PB *et al.* Complications of cone biospy related to the dimensions of the cone and the influence of prior colposcopic assessment. *Br J Obstet Gynaecol* 1985; **92**: 158.

17 Howell R, Hammond R, Pryse-Davies J. The histologic reliability of laser cone biopsy of the cervix. *Obstet Gynecol* 1991; **77**: 905.

18 Ferenczy A, Choukroun D, Falcone T *et al.* The effect of cervical loop electrosurgical excision procedure on subsequent pregnancy outcome: North America experience. *Am J Obstet Gynecol.* 1995; **172**: 1246.

19 Spitzer M, Chernys AE, Seltzer VL. The use of large-loop excision of the transformation zone in an inner-city population. *Obstet Gynecol* 1993; **82**: 731.

# 12: Glandular Lesions: An Increasing Problem

A. Ferenczy

## Summary

The objective of this study was to review current data on the natural history of endocervical adenocarcinoma, through review of literature.

The results showed that the peak incidence of cervical adenocarcinoma reached a plateau in the 1970s; the incidence more than doubled among younger women in many countries. Epidemiological–clinical–viral correlates support the notion that the pathogenesis of adenocarcinoma and squamous cell carcinomas of the uterine cervix is similar. Cervical cytology is relatively insensitive for detecting adenocarcinoma and its precursor, adenocarcinoma-*in-situ* (AIS). Since human papillomavirus (HPV), particularly type 18, is most likely involved as an aetiological agent of cervical adenocarcinomas, reliable tracing techniques combined with cervical cytology to identify this virus are warranted.

In conclusion, the relative rarity of this condition warrants multicentre-type studies combining molecular biology and epidemiology. The study should be extended to factors other than HPV that could have interactive effects on pathogenesis. The role of sex steroid hormones is particularly important to investigate. The results of studies may improve the classification of glandular cell abnormalities proposed by the Bethesda system, including the clinical relevance of the Bethesda system's atypical gland cells of undetermined significance (AGUS).

*Correspondence*: Professor Alex Ferenczy, Department of Pathology, Sir Mortimer B. Davis Jewish General Hospital, 3755 Côte Ste Catherine Road, Montreal, Quebec, Canada H3T 1E2.

## Epidemiology

Adenocarcinomas and adenosquamous carcinomas of the uterine cervix are becoming an increasingly important issue in gynaecology. They represent approximately 10% of all tumours of the cervix, with some evidence from clinical studies that this proportion has been increasing over time [1–6]. For example, in one earlier series, the proportion of adenocarcinomas was 8.2% during 1969–1978 but 18.6% during 1979–1980. These figures, however, do not derive from population-based series and may be subject to referral biases. Also, it has been problematic to determine the extent to which relative increases in adenocarcinomas and adenosquamous carcinomas reflect real increases, decreases in squamous cell carcinomas or changes in morphological classification during the past three decades.

However, several population-based studies confirm an increase in cervical adenocarcinoma over time, particularly in young women. Proportional incidence ratios from Los Angeles contained an 8% increase per year of invasive adenocarcinomas between 1972 and 1982 among women aged 35 years and younger [7]. At the same time, the rates of adenocarcinomas in older women as well as squamous cell carcinomas decreased appreciably. Increases in adenocarcinoma rates among younger women were most noticeable in those of the middle to upper socioeconomic strata. The time trend data were confirmed by Schwartz and Weiss [8], who examined data on a nationwide basis from the Surveillance, Epidemiology, and End Results (SEER) programme. They found a twofold increase between 1973 and 1982 among women less than 35 years of age, representing an annual incidence of 10%. Using SEER data through 1985, Devesa *et al.* [9] showed that the increase in cervical adenocarcinoma rates among those women less than 35 years old reached maximum levels during the 1970s.

Two surveys in Europe have corroborated the increases in the incidence of cervical adenocarcinomas among young women. According to data from three cancer registries in the UK, the incidence of adenocarcinomas increased from 2.4/million women aged 20–34 years old between 1968 and 1972 to 4.7/million women between 1978 and 1982. During the same period, squamous cell carcinomas among young and older women increased and drastically decreased, respectively [10]. Similarly, in Norway, squamous cell carcinomas decreased by 30 between 1970 and 1984, while adenocarcinomas increased by 38%, especially in women aged 20–34 years old during the same period [11]. Data from two major oncology centres in Australia showed a doubling in relative incidence of adenocarcinoma and adenosquamous carcinoma between the 1970s and 1980s, and account for 21.5% and 24%, respectively, of all cervical cancers [12].

There may be a number of non-aetiological explanations for the changing incidence rates. These include increased detection of early, asymptomatic lesions, improved cytodiagnosis and histological classifications over time, and increased hysterectomy rates.

## Age and racial trends

These are difficult to assess because the clinical studies may not all be representative. For example, in one study the rate of increase with age was identical for both squamous cell and adenocarcinomas prior to age 34, whereas the rate of increase declined with age for squamous cell cancer but not for adenocarcinomas [11]. In another study, such trends were not observed [13]. There is a possible but not proven predilection for adenocarcinoma among Asians [13].

## Risk factors

There are not too many well-designed studies focusing on the aetiology of adenocarcinomas [14–16]. In those in which this issue was well-evaluated, risk factors were similar to the epidemiology of cervical squamous cell carcinomas, including three or more births, early age at first intercourse, multiple sexual partners and history of sexually transmitted diseases (STDs). There is increasing evidence supporting the hypothesis of a hormone–adenocarcinoma relationship. Whether hormonal factors are aetiologically related to the development of cervical adenocarcinomas is not clear, however. Adenocarcinomas are encountered in pregnant women [17]; associations between oral contraceptive (OC) use and the occurrence of adenocarcinoma/hyperplasia has been noted [18–22] and adenocarcinomas often contain $E_2$ and P receptors [23]. While earlier studies failed to show a link between OC use and a higher risk of developing cervical adenocarcinoma, in three case-controlled studies with appropriate controls, an increased risk of cervical carcinomas or adenosquamous carcinomas was found among OC users (Table 12.1) [22,24,25]. In one study, the risk rose with duration of use, with a threefold increased risk in users of 10 or more years compared to non-users [24]. In the other study, ever

Table 12.1 Relationship between oral contraceptive use and adenocarcinoma of cervix.

|  | Relative risk/years of use | |
|---|---|---|
|  | < 5 years | > 10 years |
| Brinton et al. (1986) [24] | 1.4 | 3.0 |
| Brinton et al. (1990) [25] | 2.6 | 1.8 |
| Ursin et al. (1994) [22] | 1.7 | 4.4 |

use was associated with twice as great a risk of adenocarcinoma and the highest risk (4.4) was observed for OC use for more than 12 years [22]. Moreover, OC users were at persistently higher risk compared with non-users, even after adjustment for confounding factors [25].

How OCs might result in adenocarcinomas is unknown. Experimentally, progestational agents were shown to be tumorigenic in nude mice when baby rat kidney cells were infected by HPV types 16 and cellular oncogenes were activated [26]. Progestogens appear to compete for glucocorticoid receptor element in HPV DNA, resulting in impairment of viral regulatory region. Because microglandular endocervical hyperplasia (MEH) has been linked to either endogenous (pregnancy) or exogenous (OCs) progestational stimulation, MEH was considered to represent possible precursor lesions of adenocarcinoma. However, histological continuity between these two conditions is not observed and a recent case-controlled study failed to demonstrate statistically significant differences between MEH with and without a history of progestational exposure [27].

Cigarette smoking and dietary factors, such as β-carotene, vitamin C, and folate, have not been linked with cervical adenocarcinoma risk [28]. In two case-controlled studies, there was no indication that the effect of OCs was due to life-time number of cervical smears [22,24].

## Effect of screening

In general, screening has not been highly effective in detecting cervical adenocarcinomas [29]. However, two epidemiological studies noted increasing risks with longer smear intervals and with ever receiving a Papanicolaou (Pap) smear [14,30]. Also, higher false-negative rates are reported for patients with adenocarcinomas than for their squamous cell counterparts [31,32]. This issue is particularly important, as a high proportion of rapidly progressing tumours are likely to be adenocarcinomas [33].

## HPV infection and gland cell neoplasms of cervix

Current data derived from molecular hybridization techniques suggest a strong association of HPV with cervical adenocarcinoma. Several studies using *in situ* hybridization, Southern blot and polymerase chain reaction (PCR) methods localized HPV DNA in cervical adenocarcinomas (Table 12.2). The prevalence of HPV DNA in these lesions ranges from 0 to 60% using *in situ* hybridization, from 31 to 42% using PCR and from 53 to 88% using Southern blot hybridization. HPV 18 is the predominant type in most studies, whereas HPV 16 is the prevailing type in squamous cell carcinomas. The relatively high prevalence of HPV DNA in adenocarcinomas corroborates the findings from

**Table 12.2** Prevalence of human papillomavirus (HPV) 18 versus 16 in cervical adenocarcinomas by method of detection.

| Method | Adenocarcinoma | | Adenosquamous cell Ca | |
|---|---|---|---|---|
| | HPV 18(%) | HPV 16(%) | HPV 18(%) | HPV 16(%) |
| *In situ* | 14–56 | 2–18 | 13–19 | 19–26 |
| PCR | 6–27 | 15–25 | ND | ND |
| Southern blot | 59 | 24 | ND | ND |

Ca, Carcinoma; PCR, polymerase chain reaction; ND, not detected.

case-control studies, indicating a relationship between HPV infection and cervical adenocarcinoma [14,15].

## Precursors of adenocarcinoma

Adenocarcinoma-*in-situ* (AIS) is considered as a precursor lesion that may progress to invasive adenocarcinoma. The evidence for this contention includes cytological features which are similar in both conditions; AIS is often contiguous to invasive cancer, the peak incidence occurs about 5–8 years earlier than that of invasive carcinoma [34] and there has been a high rate of HPV DNA detection in coexistent cases of invasive and AIS (54–100%) with often the same HPV types [34,35]. Also, as in invasive disease, in AIS, HPV type 18 is predominant (Table 12.3).

Whether the so-called endocervical glandular dysplasia has precursor potential is unclear. Most studies showed no clinical or histological correlation

**Table 12.3** Prevalence of human papillomavirus (HPV) DNA in cervical adenocarcinoma-*in-situ* (AIS) with and without invasive cancer and glandular dysplasia by *in situ* hybridization.

| Authors | AIS | | | | Glandular dysplasia | |
|---|---|---|---|---|---|---|
| | With invasive adenocarcinoma | | Without invasive adenocarcinoma | | | |
| | HPV 18 (%) | HPV 16 (%) | HPV 18 (%) | HPV 16 (%) | HPV 18 (%) | HPV 16 (%) |
| Tase *et al.* (1989) [34] | 46 | 27 | 50 | 20 | | |
| Farnsworth *et al.* (1989) [35] | 75 | 25 | 54 | 31 | 0 | 0 |
| Leary *et al.* (1991) [36] | | | 37 | 33 | 31 | 15 |
| Tase *et al.* (1989) [37] | | | | | 6 | 0 |

with AIS or invasive adenocarcinoma; morphologically such lesions resemble reactive atypia or hyperplasia or tuboendometrial epithelium rather than dysplasia, and HPV DNA is seldom or not found, in spite of a high rate (64%) of HPV 18/16 positivity in the coexistent AIS/invasive adenocarcinoma or cervical intraepithelial neoplasia (CIN) [35–37]. It should be realized that the glandular epithelium does not accept productive-type HPV infections, thus the morphological alternations commonly found in early squamous intraepithelial lesions, i.e. koilocytotic atypia, are lacking in endocervical gland cells (Table 12.3).

In most series, AIS is associated with squamous intraepithelial lesions (SIL)/CIN in over 50% of the cases and in 63% of coexistent lesions, HPV DNA is found [34]. It may be that both the squamous and glandular lesions develop from subcolumnar reserve cells infected by HPV 18 or 16 through a process of bidirectional differentiation.

## Colposcopy/histology/cytology

The majority of AIS cases are not grossly visible, nor are appreciable with the colposcope [38] and produce no clinical symptoms or signs such as vaginal bleeding. Only occasionally, there is a granular surface erosion with some nodularity. AIS involves the transformation zone in over two-thirds of cases and is multifocal only occasionally [38,39].

Histologically, both invasive and *in situ* forms may be classified as endocervical type, endometrioid type, intestinal type, mixtures of the above, mucoepidermoid, clear cell type, adenoid basal cell carcinoma, adenoid cystic carcinoma, adenoma malignum and glassy cell carcinoma. There is no compelling evidence that the histological classification can be reproduced in cytology or helps cytological detection. In fact, most cytopathologists simply divide endocervical gland cell neoplasms into well-differentiated and poorly differentiated AIS and invasive cancer [40].

Endocervical cytology is difficult; false-negative rates in large series range from 14% [2] through 42% [2] to 100% [40]. Many cases are missed because of severe inflammation and necrosis and many AIS cases are in fact discovered because of coexistent SIL.

## Endocervical atypia

Another problematic area in endocervical cytology revolves around the so-called endocervical atypia. Unfortunately, the Bethesda system failed to define clearly the diagnostic criteria of the AGUS category other than referring to cytological alterations intermediate between reactive changes and AIS. It is noteworthy that approximately 50% of AGUS smears may be associated with clinically significant cervical lesions, including SIL, AIS and invasive adenocarcinoma [41]. False positives may be due to polyps, tubal metaplasia, endocervical cell repair and overzealous sampling of the endocervical canal with endocervical cytobrush.

Because in most instances accurate prediction is not possible on cytological grounds, further investigations must include colposcopy and multiple punch biopsies, together with endocervical curettage. The final diagnosis depends on a diagnostic cone biopsy.

## The microinvasive adenocarcinoma controversy

Although progression of AIS to frankly invasive carcinoma probably occurs via a microinvasive stage, the critieria for selection of cases are too ambiguous precluding its diagnosis and thus data on its natural history are lacking. Indeed, back-to-back glands, glandular extensions beyond normal depth of gland clefts and destruction of basement membrane in association with inflammatory reaction at stromal gland interface are features with are encountered both in AIS and frank invasive carcinoma as well as in hyperplastic and inflammatory conditions of the endocervical epithelium.

## Invasive adenocarcinoma: clinical outcome

In a number of studies in which the stage of disease at diagnosis was controlled for, a poorer prognosis has been associated with adenocarcinomas versus their squamous cell variants [42]. The observations are consistent with the fact that adenocarcinomas are difficult to detect by cytology, usually have a large volume at diagnosis, their growth pattern is often endophytic (barrel-shaped) and they have a propensity for early lymphatic and haematogenous metastases. HPV type 18 rather than 16 predominates in adenocarcinomas. HPV 18 has a higher ($\pm 100\%$) integration rate then type 16 [43]. This physical state may lead to higher rates of viral deregulation, enhanced expression of viral oncoproteins ($E_6$, $E_7$), greater cell proliferation and a worse prognosis than cervical carcinomas in general. Several investigators noted a worse prognosis for patients with HPV-negative lesions [44,45].

## References

1 Davis JR, Moon LB. Increased incidence of adenocarcinoma of the uterine cervix. *Obstet Gynecol* 1975; **45**: 79.
2 Gallup DG, Abell MR. Invasive adenocarcinoma of the uterine cervix. *Obstet Gynecol* 1977; **49**: 596.
3 Shingleton HM, Gore H, Bradley DH *et al*. Adenocarcinoma of the cervix. I. Clinical evaluation and pathologic features. *Am J Obstet Gynecol* 1981; **139**: 799.

4 Tamimi HK, Figge DC. Adenocarcinoma of the uterine cervix. *Gynecol Oncol* 1982; **13**: 335.

5 Vesterinen E, Forss M, Nieminen U. Increase of cervical adenocarcinoma: a report of 520 cases of cervical carcinoma including 112 tumors with glandular elements. *Gynecol Oncol* 1989; **33**: 49.

6 Weiss RJ, Lucas WE. Adenocarcinoma of the uterine cervix. *Cancer* 1986; **57**: 1996.

7 Peters RK, Chao A, Mack TM *et al*. Increased frequency of adenocarcinoma of the uterine cervix in young women in Los Angeles County. *J Natl Cancer Inst* 1986; **76**: 423.

8 Schwartz SM, Weiss NS. Increased incidence of adenocarcinoma of the cervix in young women in the United States. *Am J Epidemiol* 1986; **124**: 1045.

9 Devesa SS, Young JL Jr, Brinton LA *et al*. Recent trends in cervix uteri cancer. *Cancer* 1989; **64**: 2184.

10 Chilvers C, Mant D, Pike MC. Cervical adenocarcinoma and oral contraceptives. *BMJ* 1987; **295**: 1446.

11 Eide TJ. Cancer of the uterine cervix in Norway by histologic type, 1970–84. *J Natl Cancer Inst* 1987; **79**: 199.

12 Elliott PM, Tattersall MHN, Coppleson M *et al*. Changing character of cervical cancer in young women. *BMJ* 1989; **298**: 288.

13 Anton-Culver H, Bloss JD, Bringman D *et al*. Comparison of adenocarcinoma and squamous cell carcinoma of the uterine cervix: a population-based epidemiologic study. *Am J Obstet Gynecol* 1992; **166**: 1507.

14 Kjaer SK, Brinton LA. Adenocarcinoma of the uterine cervix: the epidemiology of an increasing problem. *Epidemiol Rev* 1993; **15**: 486.

15 Parazzini F, La Vecchia C, Negri E *et al*. Risk factors for adenocarcinoma of the cervix: a case-control study. *Br J Cancer* 1988; **57**: 201.

16 Kvale G, Heuch I, Nilssen S. Reproductive factors and risk of cervical cancer by cell type. A prospective study. *Br J Cancer* 1988; **58**: 820.

17 Drew NC. Adenocarcinoma *in situ* of the cervix uteri associated with cervical intraepithelial neoplasia in pregnancy. Case report. *Br J Obstet Gynaecol* 1984; **91**: 498.

18 Chumas JC, Nelson B, Mann WJ *et al*. Microglandular hyperplasia of the uterine cervix. *Obstet Gynecol* 1985; **66**: 406.

19 Czernobilsky B, Kessler I, Lancet M. Cervical adenocarcinoma in a woman on long-term contraceptives. *Obstet Gynecol* 1974; **43**: 517.

20 Dallenbach-Hellweg G. On the origin and histological structure of adenocarcinoma of the endocervix in women under 50 years of age. *Pathol Res Pract* 1984; **179**: 38.

21 Taylor HB, Irey NS, Norris HJ. Atypical endocervical hyperplasia in women taking oral contraceptives. *JAMA* 1967; **202**: 637.

22 Ursin G, Peters RK, Henderson BE *et al*. Oral contraceptive use and adenocarcinoma of cervix. *Lancet* 1994; **344**: 1390.

23 Ford LC, Bereks JS, Lagasse LD *et al*. Estrogen and progesterone receptor sites in malignancies of the uterine cervix, vagina and vulva. *Gynecol Oncol* 1983; **15**: 27.

24 Brinton LA, Huggins GR, Lehman HF *et al*. Long-term use of oral contraceptives and risk of invasive cervical cancer. *Int J Cancer* 1986; **38**: 339.

25 Brinton LA, Reeves WC, Brenes MM *et al*. Oral contraceptive use and risk of invasive cervical cancer. *Int J Epidemiol* 1990; **19**: 4.

26 Pater A, Bayatpour M, Pater MM. Oncogenic transformation by human papillomavirus type 16 deoxyribonucleic acid in the presence of progesterone or progestins from oral contraceptives. *Am J Obstet Gynecol* 1990; **162**: 1099.

27 Greeley C, Schroeder S, Silverberg SG. Microglandular hyperplasia of the cervix: a true 'pill' lesion? *Int J Gynecol Pathol* 1995; **14**: 50.

28 Potischman N. Nutritional epidemiology of cervical neoplasia. *J Nutr* 1993; **123**: 424.

29 Nieminen P, Kallio M, Hakama M. The effect of mass screening on incidence and mortality of squamous and adenocarcinoma of cervix uteri. *Obstet Gynecol* 1995; **85**: 1017.

30 Herrero R, Brinton LA, Reeves WC *et al*. Screening for cervical cancer in Latin America: a case-control study. *Int J Epidemiol* 1992; **21**: 1050–1056.

31 Kjellgren O. The diagnostic accuracy of the vaginal smear in cancer of the uterine cervix. *Acta Obstet Gynecol Scand* 1995; **34**: 249.

32 Rylander E. Negative smears in women developing invasive cervical cancer. *Acta Obstet Gynecol Scand* 1977; **56**: 115.

33 Hadjimichael O, Janerich D, Lowell DM *et al*. Histologic and clinical characteristics associated with rapidly progressive invasive cervical cancer: a preliminary report from the Yale Cancer Control Research Unit. *Yale J Biol Med* 1989; **52**: 345.

34 Tase T, Okagaki T, Clark BA *et al*. Human papillomavirus DNA in adenocarcinoma *in situ*, microinvasive adenocarcinoma of the uterine cervix and coexisting cervical squamous intraepithelial neoplasia. *Int J Gynecol Pathol* 1989; **8**: 8.

35 Farnsworth A, Laverty C, Stoler MH. Human papillomavirus messenger RNA expression in adenocarcinoma *in situ* of the uterine cervix. *Int J Gynecol Pathol* 1989; **8**: 321.

36 Leary J, Jaworski R, Houghton R. *In-situ* hybridization using biotinylated DNA probes to human papillomavirus in adenocarcinoma-*in-situ* and endocervical glandular dysplasia of the uterine cervix. *Pathology* 1991; **23**: 85.

37 Tase T, Okagaki T, Clark BA *et al*. Human papillomavirus DNA in glandular dysplasia and microglandular hyperplasia: presumed precursors of adenocarcinoma of the uterine cervix. *Obstet Gynecol* 1989; **73**: 1005.

38 Duggan MA, Benoit JL, McGregor SE *et al*. Adenocarcinoma *in situ* of the endocervix: human papillomavirus determination by dot blot hybridization and polymerase chain reaction amplification. *Int J Gynecol Pathol* 1994; **13**: 143.

39 Ostor AG, Pagano R, Davoren RAM *et al*. Adenocarcinoma *in situ* of the cervix. *Int J Gynecol Pathol* 1984; **3**: 179.

40 Pacey NF. Glandular neoplasms of the uterine cervix. In: Bibbo M (ed) *Comprehensive Cytopathology*. Philadelphia: WB Saunders, 1991, pp 231–256.

41 Goff BA, Atanasoff P, Brown E *et al*. Endocervical glandular atypia in Papanicolaou smears. *Obstet Gynecol* 1992; **79**: 101.

42 Hopkins MP, Morley GW. A comparison of adenocarcinoma and squamous cell carcinoma of the cervix. *Obstet Gynecol* 1991; **77**: 912.

43 Cullen AP, Reid R, Campion M *et al*. Analysis of the physical state of different human papillomavirus DNAs in intraepithelial and invasive cervical neoplasm. *J Virol* 1991; **65**: 606.

44 Higgins GD, Davy M, Roder D *et al*. Increased age and mortality associated with cervical carcinomas negative for human papillomavirus RNA. *Lancet* 1991; **338**: 910.

45 De Britton RC, Hildesheim A, De Lao SL *et al*. Human papillomaviruses and other influences on survival from cervical cancer in Panama. *Obstet Gynecol* 1993; **81**: 19.

# 13: Papillomavirus Infection and Neoplasia in Women Infected with Human Immunodeficiency Virus

T. C. Wright, Jr

## Introduction

Infection with human immunodeficiency virus (HIV) has reached epidemic proportions in much of the world, including the USA. The World Health Organization (WHO) Global Programme on Acquired Immunodeficiency Syndrome (AIDS) estimated in December 1995 that there were 16.9 million HIV-infected adults in the world [1]. As of that date, 1 292 890 cases of AIDS in children and adults had been reported in the WHO Global Programme on AIDS. However, the number of AIDS cases reported to the WHO is low because of underdiagnosis, reporting delay and incomplete reporting, and it is estimated that 6 million adult and paediatric cumulative AIDS cases had occurred throughout the world as at the end of 1995. [1]. There are an estimated 650 000–950 000 HIV-infected people currently living in the USA and, as of October 1996, AIDS had been diagnosed in 548 000 persons in the USA [2]. Of these people, 343 000 have died and HIV infection has become the leading cause of death for both men and women aged 25–44 [3].

Over the last decade there has been a dramatic change in the proportion of patients being diagnosed with AIDS who are women. During the early years of the epidemic (from 1983 to 1987), women accounted for approximately 8% of all reported cases of AIDS; however, from 1987 to 1995, women accounted for 17.5% of reported cases of AIDS in the USA [4]. Similar increases have been reported from other parts of the world. In 1990 it was estimated that approximately 25% of HIV-infected people worldwide were women, whereas by 1992 that proportion had risen to 40% [5]. In the future it is expected that

*Correspondence*: Dr Thomas C. Wright, Jr, College of Physicians and Surgeons of Columbia University, Division of OB/Gyn Pathology, Room 16-402 P&S, 630 W 168th St., New York, NY 10032, USA.

the number of HIV-infected women will surpass the number of HIV-infected men. In New York City, approximately 1% of women giving birth were HIV-seropositive in 1994. However, much higher rates are detected in selected groups of women (M.A. Chiasson, personal communication). For example, up to 53% of women attending certain methadone maintenance clinics in New York City were HIV-seropositive in 1992, and figures from the New York City Department of Health HIV seroprevalence surveys estimate that 2.6% of runaway adolescent girls living in shelters are HIV-infected, as are 20% of women entering prison for the first time and 5.6% of black females attending City-run sexually transmitted disease (STD) clinics.

## Invasive cervical cancers in HIV-infected women

The first suggestion that there may be an association between cervical cancer and HIV infection came from several case reports of rapidly progressive invasive cervical cancers that developed in HIV-infected women. The first of these case reports was by Rellihan *et al.*, who described a 32-year-old HIV-infected woman who developed a moderate to poorly differentiated stage IIb invasive squamous cell carcinoma of the cervix and died, despite therapy 5 months after diagnosis [6]. Shortly after this report another was published describing a 25-year-old HIV-infected woman with stage IIIb invasive squamous cell carcinoma of the cervix [7]. This patient also died 5 months after diagnosis. These case reports of invasive cervical cancer in HIV-infected women were quickly followed by a case series of young women with invasive cervical cancer at the State University of New York (SUNY) at Brooklyn [8]. In this case series, 19% of women under the age of 50 who were diagnosed with invasive cervical cancer at SUNY, Brooklyn were HIV-infected. In that study many of the HIV-infected women were young, and for most, invasive cervical cancer was the first manifestation of their HIV infection. In addition, most of the cervical cancers in the seropositive group were bulky, high-stage tumours and were associated with a poor prognosis.

Based on these isolated case reports and the one case series from Brooklyn, the Centers for Disease Control and Prevention (Atlanta, GA) included invasive cervical cancer in the expanded 1993 surveillance case definition of AIDS [9]. A recent review of the New York City AIDS case surveillance data has identified 71 HIV-infected women with invasive cervical cancer in New York City. By using an estimate of 31 000 HIV-infected women in New York City, and age/race-specific incidence rates for cancer, it has been estimated that the observed : expected invasive cervical cancer incidence rate is 2.28 (95% confidence interval, 1.9–3.0) for HIV-infected women 25–49 years of age in New York City [10]. However, the impact of invasive cervical cancer as a cause of death in HIV-infected women remains relatively low. Vital statistic data from the USA indicate that HIV infection is currently having little impact on death rates from invasive cervical cancer in regions such as New York and northern New Jersey where HIV infection is common [11]. For example, analysis of death rates in New York city from 1983 to 1992 has failed to demonstrate an increase in the number of deaths from invasive cervical cancer in women of any age group [12]. Table 13.1 includes the results of most reported studies that have examined the prevalence of invasive cervical cancer among HIV-infected women. The women included in these studies were enrolled from a variety of geographic sites and clinical settings and were screened for the prevalence of cervical disease using either cytology alone or a combination of cytology and colposcopy. In only one of the 22 studies were invasive cervical cancers detected among the HIV-infected women screened.

In addition to invasive cervical cancer there is also concern that invasive vulvar cancer may be more common in HIV-infected women. Recently, we published a case report of two HIV-infected women with vulvar intraepithelial neoplasia who subsequently went on to develop invasive vulvar cancer, [13]. A similar report has come from Italy by Giorda *et al*. [14].

## Squamous intraepithelial lesions (SIL) in HIV-infected women

There are now numerous studies which have clearly documented an association between HIV infection and cervical cancer precursors (SIL). Early studies of cervical disease in HIV-infected women compared cytological findings among HIV-seropositive women with those in control populations of HIV-seronegative women. These studies have been reported from the USA, the UK, Zaire, Kenya and Italy. In almost all of these studies a higher prevalence of cytological abnormalities was detected among women infected with HIV than among the various control groups (Table 13.2). These cytological studies reported abnormal Papanicolaou (Pap) smear prevalence to be 52–63% among HIV-seropositive women. The prevalence of cytological abnormalities in the HIV-seropositive group is up to 12.5 times that observed among the control HIV-seronegative women in these studies.

Even though the results of the cytological studies comparing prevalence of cervical disease in HIV-infected and HIV-uninfected women have been remarkably similar, there has been concern that these studies have not actually confirmed the presence of cervical disease in HIV-infected women, and that they may not reflect the true prevalence of cervical cancer precursor lesions in this population. Therefore, two recent studies have used a combination of colposcopy and cytology to screen cohorts of HIV-infected and HIV-uninfected women for cervical disease [15,16]. The largest of these colposcopic studies is a multicentre study which we have referred to as the New York Cervical Disease Study (NYCDS) [15]. The key feature of this study is that all

**Table 13.1** Prevalence of cervical cancer in human immunodeficiency virus (HIV)-seropositive women.

| Reference | Location | Population studied | No. of HIV-seropositive women | Detection method | No. of cancers |
|---|---|---|---|---|---|
| Bryne et al. | London, UK | STD clinic | 19 | Cytology | 0 |
| Provencher et al. | Miami, USA | Voluntary HIV testing | 201 | Cytology | 0 |
| Schrager et al. | Bronx, USA | HIV heterosexual transmission study | 35 | Cytology | 0 |
| Vermund et al. | Bronx, USA | Methadone maintenance | 51 | Cytology | 0 |
| Carpenter et al. | Rhode Island, USA | HIV clinic | 100 | Cytology | 0 |
| Schafer et al. | Berlin, Germany | Prostitutes | 111 | Cytology | 5 |
| Maiman et al. | Brooklyn, USA | HIV clinic | 32 | Colpo/cytology | 0 |
| Marte et al. | Chicago and NYC, USA | Ambulatory care clinic | 135 | Cytology | 0 |
| Kreiss et al. | Nairobi, Kenya | Prostitutes | 42 | Cytology | 0 |
| Laga et al. | Kinshasa, Zaire | Prostitutes | 41 | Cytology | 0 |
| Spinillo et al. | Pavia, Italy | ID clinic | 75 | Colpo/cytology | 0 |
| Conti et al. | Milan, Italy | Former IVDU | 273 | Colpo/cytology | 0 |
| Smith et al. | London, UK | HIV and methadone clinics | 43 | Cytology | 0 |
| Maggwa et al. | Kenya | Family planning | 205 | Cytology | 0 |
| Gentile et al. | Bologna, Italy | HIV clinic | 32 | Colpo/cytology | 0 |
| Wright et al. | New York, USA | HIV and methadone clinics | 398 | Colpo/cytology | 0 |
| Korn et al. | San Francisco, USA | HIV clinic | 52 | Colpo/cytology | 0 |
| Johnstone et al. | Edinburgh, UK | Drug-related HIV | 92 | Cytology | 0 |
| Tweddel et al. | Philadelphia, USA | HIV clinic | 21 | Colpo/cytology | 0 |
| Seck et al. | Senegal | ID clinic | 14 | Cytology | 0 |
| Klein et al. | New York, USA | Methadone clinics, IVDU partner | 114 | Cytology | 0 |
| Heard et al. | Paris, France | Gynaecological outpatient service | 99 | Cytology | 0 |

STD, sexually transmitted disease; ID, infectious disease; IVDU, intravenous drug user.
Data from references 15, 16, 22, 23, 28–45.
From Wright and Sun [46] with permission.

**Table 13.2** Prevalence of cytological abnormalities in human immunodeficiency virus (HIV)-seropositive and HIV-seronegative women.

| Reference | Location | Population studied | HIV-seropositive women | | HIV-seronegative women | |
|---|---|---|---|---|---|---|
| | | | No. of women | Abnormal Pap smears (%) | No. of women | Abnormal Pap smears (%) |
| Provencher et al. | Miami, USA | Requesting screening | 201 | 63 | 213 | 5 |
| Schrager et al. | Bronx, USA | Heterosexual transmission | 35 | 31 | 23 | 4 |
| Feingold et al. | Bronx, USA | Methadone clinic | 35 | 40 | 32 | 9 |
| Vermund et al. | Bronx, USA | Methadone clinic | 51 | 33 | 49 | 13 |
| Marte et al. | Chicago and NYC, USA | HIV clinics | 135 | 26 | Clinics* | 6 |
| Laga et al. | Kinshasa, Zaire | Prostitutes | 41 | 27 | 41 | 3 |
| Kreiss et al. | Nairobi, Kenya | Prostitutes | 42 | 26 | 21 | 24 |
| Maggwa et al. | Kenya | Family planning | 205 | 5 | 3853 | 2 |
| Smith et al. | London, UK | HIV and methadone clinic | 43 | 35 | 43 | 19 |
| Conti et al. | Milan, Italy | IVDU | 273 | 42 | 161 | 8 |
| Wright et al. | New York, USA | Methadone/STD/HIV clinic | 398 | 30 | 357 | 8 |
| Johnstone et al. | Edinburgh, UK | IVDU and IVDU partners | 92 | 38 | 157 | 22 |
| Seck et al. | Senegal | ID clinic and partners HIV(+) | 14 | 43 | 50 | 6 |

Pap, Papanicolaou; IVDU, intravenous drug user; STD, sexually transmitted disease; ID, infectious disease.
* The prevalence of cytological abnormalities in HIV-seropositive women in this study was compared to the overall prevalence of cytological abnormalities in women attending the gynaecological outpatient clinics at the institutions involved in this study.
Data from references, 15–17, 29–31, 34–36, 38, 39, 41, 43.
From Wright and Sun [46] with permission.

women, irrespective of their cervical disease status, undergo a complete gynaecological examination including colposcopy, cytology and the collection of samples for human papillamavirus (HPV) DNA testing at 6-month intervals. The NYCDS detected biopsy-confirmed, low-grade cervical intraepithelial neoplasia (CIN) in 13% of 398 HIV-seropositive women compared to 4% of 307 seronegative women ($P > 0.001$). High-grade CIN (CIN II–III) was detected in 7% of HIV-seropositive women compared to 1% of HIV-seronegative women ($P > 0.001$). Similar results have been reported by Conti *et al.* from Italy; they colposcopically detected CIN in 42% of 273 HIV-infected women compared to 8% of 161 HIV-uninfected women [16].

These studies clearly indicate that there is a high burden of cervical cancer precursors in HIV-infected women and that much of this disease is histologically high-grade. However, it is also clear that an 'epidemic' of invasive cancer is not occurring in HIV-infected populations. Nevertheless, as new antiretroviral therapies and better prophylaxis begin to extend these women's lives, more cases of cervical cancer can be expected because of the high prevalence of high-grade cervical cancer precursors in HIV-infected women.

## Risk factors for the development of CIN in HIV-infected women

Relatively few studies have investigated whether the high prevalence of CIN in HIV-infected women is due to an increase in high-risk behaviours or biological risk factors for CIN, or is a direct result of infection with HIV. To help address this issue we have analysed demographic and CIN risk factor information in HIV-infected and uninfected women enrolled in the NYCDS [5]. Biopsy-confirmed CIN in this cohort of women was significantly associated with HIV-seropositivity, CD4+ T-lymphocyte counts less than 200 cells/µl, a history of treatment for CIN, a history of genital warts, detection of HPV DNA in cervicovaginal lavages using polymerase chain reaction and L1 open reading frame consensus primers, and age greater than 34 years. In a multivariate analysis, four variables were found to be associated with CIN. These were cervicovaginal HPV infection, HIV-seropositivity, CD4+ T-lymphocytes less than 200 cells/µl, and age greater than 34. These findings suggest that HIV infection and HIV-associated immunosuppression are significant risk factors for the development of CIN.

## Anogenital HPV infections in HIV-infected women

A number of studies have analysed the prevalence of anogenital HPV infections in HIV-infected women (Table 13.3). In the first study to analyse HPV infections in HIV-seropositive women, Feingold *et al.* [17] analysed cervical vaginal lavages from 35 HIV-infected women and 32 HIV-uninfected women

**Table 13.3** Studies of human papillomavirus (HPV)-infection in human immunodeficiency virus (HIV)-seropositive women.

| Author | Clinical performance site | | Methods of HPV detection and typing | |
|---|---|---|---|---|
| | Location | Setting | Sample collection | HPV detection |
| Feingold et al. | Bronx, USA | Methadone, IVDU partner | Cervicovaginal lavage | Southern blot |
| Kreiss et al. | Nairobi, Kenya | Prostitutes | Cervical swabs | Dot and Southern blot |
| Laga et al. | Kinshasha, Zaire | Prostitutes | Cervicovaginal lavage | Dot and Southern blot |
| ter Meulen et al. | Tanzania | Gyn inpatients | Cervical swabs | PCR |
| Johnson et al. | Washington, DC, USA | ID clinics | Cervical swabs | Dot blot (ViraPap) |
| Smith et al. | London, UK | Gyn and ID clinics | Cervical smears | Southern blot |
| Williams et al. | San Francisco, CA, USA | IVDU, methadone clinics | Cervical swabs | Dot blot/L1 PCR |
| Sun et al. | New York, NY, USA | ID clinics, methadone clinics | Cervicovaginal lavage | L1 PCR |
| Vernon et al. | Kinshasha, Zaire | Prostitutes | Cervicovaginal lavage | Dot blot (Virapap) |
| Seck et al. | Dakar, Senegal | ID clinics | Cervical swabs | L1 PCR/Southern blot |

Data from references 17–20, 35, 36, 38, 43, 47, 48.
From Wright and Sun [46] with permission.
IVDU, intravenous drug user; Gyn, gynaecology; ID, infectious disease; PCR, polymerase chain reaction.

using Southern blot hybridization. HPV DNA was detected in 49% of the lavages from HIV-seropositive women, compared to 25% of those from the HIV-seronegative women ($P < 0.05$). Similarly, higher rates of HPV infection among HIV-infected women have been confirmed by other studies from both Africa and North America. For example, using PCR with LI consensus primers, Sun et al. [18] detected HPV DNA in 60% of the HIV-seropositive women enrolled in the NYCDS compared to 36% of the HIV-seronegative women. Williams et al. [19] from San Francisco detected HPV DNA using a PCR-based method in 57% of cervical swabs from HIV-seropositive women compared to 13% of the swabs from HIV-seronegative women.

One of the problems with interpreting the HPV studies listed in Table 13.3 is that the prevalence of CIN in the HIV-infected and HIV-uninfected women was frequently not determined. Therefore, it is unclear whether the increase in HPV infections observed among HIV-infected women can be attributed entirely to an increase in clinically expressed HPV infections (e.g. CIN and genital warts) or whether latent HPV infections are also increased. To investigate this question, Sun et al. analysed HPV data from the NYCDS in which women underwent colposcopy at the same time that the sample for HPV DNA testing was obtained [18]. Data from this study indicate that latent HPV infections as well as clinically expressed HPV infections are significantly increased in HIV-seropositive women compared to HIV-seronegative women ($P < 0.001$ for both).

When assessing risk factors for the increase in HPV infection observed among HIV-seropositive women, Sun et al. found that the detection of HPV DNA in cervicovaginal lavages was significantly associated with younger age, not being currently married, a history of previous CIN, HIV-seropositivity and CD4+ T-lymphocyte counts of less than 200 cells/µl. Using a multivariate model, it was found that young age, not being currently married, HIV-seropositivity and CD4+ T-lymphocyte counts of less than 200 cells/µl remained associated with HPV, even after controlling for other variables. To investigate more fully associations between HIV immunosuppression and HPV infections, Sun et al. [18] used additional regression models. The results of these studies indicated that HIV infection per se remains a risk factor for anogenital HPV infection in women even after controlling for HPV infection. However, it has not been elucidated whether this association is due to direct molecular interactions between HIV and HPV or whether it is simply due to HIV-associated immunosuppression.

Some studies have suggested that the distribution of HPV types differs among women who are HIV-infected and uninfected. For example, Feingold et al. have detected HPV 18 in 14% of HIV-infected women, which is considerably higher than reported in women in the general population [17]. In addition, Johnson et al. found an increasing prevalence in HPV infection as the

CD4+ T-lymphocyte count dropped in HIV-infected women [20]. For example, HPV 18 was detected in 5% of HIV-seropositive women with CD4 counts above 200 cells/µl compared to 50% of those with CD4 counts less than 200 cells/µl. However, Sun *et al.* detected no significant differences in the relative proportions of different types of HPV that were obseved between HIV-seropositive and HIV-seronegative women enrolled in the NYCDS, which included many more women than the other studies combined. For example, HPV 16 and 18 comprised 20% of the identifiable HPV types in HIV-seropositive women and 21% those from HIV-seronegative women. HPV 6 and 11, combined, comprised 12% of the identifiable HPV types in HIV-seropositive women compared to 11% in seronegative women. Sun *et al.* also found that the HPV types associated with low-grade CIN (CIN I) were relatively similar in HIV-seropositive and HIV-seronegative women. However, differences were observed in the HPV types associated with high-grade CIN (CIN II–III) in the two groups. High-grade CIN in HIV-infected women was more commonly associated with members of the 30s and 50s HPV groups than is high-grade CIN in HIV-seronegative women.

Anal HPV infections are also increased in HIV-infected women. Williams *et al.* detected HPV DNA using the Virapap/Viratype method in 32% of anal swabs from HIV-seropositive women compared to 14% of those from HIV-seronegative women [19]. Using PCR with LI (consensus) primers, 77% of the anal specimens from the same HIV-seropositive group were HPV DNA-positive, as were 56% of those from the HIV-seronegative women. Recently we assessed anal HPV infections and cytological abnormalities in women enrolled in the NYCDS [21]. Anal swabs were analysed for the presence of HPV DNA using the Hybrid Capture DNA Assay and probes for both low-risk and high-risk HPV types. Using the Hybrid Capture assay, HPV DNA was detected in 29% of the anal samples from the HIV-seropositive women compared to only 2% of the samples from the HIV-seronegative women ($P < 0.001$). In addition, there was a higher prevalence of anal cytological abnormalities among the HIV-infected group. Twenty-six per cent of the 102 HIV-seropositive women compared to 6% of the 96 HIV-seronegative women had some level of anal cytological abnormality. Five per cent of the anal smears from the HIV-seropositive group and 1% of those from the seronegative group had low-grade anal intraepithelial neoplasia.

## Screening for cervical disease in HIV-infected women

Because of the high prevalence of cervical cancer precursors and increased risk for the development of invasive cervical cancer identified in HIV-infected women, it is clear that these women need to be carefully screened for the presence of cervical disease. However, there continues to be controversy over

**Table 13.4** Centers of Disease Control Recommendations for Papanicolaou (Pap) smear screening of human immunodeficiency virus (HIV)-infected women.

Women who are HIV-infected should be advised to have a comprehensive gynaecological examination, including a Pap smear, as part of their initial medical evaluation

If initial Pap smear results are within normal limits, at least one additional Pap smear should be obtained in approximately 6 months to rule out the possibility of false-negative results on the initial Pap smear

If the repeat Pap smear is normal, HIV-infected women should be advised to have a Pap smear obtained annually

If the initial or subsequent Pap smear shows severe inflammation with reactive squamous cellular changes, another Pap smear should be collected within 3 months

If the initial or follow-up Pap smear shows SIL (or equivalent) or ASCUS, the women should be referred for colposcopic examination of the lower genital tract and, if indicated, colposcopically directed biopsies

From Wright and Sun [46] with permission.
SIL, Squamous intraepithelial lesion; ASCUS, atypical squamous cells of undetermined significance.

how best to screen HIV-infected women. Although one early study of the sensitivity and specificity of Pap smears in HIV-infected women reported an extremely high false-negative rate in this population [22], other studies have failed to confirm significant differences in the performance of cytological screening between HIV-infected women and women in the general population [15,23–24]. Therefore, suggestions that all HIV-infected women should undergo routine colposcopy do not appear to be warranted at this time. In addition, concern has been expressed that colposcopic screening may actually result in the overdiagnosis of CIN and perhaps overtreatment of this population [25]. Current recommendations from the Centers for Disease Control and Prevention are that HIV-infected women be monitored for cervical disease using frequent Pap smears rather than colposcopy (Table 13.4) [26]. It should be stressed, however, that in our opinion, mild degrees of cytologic atypia (atypical squamous cells of undetermined significance or ASCUS) should be considered indications for colposcopy in HIV-infected women. This recommendation is based on a recent study in which we compared the prevalence of CIN among HIV-infected and uninfected women with ASCUS Pap smears [27]. Coexistent CIN was detected by colposcopically directed biopsy in 38% of the HIV-infected women with mild cytological atypia, compared to 14% of HIV-uninfected women.

## Summary

It appears that there is a very high prevalence of CIN in HIV-infected women and that much of the CIN is high grade. In addition, there are high rates of both cervical and anal HPV infections in HIV-infected women, suggesting that these women may be at high risk for the development of cervical cancer and should be monitored very carefully.

## References

1 WHO. The current global situation of the HIV/AIDS pandemic. World Health Organization. Global Program on AIDS.
2 CDC. HIV/AIDS Surveillance Report. Centers for Disease Control, Vol. 7, No. 2.
3 Curran JW. *Pneumocystis* pneumonia – Los Angeles. From the CDC. *JAMA* 1996; **276**: 1020–1022.
4 CDC. Update: AIDS among women – United States. *JAMA* 1995; **273**: 7678.
5 AIDS in the world, 1992. *JAMA* 1992; **268**: 445–446.
6 Rellihan MA, Dooley DP, Burke TW, Berkland ME, Longfield RN. Rapidly progressing cervical cancer in a patient with human immunodeficiency virus infection. *Gynecol Oncol* 1990; **36**: 435–438.
7 Schwartz LB, Carcangiu ML, Bradham L, Schwarz PE. Rapidly progressive squamous cell carcinoma of the cervix coexisting with human immunodeficiency virus infection: clinical opinion. *Gynecol Oncol* 1991; **41**: 255–258.
8 Maiman M, Fruchter RG, Guy L, Cuthill S, Levine P, Serur E. Human immunodeficiency virus infection and invasive cervical carcinoma. *Cancer* 1993; **71**: 402–506.
9 CDC. Revised classification system for HIV infection and expanded surveillance case definition for AIDS among adolescents and adults. *MMWR* 1993; **41**: 1–20.
10 Chiasson M. Death rates from cervical cancer in New York City. 1993. (Personal communication.)
11 Rabkin C, Biggar R, Baptiste M, Abe T, Kohler B, Nasca P. Cancer incidence trends in women at high risk of human immunodeficiency virus (HIV) infection. *Int J Cancer* 1993; **55**: 208–212.
12 Chiasson MA, Wright TC. The gynecologic manifestations of HIV. In: Mandel G (ed) *Atlas of Infectious Disease*. Edinburgh: Churchill Livingstone, 1993.
13 Wright TC, Koulos JP, Liu P, Sun X-W. Invasive vulvar carcinoma in two women infected with human immunodeficiency virus. *Gynecol Oncol* 1995; **60**: 500–503.
14 Giorda G, Vaccher E, Volpe R, DePiero G, Tirelli U, Scarabello C. An unusual presentation of vulvar carcinoma in a HIV patient. *Gynecol Oncol* 1992; **44**: 191–194.
15 Wright TCJ, Ellerbrock TV, Chiasson MA, Sun XW, Van de Vanter N. Cervical intraepithelial neoplasia in women infected with human immunodeficiency virus: prevalence, risk factors, and validity of Papanicolaou smears. *Obstet Gynecol* 1994; **84**: 591–597.
16 Conti M, Agarossi A, Parazzini F *et al*. HPV, HIV infection, and risk of cervical intraepithelial neoplasia in former intravenous drug abusers. *Gynecol Oncol* 1993; **49**: 344–348.
17 Feingold AR, Vermund SH, Burk RD *et al*. Cervical cytologic abnormalities and papillomavirus in women infect with human immunodeficiency virus. *J AIDS* 1990; **3**: 896–903.
18 Sun X-W, Ellerbrock RV, Lungu O, Chiasson MA, Bush RJ, Wright TC. Human papillomavirus infection in human immunodeficiency virus-seropositive women. *Obstet Gynecol* 1995; **85**: 680–686.
19 Williams AB, Darragh TM, Vranizan K, Ochia C, Moss AR, Palefsky JM. Anal and

cervical human papillomavirus infection and risk of anal and cervical epithelial abnormalities in human immunodeficiency virus-infected women. *Obstet Gynecol* 1994; **83**: 205–211.

20 Johnson JC, Burnett AF, Willet GD, Young MA, Doniger J. High frequency of latent and clinical human papillomavirus cervical infections in immunocompromised human immunodeficiency virus-infected women. *Obstet Gynecol* 1992; **79**: 321–327.

21 Hillemanns P, Ellerbrock TC, McPhillips S *et al*. Prevalence of anal cytologic abnormalities and anal human papillomavirus infections in HIV-seropositive women. *AIDS* 1996; (in press).

22 Maiman M, Tarricone N, Vieira J, Suarez J, Serur E, Boyce JG. Colposcopic evaluation of human immunodeficiency virus-seropositive women. *Obstet Gynecol* 1991; **78**: 84–88.

23 Korn A, Autry M, DeRemer P, Tan W. Sensitivity of the Papanicolaou smear in human immunodeficiency virus-infected women. *Obstet Gynecol* 1994; **83**: 401–404.

24 Fink MJ, Fruchter RG, Maiman M *et al*. The adequacy of cytology and colposcopy in diagnosing cervical neoplasia in HIV-seropositive women. *Gynecol Oncol* 1994; **55**: 133–137.

25 Wright TC. Cervical disease in HIV-infected women: prevalence, pathogenesis, detection, and treatment. In: Luesley D, Jordan J, Richart RM (eds) *Intraepithelial Neoplasia of the Lower Genital Tract*. Edinburgh: Churchill Livingstone, 1995, pp 263–277.

26 CDC. Sexually transmitted disease guidelines. *MMWR* 1993; **42**: 90–91.

27 Wright TC, Moscarelli RD, Dole P, Ellerbrock TV, Chiasson MA, Vandevanter N. Clinical significance of mild cytologic atypia on Papanicolaou smears from women infected with human immunodeficiency virus. *Obstet Gynecol* 1996; **87**: 515–519.

28 Byrne MA, Moller BR, Taylor-Robinson D *et al*. The effect of interferon on human papillomaviruses associated with cervical intraepithelial neoplasia. *Br J Obstet Gynaecol* 1986; **93**: 1136.

29 Provencher D, Valme B, Averette HE *et al*. HIV status and positive Papanicolaou screening: identification of a high-risk populations. *Gynecol Oncol* 1988; **31**: 184–188.

30 Schrager LK, Friedland GH, Maude D *et al*. Cervical and vaginal squamous cell abnormalities in women infected with human immunodeficiency virus. *J AIDS* 1989; **2**: 570–575.

31 Vermund SH, Kelley KF, Klein RS *et al*. High risk of human papillomavirus infection and cervical squamous intraepithelial lesions among women with symptomatic human immunodeficiency virus infection. *Am J Obstet Gynecol* 1991; **165**: 392–400.

32 Carpenter CCJ, Mayer KH, Stein MD, Leibman BD, Fisher A, Fopre T. Human immunodeficiency virus infection in North American women: experience with 200 cases and a review of the literature. *Medicine* 1991; **70**: 307–325.

33 Schafer A, Friedmann W, Meilke M, Schwartlander B, Koch MA. The increased frequency of cervical dysplasia–neoplasia in women infected with the human immunodeficiency virus is related to the degree of immunosuppression. *Am J Obstet Gynecol* 1991; **164**: 593–599.

34 Marte C, Kelly P, Cohen M *et al*. Papanicolaou smear abnormalities in ambulatory care sites for women infected with immunodeficiency virus. *Am J Obstet Gynecol* 1992; **166**: 1232–1237.

35 Kreiss JK, Kiviat NB, Plummer FA *et al*. Human immunodeficiency virus, human papalliomavirus, and cervical intraepithelial neoplasia in Nairobi prostitutes. *Sex Transm Dis* 1992; **19**: 54–59.

36 Laga M, Icenogle JP, Marsella R *et al*. Genital papillomavirus infection and cervical dysplasia – opportunistic complications of HIV infection. *Int J Cancer* 1992; **50**: 45–48.

37 Spinillo A, Tenti P, Zappatore R *et al*. Prevalence, diagnosis and treatment of lower

genital neoplasia in women with human immunodeficiency virus infection. *Eur J Obstet Gynecol Reprod Biol* 1992; **43**: 235–241.

38  Smith J, Kitchen V, Botcherby M *et al*. Is HIV infection associated with an increase in the prevalence of cervical neoplasia? *Br J Obstet Gynaecol* 1993; **100**: 149.

39  Maggwa BN, Hunter DJ, Mbugua S, Tukei P, Mati JK. The relationship between HIV infection and cervical intraepithelial neoplasia among women attending 2 family planning clinics in Nairobi, Kenya. *AIDS* 1993; 7: 733–738.

40  Gentile G, Formelli G, Costigliola P, Busacchi P, Pelusi G. Cervical intraepithelial neoplasia in HIV seropositive patients. *Eur J Gynaecol Oncol* 1993; **14**: 246–248.

41  Johnstone FD, McGoogan E, Smart GE, Brettle RP, Prescott RJ. A population-based, controlled study of the relation between HIV infection and cervical neoplasia. *Br J Obstet Gynaecol* 1994; **101**: 986–991.

42  Tweddel G, Heller P, Cunnane M, Multhaupt H, Roth K. The correlation between HIV seropositivity, cervical dysplasia, and HPV subtypes 6/11, 16/18, 31/33/35. *Gynecol Oncol* 1994; **52**: 161–164.

43  Seck AC, Faye MA, Critchlow CW *et al*. Cervical intraepithelial neoplasia and human papillomavirus infection among Senegalese women seropositive for HIV-1 or HIV-2 or seronegative for HIV. *Int J STD AIDS* 1994; **5**: 189–193.

44  Klein RS, Ho GYF, Vermund SH, Fleming I, Burk RD. Risk factors for squamous intraepithelial lesions on Papanicolaou smear in women at risk for human immunodeficiency virus infection. *J Infect Dis* 1994; **170**: 1404–1409.

45  Heard I, Bergeron C, Jeannel D, Henrion R, Kazatchkine MD. Papanicolaou smears in human immunodeficiency virus-seropositive women during follow-up. *Obstet Gynecol* 1995; **86**: 749–753.

46  Wright TC, Sun X-W. Anogenital papillomavirus infection and neoplasia in immunodeficient women. *Obst Gynecol Clinics North Am* 1996; **23**: 861–893.

47  ter Meulen J, Eberhardt HC, Luande J *et al*. Human papillomavirus (HPV) infection, HIV infection and cervical cancer in Tanzania, East Africa. *Int J Cancer* 1992; **51**: 515–521.

48  Vernon SD, Reeves WC, Clancy KA *et al*. A longitudinal study of human papillomavirus DNA detection in human immunodeficiency virus type 1-seropositive and seronegative women. *J Infect Dis* 1994; **169**: 1108–1112.

# Section 3
# The Cervical Cytology Paradigm

# 14: Performance of Cytology in Screening for Precursor Lesions and Early Cancer of the Uterine Cervix

## L. G. Koss

## Summary

A brief review of the historical background of cytological screening for precursor lesions of carcinoma of the uterine cervix is presented. The principal causes of screening errors are discussed, with emphasis on laboratory performance. Proposed remedies include education of personnel and automation of screening.

## Introduction

Over 50 years have elapsed since the publication of the original paper by Papanicolaou and Traut [1,2] that led to the introduction of the concept of mass screening for precursors of carcinoma of the uterine cervix. The method was first introduced in the USA, whence it spread to Canada and to other developed countries. The history of the early events has been described elsewhere [3]. It is of interest, however, to stress that a Romanian pathologist, Aureli Babès, was the first to describe the use of direct smears for cervix cancer diagnosis in an excellent article published in *Presse Médicale* on 11 April 1928 [4].

Unfortunately, the performance of the method, first based on vaginal smears, as proposed by George Papanicolaou, and subsequently on direct sampling of the uterine cervix by means of a scraper, described by J. Ernest Ayre in Canada [5] has never been tested in a double-blind study. Because early on the smears have been shown to detect precancerous lesions of the uterine cervix not visible to the naked eye, the paramount task of health officials was to

*Correspondence*: Dr Leopold Koss, Department of Pathology, Montefiore Medical Center, Albert Einstein College of Medicine, Bronx, NY 10467, USA.

enrol as many women as possible into the cancer detection system. Neither the providers of the method—physicians and gynaecologists, nor the consumers, Well-Women, were aware of the limitations of the method. It could be shown fairly rapidly that in some screened populations the rate of invasive cancer of the uterine cervix fell significantly, although complete eradication of this deadly disease has not been achieved in any large cohort studied to date [6,7]. In some geographical areas with extensive screening the successes have not been shared, although the reasons for failure have not been appropriately analysed [8]. On balance, the achievements of the method were very positive, with numerous lives saved. A recent consensus development conference convened by the National Cancer Institute (USA) has stressed that the cervical smear is still the best method of prevention of cervical carcinoma [9]. The negative aspects of screening – the development of invasive cancer in screened women – have only recently become the subject of a major debate, particularly in the USA, although many publications in the 1960s and 1970s stressed the failures of cytology in many cases [10–12]. To my knowledge, there are no statistical data to determine the exact rate of failures of cytological screening in any given geographical area or country. The failure rates in individual laboratories have been published and will be the subject of Chapter 17.

## Causes of screening failure

There are many known reasons for screening failure, but six are most important. They are:
1   Inadequate sampling.
2   Poor techniques of sample preparation.
3   Inadequate screening of smears.
4   Inadequate quality control.
5   Inadequate interpretation of cytological findings.
6   Inadequate clinical follow-up.

Any one of these factors can lead to a failure of the system, with resulting loss of life, often in young women. There is so far no evidence that the situation will change radically in the near future unless drastic steps to improve the performance of the system are undertaken.

These facts pose some important dilemmas to all those interested in the issue of cancer of the uterine cervix: cytological screening has been considered as a relatively inexpensive public health measure with significant benefits and virtually no known drawbacks. As recent events in the USA have shown, the failure rate of the cervix cancer detection system may be larger than previously thought and may lead to legal proceedings against laboratories and pathologists, adding significant costs to the system [13]. Although European health-care systems may prevent the injured women from resorting to judicial approaches and the laboratories and the cytologists may be protected by the doctrine *errare humanum est* (to err is human), I am not sure how much longer the current situation will continue. The prevailing winds go from west to east. In my judgement there are only two possible solutions to the dilemma.

## Remedies

One approach is to make the failures of the cancer detection system known to the public and inform the women that the cervical smear is effective in most cases but may fail in some. The advantage of this approach is to maintain current policies and keep the costs of the test low. The potential disadvantage is the loss of lives and the danger that women, upon learning about the failures of the system, will not present themselves for screening.

The alternative approach is to make the system more effective by better training, better screening and better quality control. The use of new automated instruments may significantly improve the performance of the cytology laboratory [14]. By adopting these approaches the costs of screening will increase but this increase will have to be weighed against the number of additional lives saved. It is evident that major policy decisions will have to be made by health officials in adopting either one of these options.

## References

1 Papanicolaou GN, Traut HF. *Diagnosis of Uterine Cancer by the Vaginal Smear*. New York: Commonweath Fund, 1943.
2 Papanicolaou GN, Traut HF. The diagnostic value of vaginal smears in carcinoma of the uterus. *Am Obst Gynecol* 1943; **42**: 193–206.
3 Koss LG. *Diagnostic Cytology and its Histopathologic Bases*, 4th edn. Philadelphia: JB Lippincott, 1992.
4 Babès A. Le diagnostique du cancer du col uterin par les frottis. *Presse Med* 1928; **36**: 451–454.
5 Ayre JE. Selective cytolgy smear for diagnosis of cancer. *Am J Obstet Gynecol* 1947; **53**: 609–617.
6 Anderson GH, Boyes DA, Benedet JL *el al*. Organization and results of the cervical cytology screening programme in British Columbia, 1955–1985. *BMJ* 1988; **296**: 975–978.
7 Hakama M, Louhivuori K. A screening programme for cervical cancer that worked. *Cancer Surv* 1988; 7: 403–416.
8 Raffle AE, Alden B, Mackenzie EFD. Detection rates for abnormal cervical smears: what are we screening for? *Lancet* 1995; **345**: 1469–1474.
9 NIH Consensus Development Conference on Cervical Cancer, April 1–3, 1996. Press release, National Institutes of Health, Bethesda, MD, USA.
10 Foltz AM, Kelsey JL. The annual Pap test: a dubious policy success. *Heatlh Soc* 1978; **56**: 426–462.
11 Rylander E. Cervical cancer in women belonging to cytologically screened population. *Acta Obstet Gynecol Scand* 1976; **55**: 361–366.

12 Rylander E. Negative smears in women developing invasive cancer. *Acta Obstet Gynecol Scand* 1977; **56**: 115–118.

13 Sabella JD. Pathology claims up – liability premiums to follow. *CAP Today* 1993; 7: 39.

14 Hematology and Pathology Devices Panel of the Medical Devices Advisory Committee to FDA. *Transcript of Proceedings*. Federal Department of Health and Human Services, Rockville, MD, 1995.

# 15: The Bethesda System (TBS): Advantages and Pitfalls

## A. Ferenczy

## Summary

The objective of this study was to review the rationale for developing the Bethesda System (TBS) for reporting cervicovaginal cytological diagnoses.

The Division of Cancer Prevention and Control of the National Cancer Institute (NCI) in Bethesda, MD, USA, convened in December 1988 a workshop of consultants, expert in their respective fields of interest as related to cervicovaginal cytopathology. The 1988 TBS was revised and simplified at the following 1991 NCI workshop and criteria were established for specific entities as well as for specimen adequacy. Furthermore, because of uncertainties surrounding an atypical squamous cell of undetermined significance (ASCUS) diagnosis, leading to overclassification as low-grade squamous intraepithelial lesion (LGSIL) and overtreatment, the NCI invited experts in 1992 for the purpose of developing interim guidelines for the management of women with positive tests using TBS, including ASCUS and LGSIL smears. At the same time, major efforts are being made to determine the clinical value of combining cytology with ancillary techniques such as viral testing in the cost-effective management of patients with minor-grade cytological abnormalities. Another means of improving on diagnostic performance indices and reducing false-negative readings focuses on the use of computers for automated image analysis technology.

The 1991 workshop participants unanimously recommended the following:

1 The Papanicolaou classification of reporting is not acceptable in the modern practice of diagnostic cytopathology.

*Correspondence*: Professor Alex Ferenczy, Department of Pathology, Sir Mortimer B. Davis Jewish General Hospital, 3755 Côte Ste Catherine Road, Montreal, Quebec, Canada H3T 1E2.

**2**  TBS should serve as a guidance for cytopathology reports of cervicovaginal specimens.

**3**  The cytopathology report should include a statement on the adequacy of specimens for diagnostic evaluation.

Acceptance of TBS has received support from a large number of professional societies and the federal Clinical Laboratory Improvements Amendments (CLIA-88) requires its use in the USA. As such, TBS provides for standardized nomenclature to allow regional, national analyses and comparisons among laboratories, which in turn can be used for quality control by registries. Also, the classification to the two- versus three-grading categories of cervical cancer precursors, i.e. low- and high-grade SILs, has the potential to achieve greater diagnostic concordance between observers. However, TBS fails to provide microscopic criteria for defining first, what represents a 'satisfactory but limited by (SBLB) absence of transformation zone (TZ) components' smear; and second, the ASCUS/AGUS category. These drawbacks led to an increased number of repeat Pap smears (4%) and overclassification (15%), respectively, and an increase in unnecessary colposcopies and inappropriate use of health care funds. This is particularly true, as current data in the literature do not seem to support the hypothesis of improved diagnostic accuracy in the presence versus absence of TZ components and the ASCUS/LGSIL categories account for the largest volume of patients who require evaluation.

The 1992 guidelines have to be considered interim because they are subject to modification as new data become available with respect to the natural history of minor-grade lesions of the cervix. Also, the guidelines do not make the diagnosis of ASCUS/LGSIL easier than in the past. The recent data generated from viral studies suggest that human papillomavirus (HPV) DNA testing may be an effective adjunct to cervical cytology in the diagnosis and cost-effective management of patients with borderline ASCUS/LGSIL Papanicolaou (Pap) smears. Published studies on the clinical value of automated cytology in quality assurance suggest this technique has the potential of improving the sensitivity of disease detection over manual reading by 50%. However, at present this approach appears to have a less cost-effective profile for rescreening for quality control purposes than the 100% rapid manual research approach.

TBS for reporting cervicovaginal cytological diagnoses provides for a uniform format and standardization of terminology based on current understanding of cervical cancer and its precursors. TBS is supported by major professional societies and national health agencies and is used by most laboratories in the USA and, increasingly, worldwide. So far, TBS has not provided help to the challenging management categories classified as ASCUS and LGSIL. Recent advances made in ancillary diagnostic techniques such as HPV typing may help to clarify the confusing issue of appropriate management of patients with borderline or minor-grade cytological abnormalities.

The NCI-generated guidelines for the management of women with ASCUS/ LGSIL should be considered interim as they are subject to modification as new clinical data on the clinical significance of minor-grade lesions become available.

## Introduction

It has been generally recognized and accepted that precursor lesions to invasive cancer of the cervix comprise a morphological and biological spectrum of changes ranging from mild dysplasia to carcinoma-*in-situ*. A unifying generic term, cervical intraepithelial neoplasia was suggested to emphasize the continuum concept [1]. However, in recent years a strong link between precursors and invasive cancer with HPV and, in particular, between HPV types and cancer have indicated that cancer precursors segregate into biologically heterogeneous low-grade-type lesions and a homogeneous-type high-grade lesion [2]. The former manifests as a productive HPV infection and is associated with diploid–polyploid to aneuploid DNA content, low to high oncogenic risk HPV types and, while most regress, some may progress to high-grade lesions. The latter is associated with non-productive-type HPV infections, contains generally aneuploid nuclear DNA values and high oncogenic risk HPV types. The latter have an enhanced ability to integrate into host cells' genome and have high rates of progression to invasive carcinoma.

The Bethesda System (TBS) for reporting cervicovaginal cytological diagnoses was initially developed in a December 1988 workshop sponsored by the NCI [3]. The basic rationale for the new classification was to offer a uniform, standardized terminology based on current understanding of the natural history of cervical cancer precursors. More specifically, TBS resulted from the perception of deficiencies in traditional reporting systems for cervicovaginal smears. These were:

1   Lack of uniform reporting of cervicovaginal laboratories among laboratories in the USA, with different synonyms and lack of convertibility among the various reporting systems.
2   Traditional systems failed to reflect modern understanding of the natural history of cervical neoplasia.
3   Lack of standardization for reporting non-neoplastic conditions.
4   Lack of precise correlation with histological terminology.

The main goal of TBS was to enhance communication between cytopathologists and clinicians, leading hopefully to better correlation of cytological, colposcopic and histological impressions. It is expected that as experience with TBS grows, it may eventually help to provide:

1   Better cytologic–histologic correlation.
2   Useful information for patient management.

**3**  Improved reproducibility in classifying cancer precursor lesions.

**4**  Standardized nomenclature to allow regional, national analyses and comparisons among laboratories which in turn can be used for quality control by registries.

**5**  Better understanding of the new HPV–cervical neoplasia concept.

Some of these objectives have been attained; others are subject to debate (see below). In response to criticisms by major clinical groups and investigators, TBS was revised and simplified in a 1991 NCI workshop (Table 15.1) [4]. It is likely that it will be refined further as new data are generated. In the meantime, TBS has received support from a large number of professional societies and the federal CLIA-88 require its use in the USA. Today, over 80% of the cytology laboratories report their diagnoses using TBS [5]. TBS has three parts: a statement regarding the adequacy of the specimens, a general category for the diagnosis, and a descriptive diagnosis [6]. The unique features of TBS are:

**1**  The atypical or class II category is removed.

**2**  A streamlined two-tier system for reporting squamous intraepithelial lesions replaces the traditional (CIN 1–3) or four (mild–moderate–severe dysplasia/carcinoma-*in-situ*) class system to emphasize that the lesions are squamous in nature on the one hand and have the uncertain biological outcome of morphologically low-grade lesions on the other.

**3**  It includes HPV effects into SILs and eliminates terms such as koilocytotic atypia.

**The controversial features of TBS**

**1**  It fails to provide precise microscopic criteria for defining what represents an adequate smear, particularly the SBLB absence of TZ cell components smear. The rationale for a statement on smear adequacy has been to encourage clinicians to sample the TZ, the seat of precursor lesions, and at least in theory reduce false-negative smears due to sampling error. However, there has been no prospective randomized study to determine whether adequacy implies a decrease in both the incidence and mortality due to cervical cancer. As a result, SBLB has little, if any clinical value. In fact, recently published studies suggest that absence of TZ (endocervical and squamous metaplastic cells) has no demonstrable negative impact on the diagnostic accuracy of cervical cancer precursor lesions [7]. On the other hand, the SBLB category may have legal implications, at least in North America.

**2**  Lack of precisely defining the ASCUS category. Although ASCUS should include squamous cell abnormalities greater in severity than those associated with reactive changes, until consensus-derived visual (microscopic) criteria are provided to distinguish LGSIL from repair-related atypia, the term ASCUS is

**Table 15.1** The 1991 Bethesda system.

**Adequacy of the specimen**
Satisfactory for evaluation
Satisfactory for evaluation but limited by . . . (specify reason)
Unsatisfactory for evaluation

**General categorization (optional)**
Within normal limits
Benign cellular changes: see descriptive diagnosis
Epithelial cell abnormality: see descriptive diagnosis

**Descriptive diagnosis**
BENIGN CELLULAR CHANGES
*Infection*
*Trichomonas vaginalis*
Fungal organisms morphologically consistent with *Candida* spp.
Predominance of coccobacilli consistent with *Actinomyces* spp.
Cellular changes associated with herpes simplex virus
Other
*Reactive changes*
Reactive cellular changes associated with:
   Inflammation (including atypia of repair)
   Atrophy with inflammation (atrophic vaginitis)
   Radiation
   Intrauterine contraceptive device
   Other
*Epithelial cell abnormalities*
Squamous cell: atypical squamous cells of undetermined significance: qualify.
Low-grade squamous intraepithelial lesion, encompassing HPV mild dysplasia/CIN I.
High-grade squamous intraepithelial lesion, encompassing moderate and severe dysplasia,
   CIS/CIN II and CIN III.
Squamous cell carcinoma
Glandular cell
   Endometrial cells, cytologically benign, in a post-menopausal woman
   Atypical glandular cells of undetermined significance: qualify
   Endocervical adenocarcinoma
   Endometrial adenocarcinoma
   Extrauterine adenocarcinoma
   Adenocarcinoma, not otherwise specified
Other malignant neoplasma: specify
   Hormonal evaluation (applies to vaginal smears only)
   Hormonal pattern compatible with age and history
   Hormonal pattern incompatible with age and history: specify
   Hormonal evaluation not possible due to. . . (specify)

HPV, Human papillomavirus; CIN, cervical intraepithelial neoplasia; CIS, carcinoma-*in-situ*.

likely to lead to overclassification, and unnecessary colposcopic examination. In fact, the rate of abnormal smears and in particular, the LGSIL category has increased from pre-TBS (4%) to post-TBS (15%) [8].

**3** Lack of clearly distinguishing cellular changes due to inflammation from true koilocytosis (nuclear atypia with haloes) is likely to lead to a further increase in the number of LGSIL smears [9,10].

**4** Incorporating HPV/koilocytosis in LGSIL may result in treatment of a substantial number of women who could be simply followed by repeat smears [11].

**5** If TZ cellular components are indeed important to improve diagnostic yield, the system should provide a qualitative and quantitative definition of a completely satisfactory smear.

**6** The term atypical glandular cells of undetermined significance (AGUS) is confusing and, like ASCUS, difficult to apply to clinical management. Because of lack of consensus-type visual criteria to separate the reactive from the neoplastic processes, danger exists for overclassification as adenocarcinoma-*in-situ* or invasive adenocarcinoma of endocervix.

It is clear that TBS will need further refinement. It is also clear that classifications, regardless of how simplified they are, do not make cytopathologists better diagnosticians. However, TBS is the best classification we have currently, reflecting progress made in our understanding of the natural history of cervical cancer precursors [12]. It serves as a basis for developing a unified system of reporting cytopathological diagnoses in an effort to create nationwide quality assurance programmes and interlaboratory communication systems. The rationale for key decisions proposed in the system can be outlined below:

**1** Koilocytosis and CIN I (mild dysplasia or dyskaryosis) are grouped together as LGSIL, because a large number of studies showed a lack of inter- and intraobserver reproducibility in distinguishing between HPV-associated changes and CIN I. Furthermore, prospective and retrospective epidemiological studies combined with HPV typing and ploidy analyses showed that the above lesions have similar rates of progression ($\pm 15\%$); and both their ploidy and viral contents are heterogeneous, mainly ranging from diploidy to aneuploidy and low to high oncogenic risk HPV types, respectively. Because of the biological heterogeneity of LGSIL, management strategies depend on a number of features, including patients' demographic characteristics, viral type and ploidy of lesional epithelium [2].

**2** Lesions designated traditionally as CIN II (moderate dysplasia) and CIN III (severe dysplasia–carcinoma-*in-situ*) are grouped together as high-grade SIL because it is impossible to distinguish reproducibly among the traditional terms; they form a homogeneous group as they all have aneuploid DNA values, a similar mix of HPV types and relatively high progression rates to invasion

[1,2]. As a result, their management is similar – conservative excisional therapy.

**3** The frequency of the diagnostic category of ASCUS should not exceed two to three times the rate of SIL or account for more than 5% of cytological diagnoses because koilocytotic atypia and benign alterations due to other known agents have been excluded from this group.

**4** Management of abnormal cytology should centre on the prevention of invasive cervix carcinoma using the most cost-effective approach possible [13]. As new data on the natural history of HPV-related cervical lesions become available and familiarity with TBS increases, new management options for patients with abnormal cytology will be developed. In this regard, ancillary techniques using viral testing, cervicography or automated cytology may be useful tools to improve on diagnostic performance indices as well as quality assurance of cervical cytology [14]. Current management of patients with abnormal Pap smears should focus on combined information on the risk factors for cervical carcinoma, category of cytopathology report, reliability for follow-up and visual inspection of the cervix. It should be realized that a negative Pap smear report has no clinical meaning in the face of a clinically suspicious-looking cervix.

### Definitions of disease categories

An ASCUS diagnosis should include only those squamous cell abnormalities that are greater than those associated with reactive changes, but fail to demonstrate a definite SIL. By definition, ASCUS is not equivalent to squamous atypia or class II used in the Papanicolaou classification system. In TBS, clearly reactive changes are categorized as benign.

LGSIL encompasses cellular changes of HPV as well as CIN I or mild dysplasia or still mild dyskaryosis.

High-grade SIL encompasses moderate to severe dysplasia to carcinoma-*in-situ* or CIN II and CIN III.

AGUS encompasses changes involving either endometrial or endocervical cells. If possible, the origin of the cells should be specified, such as 'atypical endometrial cells of undetermined significance' or 'AGUS, favour endometrial origin'. If the cell type cannot be specified, it is classified as AGUS alone. No criteria are established to separate the reactive from the neoplastic processes. In cases of atypical endocervical cells, nuclear atypia exceeds obvious reactive changes, but falls short of definite evidence of invasive adenocarcinoma. If possible, the nature of the changes should be qualified, such as 'AGUS favour reactive or premalignant/malignant'.

## References

1 Richart RM. Cervical intraepithelial neoplasia. In: Sommers SC (ed) *Pathology Annual.* New York: Appleton-Century-Crofts, 1973, pp 301–328.

2 Ferenczy A, Jenson AB. Tissue effects and host response: the key to the rational triage of cervical neoplasia. In: Lorincz A (ed) *Obstetrics and Gynecology Clinics of North America.* Philadelphia: WB Saunders, 1996, in press.

3 National Cancer Institute Workshop. The 1988 Bethesda system for reporting cervical/vaginal cytological diagnoses. *JAMA* 1989; **262**: 931.

4 Broder S. Rapid communication – the Bethesda system for reporting cervical/vaginal cytologic diagnoses – report of the 1991 Bethesda workshop. *JAMA* 1992; **267**: 1892.

5 Davey DD, Nielsen ML, Rosenstock W *et al.* Terminology and specimen adequacy in cervicovaginal cytology: the College of American Pathologists' interlaboratory comparison experience. *Arch Pathol Lab Med* 1992; **116**: 903.

6 Kurman RJ, Solomon D. *The Bethesda System for Reporting Cervical/vaginal Cytologic Diagnoses: Definitions, Criteria and Explanatory Notes for Terminology and Specimen Adequacy.* New York: Springer-Verlag, 1994.

7 Ferenczy A, Robitaille J, Franco E, Arseneau J, Richart RM, Wright TC. Conventional cervical cytologic smears vs. Thin-Prep smears. A paired comparison study on cervical cytology. *Acta Cytol* 1996; **40**: 1136.

8 Gordon P, Hatch K. Survey of colposcopy practices by obstetricians/gynecologists. *J Reprod Med* 1992; **37**: 861.

9 Herbst AL. The Bethesda system for cervical/vaginal cytologic diagnoses: a note of caution. *Obstet Gynecol* 1990; **76**: 449.

10 Himmelstein L. Evaluation of inflammatory atypia: a literature review. *J Reprod Med* 1989; **34**: 634.

11 Montz FJ, Bradely JM, Fowler JM *et al.* Natural history of the minimally abnormal Papanicolaou smear. *Obstet Gynecol* 1992; **79**: 328.

12 Crum CP. The Bethesda system: a perspective. *Am J Clin Pathol (Suppl)* 1991; **96**: S2.

13 The 1992 National Cancer Institute Workshop. Interim guidelines for management of abnormal cervical cytology. *JAMA* 1994; **271**: 1866.

14 Hutchinson ML. Assessing the costs and benefits of alternative rescreening strategies. *Acta Cytol* 1996; **40**: 4.

# 16: Quality Assurance in Cervical Cytopathology

## M. E. Sherman

## Introduction

Cervical cancer screening is a complex, multistep process that may fail at any point in the sequence between obtaining a cytological sample and providing appropriate patient management. In the USA and elsewhere, cervical cancer fatalities are often attributable to women never having been screened rather than diagnostic error. None the less, pressure from both professional societies and the popular press has resulted in the imposition of federally mandated quality assurance procedures. The majority of these requirements are intended to minimize the rate of false-negative cytological diagnoses. However, the development of strategies to control the rate of equivocal cytological reports (referred to as atypical squamous cells of undetermined significance in the Bethesda system) has also received increasing attention.

In this review, the major recommendations of the Clinical Laboratory Improvement Amendments of 1988 (CLIA '88) are discussed [1,2]. Readers may also consult a recent review [3]. In addition, methods that have been proposed for monitoring the reporting of atypical squamous cells of undetermined significance (ASCUS) in cervical smears are also enumerated.

## Provisions of CLIA '88

CLIA '88 limits a cytotechnologist's workload to a maximum of 100 slides per day. The screening must be performed in no less than an 8-h period, adjusting for professional experience and other activities. In non-gynaecological cytology, types of preparations in which only half the surface area of a microscopic

*Correspondence*: Dr Mark Sherman, Department of Pathology, John Hopkins Hospital, 600 N Wolfe St, Baltimore, MD 21287, USA.

glass slide is used count as half a slide for workload-reporting purposes. In gynaecological cytology, thin-layer slides should probably also be counted as less than a single smear for purposes of assessing workload, but this issue should not be considered finalized until there is significant clinical experience using this technique. In addition, it has been argued that screening a two-slide case is not twice as much work as screening a one-slide case; therefore, workload limits should reflect the number of cases screened rather than the number of slides examined [4].

In the USA, all slides that are interpreted by cytotechnologists as benign cellular changes or abnormal (including ASCUS) are referred to a cytopathologist for final diagnosis. Consequently, many cytopathologists expend a great deal of effort reviewing cases that are benign or show minimal cytological abnormalities rather than examining cases that display unequivocal cervical cancer precursors.

Current standards of practice in the USA require that a qualified cytotechnologist or pathologist rescreen 10% of smears diagnosed as normal by each screener. Although this practice has been criticized since its inception, it remains an entrenched part of cytopathology practice in the USA. The futility of the 10% rescreen in identifying unqualified cytotechnologists was described over two decades ago by Dr Myron Melamed in his presidential address to the American Society of Cytology [5]. In the model presented, a 10% false-negative rate was considered satisfactory and a 25% false-negative rate was considered unacceptable. Based on a 10% random rescreen of negative smears, the number of years required to determine that a screener's performance was unsatisfactory was estimated. The model predicted that in a hypothetical population with a rate of positive smears of 5 per 1000, a cytotechnologist whose performance was unsatisfactory would not be discovered until he or she had screened 132 000 cases. Based on a workload of 10 000 screened cases per year, this would require over 13 years. In a population with a lower rate of positive cases, the period of time required would be even longer. Therefore, it was concluded that the practice of rescreening 10% of negative smears contributes little, if anything, to ensuring quality performance.

Another CLIA mandate is that laboratories review all negative smears obtained within 5 years of a diagnosis of a high-grade squamous intraepithelial lesion (SIL). Based on our experience, this practice may have significant educational benefit for both cytotechnologists and pathologists. In a retrospective search of the cytopathology files of a large teaching hospital spanning a 30-year period, we identified 18 patients with high-grade SIL and 2 with carcinoma who had received at least three negative smear reports prior to diagnosis [6]. The patients had a median of 9.5 smears each, obtained 93.5 months on average prior to colposcopy. On careful rescreening, we identified a missed SIL in 28 (23%) of the 123 slides that were originally interpreted as negative. An additional 37 (30%) slides were interpreted as ASCUS on review and 17 (14%) were judged unsatisfactory. In 7 women, multiple false-negative smears were identified (reported as normal, but SIL on review), in 7 multiple unsatisfactory smears were found and in 7 there were at least two smears without transformation zone sampling. In addition, a previously unrecognized variant of atypical squamous metaplasia was recognized as an antecedent to the diagnosis of high-grade SIL in some women. The cells were smaller than typical metaplastic squamous cells and possessed an increased nuclear to cytoplasmic ratio with some hyperchromasia and nuclear irregularity. In some cases, the cells were hard to classify as a definite high-grade SIL, even in retrospect.

Hatem and Wilbur reported a similar experience in reviewing negative smears immediately preceding the diagnosis of high-grade SIL in 17 patients [7]. These authors reported that missed abnormalities were present in 16 (88%) of the 17 smears originally reported as normal. In 11 of 16 slides, the authors described small atypical cells which they referred to as 'atypical immature squamous metaplasia'. In another study examining the value of the 5-year review of negative slides preceding high-grade SIL, Allen *et al.* reported only a 17.5% rate of false-negative smears [8]. Because 9 (75%) of the 12 false-negative cases were discovered within 2 years of the missed abnormality, the authors advocated limiting review of negatives to the 2-year period immediately preceding the recognition of high-grade SIL.

In summary, the mandated look-backs in women with high-grade SIL have focused attention on the quality of smears and heightened awareness among cytopathologists about cytological patterns of disease that may have previously been overlooked.

Other policies mandated by CLIA '88 include maintaining annual statistics, monitoring the technical process of slide preparation and performing regular correlation of cytology and histology. In accord with the Bethesda System guidelines, it is standard practice not to provide any diagnostic interpretation in smears that are unsatisfactory due to obscuring blood, inflammation, hypocellularity or other causes.

## Quality assurance of ASCUS

In the Bethesda system, ASCUS is defined as changes exceeding those typically found in reactive cells, but which qualitatively or quantitatively fall short of a definite SIL [9]. The diagnosis of ASCUS poses a major public health problem. Rates of ASCUS vary greatly, with 10% of laboratories in the USA reporting rates exceeding 9% [10]. An underlying SIL is uncovered in 10–43% of patients with ASCUS smears. Rates of ASCUS are too high to permit colposcopy in every case, therefore guidelines have been established to control the frequency with which this diagnosis is used. According to the interim guidelines set forth by a consensus panel [11], ASCUS rates should be kept below 5% in most populations with ratios of ASCUS to SIL of about 2 : 1 or 3 : 1. Methods that have been proposed to monitor the frequency with which the ASCUS diagnosis is used include calculation of crude ASCUS rates, calculation of the ASCUS to SIL ratio, correlation of follow-up smears and biopsies in women with ASCUS and human papillomavirus testing [12].

## Acknowledgement

George Washington University has had contractual agreements with Cytyc Corp., Boxborough, MA and Digene Corp., Silver Spring, MD.

## References

1 Clinical laboratory improvement amendments of 1988: final rule. *Fed Reg* 1992; **57**: 7001–7186.
2 CLIA '88 final rule: a summary of major provisions of the final rules implementing the clinical laboratory improvement amendments of 1988. CAP, 1992.
3 Lachowicz CM, Kline TS. Quality improvement principles in cytopathology. In: Kline TS, Nguyen G (eds) *Critical Issues in Cytopathology*. New York: Igaku-Shoin, 1996, pp 42–61.
4 Melamed MR, Flehinger BJ. Editorial. Reevaluation of quality assurance in the cytology laboratory. *Acta Cytol* 1992; **36**: 461–465.
5 Melamed MR. Presidential address. Twentieth annual scientific meeting, American Society of Cytology. *Acta Cytol* 1973; **17**: 285–288.
6 Sherman ME, Kelly D. High-grade squamous intraepithelial lesions and invasive carcinoma following three negative Papanicolaou smears: screening failures or rapid progression? *Mod Pathol* 1992; **5**: 337–342.
7 Hatem F, Wilbur DC. High grade squamous cervical lesions following negative Papanicolaou smears: false negative cervical cytology or rapid progression. *Diagn Cytopathol* 1995; **12**: 135–141.
8 Allen KA, Zaleski S, Cohen MB. Review of negative Papanicolaou tests. Is the retrospective 5-year review necessary? *Am J Clin Pathol* 1994; **101**: 19–21.
9 National Cancer Institute Workshop (1991) The revised Bethesda system for reporting cervical/vaginal cytologic diagnoses: report of the 1991 Bethesda Workshop. *JAMA* 1991; **267**: 1892.
10 Davey DD, Naryshkin S, Nielsen ML *et al*. Atypical squamous cells of undetermined significance: interlaboratory comparison and quality assurance monitors. *Diagn Cytopathol* 1994; **11**: 390–396.
11 Kurman RJ, Henson DE, Herbst AL *et al*. Toward optimal laboratory use. Interim guidelines for management of abnormal cervical cytology. *JAMA* 1994; **271**: 1866–1869.
12 Sherman ME, Schiffman MH, Lorincz AT *et al*. Towards objective quality assurance in cervical cytopathology: correlation of cytopathologic diagnoses with detection of high-risk human papillomavirus types. *Am J Clin Pathol* 1994; **102**: 182–187.

# 17: Error Rates in Cervical Cancer Screening: Causes and Consequences

## L. G. Koss

## Summary

This chapter provides two definitions of false-negative smears – a narrow definition that includes only missed low- and high-grade neoplastic lesions and a broad definition that also includes atypical squamous cells of undetermined significance (ASCUS) and atypical glandular cells of undetermined significance (AGUS). The error rate is defined as the rate of false-negative smears expressed as a percentage of documented neoplastic lesions in the same cohort. Several examples of error rates are provided and the principal causes of screening errors discussed. Consequences of screening errors and possible remedies such as training of personnel and automation are briefly summarized.

## Introduction

In the absence of a double-blind initial study on the effectiveness of the cervicovaginal smear in the detection of precursors and early cancer of the uterine cervix, the error rates and their causes have been mainly studied in individual laboratories. There are also a few recent surveys of multiple laboratories, conducted in the USA [1,2]. Perhaps the most important issue at hand is the definition of an error and the manner of its calculation. For the purpose of this presentation, two definitions will be adopted:

1    A false-negative screening error in cervical cytology is a smear report of 'negative', 'within normal limits', 'benign (inflammatory) atypia' or 'no further action required' (equivalent of Papanicolaou classes I and II – benign) in women, who within 5 years or less, developed either a high-grade preinvasive

*Correspondence*: Dr Leopold Koss, Department of Pathology, Montefiore Medical Center, Albert Einstein College of Medicine, Bronx, NY 10467, USA.

lesion or invasive carcinoma, if on review the smear shows evidence of significant cytological abnormalities. Two definitions of such abnormalities can be adopted, as recently suggested by Jones [2]: the *narrow definition* includes smears that on review show cytological evidence of low-grade and high-grade preinvasive squamous lesions (cervical intraepithelial neoplasia (CIN) I–III), corresponding to glandular endocervical lesions, or invasive cancer. The *broad definition* also includes ASCUS or similar atypias of endocervical cells (AGUS), both terms introduced by the Bethesda system [3,4].

2   The errors can be calculated as a percentage of all smears screened. Because the percentage of abnormal smears in any given population studied is small (from 5 to 10% of all smears), the resulting error rate is very small and does not fully reflect the performance of a laboratory. Rather, the error rate should be defined as a percentage of documented neoplastic lesions occurring in the same cohort. It is the latter definition that has been adopted in our laboratory and is the basis of this discussion.

## Rate of errors

A pioneering paper on this subject was published by van der Graaf *et al.* [5] in 1987. They reviewed 555 cervical smears previously reported as negative or benign atypia, in women who within 3 years developed either a high-grade squamous intraepithelial lesion (CIN grade II or III) or, in 8 cases, an invasive carcinoma. Van der Graaf *et al.* documented that in 97 of the 555 initial smears, various levels of dysplasia or carcinoma were observed on review; thus the narrow definition error rate was 17.5%. This figure, however, did not include atypical and mild dysplasia smears. If these various grades of atypia were included, the broad definition false-negative rate would have risen to 163 of 555, or over 29% of smears in this cohort. Approximately 12% of the smears were considered inadequate.

This important study has led us to undertake a study of screening errors in our own laboratory. There was one significant difference between the setting of the two studies: major quality control measures have been in place in our laboratory since 1989: the smears on *all* women considered to be at risk because of clinical history or other data have been rescreened by a senior cytotechnologist and, if necessary, referred to a pathologist for a diagnosis [6]. For the years 1989–1991 the resulting volume of quality control smears averaged 25% of all smears (range from 11 to 40%). For the years 1989–1991, with an average quality control rescreening volume of 24%, the *primary* screening error rate (including atypias requiring colposcopic follow-up but not other forms of ASCUS or AGUS, and all CIN lesions) was about 5% of lesions. In all these cases correct reports were issued. For the remaining patients no such quality control measures could be conducted but occasional additional screening errors came to our attention with the passage of time: in nearly all such cases some form of previously overlooked atypia was observed. It has been estimated that in our laboratory with extensive quality control the total primary false-negative screening rate is by broad definition about 10% of lesions, with half of the errors corrected on quality control rescreening [6]. To document the accuracy of this figure a total second rescreening of all smears would have been required.

Several other studies of previous negative smears on women who subsequently developed high-grade CIN or invasive cancer were reported. Among them, Gay *et al.* [7] and Sherman and Kelly [8] observed a false-negative rate of approximately 20%; in many such cases small cancer cells were overlooked on screening. This has also been my personal experience with several legal cases pertaining to women who subsequently developed invasive cervical cancer (unpublished data). In a survey of 3762 cases of women who subsequently developed a high-grade lesion or invasive carcinoma from 312 laboratories, Jones [2] reported a false-negative rate of 10.1% using the narrow definition and 19.7% using the broad definition. Davey *et al.* [1] reported that the false-negative error rate by very large groups of pathologists on prescreened smears was somewhat above 5%.

## Causes of errors

Screening of cervicovaginal smears has been repeatedly described as tedious, monotonous and time-consuming [9]. It is therefore not surprising that evidence of an abnormality, sometimes confined to only a few cells, can be overlooked, particularly if the cytotechnologist is burdened with an excessive load of work. In my estimation, on the average, about 5 min is required to screen a smear well, with some smears requiring less, and some more time. Under these conditions the maximum number of smears that a cytotechnologist can screen is 12 in an hour and 72 smears in a 6-hour working day, accounting for the necessary rest periods, less than the currently authorized (by the Centers for Disease Control) maximum of 100 smears a day. To be sure, this is an arbitrary figure based on personal experience and not on a scientific analysis of screening. Some exceptionally able, trained people can probably handle a larger volume of smears but most become extremely tired after having screened 50 smears in a day's work, which is the maximum currently authorized in our laboratory. A larger volume of work will almost inevitably lead to errors. There are two types of screening errors: errors of commission and errors of omission.

*Errors of commission* are based on misinterpretation of cytological evidence either by the cytotechnologist or by his or her professional supervisor who, in the USA and Canada, must be a board-certified pathologist. Some, but not all,

European countries also adhere to this professional standard. Most, but not all, errors of commission occur because of inadequate training or experience. In some cases the evidence itself is very difficult to interpret. As an example of errors of commission, small cancer cells may be interpreted as benign endometrial cells; many other sources of such errors have been identified [10]. In some of the most distressing cases of this type the cytotechnologist correctly identified abnormal cells, only to be overruled by her professional supervisor.

*Errors of omission* occur because the cytotechnologist either fails to notice important evidence or fails to identify it and bring it to the attention of the supervisor. Most of these errors occur because of inattention or fatigue, but some are caused by very scanty evidence of disease, confined to a few cells. Again, in some instances, inadequate training is the cause of such events.

## The consequences of screening errors

Not all screening errors are costly to the patients. In many, perhaps even most, cases of preinvasive lesions missed on initial screening, the lesion will be identified in routine follow-up rescreening. Routine colposcopy on all patients, as practised in some European centres, certainly prevents a great many of these errors from becoming serious. Still, an analysis of previous negative smears in women who developed either high-grade preinvasive lesions or invasive cancer of the uterine cervix disclosed three categories of smears. Some of the smears were adequate and, for reasons unknown, truly negative and did not contain any abnormal cells. Some smears were poorly obtained and were judged to be inadequate. In at least 20% of such smears, however, errors of commission or omission have occurred [7,8]. The principal culprit in many such cases was small cancer cells, occurring singly or in tight clusters that some observers have named syncytial clusters [11]. Sometimes the number of these difficult-to-identify cancer cells was small [8] but occasionally abundant evidence of small-cell cancer was present but not identified. In the latter cases it is clear that inattention to screening, poor recognition ability or poor training caused such errors. The error may be compounded if the lesion is located in the endocervical canal and thus not visible on a casual inspection of the uterine cervix, as is customary with primary care physicians who do not practise colposcopy.

The development of invasive cancer, let alone the loss of life to this disease, diagnosed after one or more false-negative smears is particularly painful in young patients, some of whom have small children. As is now the custom in the USA, in many such cases, legal proceedings against the laboratory, the pathologist, and usually also the physician or gynaecologist are initiated by the patient who may have been injured by treatment, or by her bereaved family, in case of death. In many such cases pre-trial settlements or jury verdicts costing from several hundred thousand to several million dollars are the outcome. Today, false-negative cervicovaginal smears are the fastest-growing segment of malpractice cases, adding enormous costs to cytological screening [12].

## The remedies

### Training of physicians responsible for cytological diagnoses

In the USA and Canada, the routine training of physicians in pathology requires that only a small segment of their time – not more than 3 months – be dedicated to cytopathology. Within recent years, a qualifying examination in cytopathology has been offered to fully trained pathologists in the USA, requiring a minimum of 1 year of additional specialized training in an approved fellowship programme. Even under such optimal circumstances, however, the exposure of trainees to the difficult art of analysis and interpretation of cervicovaginal smears is often unequal to the task at hand. In many European countries there are only the most trivial training requirements, before a physician can open a laboratory and practise cytopathology. In some countries, such as Germany, most laboratories are run by practising gynaecologists, some with minimal training and experience in the difficult art of cervicovaginal cytology. There are no data available on the error rate in such laboratories.

### Training of cytotechnologists

In reference to cytotechnologist, the situation is similar. Although in the USA and in Canada a rigidly observed training period of 1 year in an approved school is mandatory prior to a qualifying examination in cytotechnology, the situation in Europe is far less structured, with only a very few dedicated schools and few schooled cytotechnologists. In most instances the European cytotechnologists are trained 'on the job'.

Some appropriate training standards and postgraduate education may alleviate some the difficulties in the interpretation of cervicovaginal smears.

### Automation

There are two automated scanning systems recently approved for quality control by the Food and Drug Administration [13]. These systems and their performance are discussed in Chapter 30.

## References

1 Davey DD, Nilsen ML, Frable WJ *et al*. Improving accuracy in gynecologic cytology: results of the College of American Pathologists interlaboratory comparison program in cervicovaginal cytology (PAP). *Arch Pathol Lab Med* 1993; **117**: 1193–1198.

2 Jones BA. Rescreening in gynecologic cytology. Rescreening of 3762 previous cases for current high-grade squamous intraepithelial lesion and carcinoma – a College of American Pathologist Q-Probes study of 312 institutions. *Arch Pathol Lab Med* 1996; **119**: 1097–1103.

3 Kurman RJ, Solomon D. *The Bethesda System for Reporting Cervical/vaginal Smears*. New York; Springer Verlag, 1994.

4 Koss LG. The new Bethesda system for reporting results of smears of the uterine cervix. *J Natl Cancer Inst* 1990; **82**: 988–991.

5 Van der Graaf Y, Vooijs GP, Gaillard HLJ, Go DMD. Screening errors in cervical cytology smears. *Acta Cytol* 1987; **31**: 434–438.

6 Koss LG. Cervical (Pap) smear – new directions. *Cancer* 1993; **71**: 1406–1412.

7 Gay JD, Donaldson LD, Goellner JR. False-negative results in cervical cytology studies. *Acta Cytol* 1985; **29**: 1043–1046.

8 Sherman ME, Kelly D. High-grade squamous intraepithelial lesions and invasive carcinoma following the report of three negative Papanicolaou smears: screening failure or rapid progression? *Mod Pathol* 1992; **5**: 337–342.

9 Koss LG. The Papanicolaou test for cervical cancer detection. A triumph and a tragedy. *JAMA* 1989; **261**: 737–743.

10 Koss LG. *Diagnostic Cytology and its Histopathologic Bases*, 4th edn. Philadelphia J.B. Lippincott, 1992.

11 Patten SFJ. *Diagnostic Cytopathology of the Uterine Cervix* 2nd edn. New York; S. Karger, 1978.

12 Sabella JD. Pathology claims up – liability premiums to follow. *CAP Today* 1993; **7**: 39.

13 Hematology and Pathology Devices Panel of the Medical Devices Advisory Committee to FDA. Federal Department of Health and Human Services, Rockville, MD. Transcript of Proceedings. 1995.

# 18: Cervical Cancer Following Negative Smears

## E. McGoogan

## Summary

Conventional cervical screening, as with all screening programmes, has a sensitivity and specificity less than 100%. The sensitivity is limited by problems in the programme (deficiencies in organization, inappropriate screening intervals or failures to cover the whole population at risk), problems with smear-taking (inadequate sampling, preparation or fixation, histological type and site of the lesion) problems with follow-up and treament and, only to a lesser extent, problems with microscopic assessment in the laboratory. Most public attention had focused on the laboratory since there is a significant false-negative rate even in the best of laboratories but targeting the laboratory alone with ever-increasing quality control and quality assurance measures will not result in a significant increase in sensitivity of the cervical screening programme. Improvements in diagnostic accuracy of the Papanicolaou (Pap) test need to begin in the doctor's clinic with better-quality smear-taking, preparation and fixation. In the final analysis the smear-taker, in collecting and sending an appropriate sample to the laboratory, is the limiting factor in the whole screening process. Specificity is also important in screening programmes because false positives cause morbidity. The false-positive Pap smear is far more prevalent and results in additional economic costs and emotional stress to the woman. In an attempt to lower the false-negative rate, laboratories have been increasing their false-positive rate with resulting additional economic and emotional costs.

*Correspondence*: Dr Euphemia McGoogan, Department of Pathology, University of Edinburgh Medical School, Teviot Place, Edinburgh EH8 9AG, UK.

## Introduction

The aim of any screening programme is to sort out those individuals who probably have the disease from those who probably do not. Unlike a diagnostic test, screening aims to identify asymptomatic disease, does not deal with patients and is initiated by the doctor who recommends the screening test because it will do the individual good. Therefore, the chance of benefit to the individual must far outweigh the chance of harm. The report of the International Agency for Research on Cancer (IARC) working group on cervical cancer screening in 1986 [1] showed that population-based cervical screening programmes can be effective in reducing the incidence and mortality from cervical cancer. Following the relaunch of a call-and-recall population-wide cervical screening programme in the UK in 1988, a recent striking reduction in mortality has been shown [2,3] and more recently Sasieni *et al.* [4] report a drop in incidence too. In a study of 348 women with invasive cervical cancer in the UK in 1992 together with 677 age- and residence-matched controls, Sasieni *et al.* showed that the incidence would have been 57% greater in the absence of screening. In women under 70 years of age the incidence would have been 75% greater. Thus, screening prevented between 1100 and 3900 cases of invasive cancer in the UK that year and the authors calculated that, had the screening guidelines been strictly followed, an additional 1250 cases could have been prevented. Only 47% of women under 70 years of age with stage 1 B cancer had been screened. Thirteen per cent of women had been inadequately followed up following detection of an abnormality.

Conventional cervical screening, as with all screening programmes, has a sensitivity and specificity less than 100% [5]. Sensitivity is affected by a variety of factors, including failure of the programme to reach the entire population at risk; failure of the test to detect all cases; the frequency of screening missing rapidly developing cancers; failure to act on all abnormalities identified by screening and failure of treatment to cure all women identified.

Fortunately, since it is well-accepted that screening reduces the incidence and mortality from invasive cervical cancer, it is not critical to establish the exact false-negative rate. The main reasons for attempting to calculate it are to compare the quality of programmes and laboratories in different settings and to seek ways to identify and reduce deficiencies. The sensitivity of a Pap test has been variably assessed in the literature as between 6% and 55% [5].

## Sensitivity

A wide range of definitions of false-negative rate is used in publications resulting in great variations in the rates quoted. Hakama *et al.* [1] calculated a false-negative rate of between 40% and less than 10%. The technical definition of false-negative rate is the probability of a negative result in a woman who actually has a cancer or cervical intraepithelial neoplasia (CIN) presuming this is part of a population-based screening programme. Other definitions of false-negative rate may lead to an overestimate of the true rate; e.g. the proportion of women with invasive cancer who had a recent negative smear; the rate of misclassified smears in those who developed invasive cancer; and the false-negative rate in women who developed invasive cancer if the true positives which detected lesions before they became invasive are not included. Other ways of looking at false-negative rates include interlaboratory comparisons such as that described by Yobs et al. [6], which led to a rate of undercalling of high-grade SIL of between 34% and 57%. Van der Graaf and Vooijs [7] defined their test a false negative if a woman developed a confirmed lesion within 2 years of a negative smear. They calculated a rate of 17%. These variations can be explained on the basis of the different definitions of false-negative rate used, how a negative smear test is defined in different situations and how doubtful tests are handled operationally.

## Interval since last negative smear

There is considerable change in the risk of developing invasive cervical cancer with the time elapsed since the last negative smear and with the number of previous negative smears. Lynge and Poll in their chapter in the IARC report [1] calculated that women had zero risk of developing invasive cancer within 12 months of a negative test while protection falls to the level of the unscreened women by 5 years. The risk at 5 years was 48% lower for women with one previous negative smear and 62% lower if two previous negative smears. At 3 years the risk was 78% lower if one previous negative smear and 89% lower if two negative smears. Women with five negative smears had a negligible risk of developing cancer. Sasieni et al. [4] also showed that the relative protection following a negative smear was greatest in the first 12 months and fell off towards the end of the fifth year. Eddy [8] showed that screening every 2–3 years was almost as effective as every year (within 3%) but dropped off more sharply when the screening intervals extended beyond 3–5 years.

With non-organized programmes and in the early years after the introduction of organized population-based call-and-recall screening programmes, the majority of women who develop invasive cancer will not have been adequately screened. As population coverage and compliance improve, an increasing proportion of women who develop invasive cancer will have been adequately screened and may have a history of one or more negative smears. The term interval cancer has been used in these cases. This is an unfortunate term to use since cervical screening is aimed at detecting intraepithelial disease and not invasive cancer. Furthermore, it is unlikely that these cancers have developed *ab initio* since the time of the last smear. It is more likely that the Pap test has failed to detect the presence of disease.

### Rate of invasive cancer in screened women

Many published series have looked at cervical cancer diagnosis after negative cervical cytology. Mitchell and Giles [9] showed that the rate of cancer diagnosis in women whose first smear during the last 3 years was negative was 2.54 per 100 000 women per year and that the rate did not vary by age group or by endocervical status of smear. The proportion of women with invasive cancer who had a negative smear in the last 3 years was 24% overall (20% for squamous carcinoma and 33% for endocervical carcinoma). However, Mitchell *et al*. [10] showed that only 10% of women dying from cervical cancer had been adequately screened and that 70% of women were 50 years or older. Our own figures from Edinburgh for the period 1993–1995 show that there were 179 invasive cervical cancers diagnosed, 40 (22%) of which were endocervical adenocarcinomas. There were 139 diagnoses of invasive squamous carcinoma but 37 occurred in women over 65 years and outside the screening programme (Scottish cervical screening policy is for women aged 20–60 years at a 3-yearly interval). Of the 102 invasive squamous cancers which occurred in women in the screening age group, 40% had a negative smear within the last 5 years, 28% had not been screened in the last 5 years and the remainder (32%) had been identified as abnormal on screening and were follow-up or treatment failures. Thirty-one cancers were microinvasive and all these women had been screened within the last 5 years.

## Factors affecting sensitivity of the Pap smear

The potential deficiencies in the Pap test are wide-ranging and women with invasive cancer may have had a recent negative smear for a variety of reasons. Public attention has focused on the laboratory as the main source of false-negative tests but this is probably not the case [5,11]. The sensitivity of the Pap test is limited by many factors, including incorrect or inadequate sampling of the cervix, poor transfer of cellular material to the glass slide and suboptimal preparation and fixation by the smear-taker and, to a lesser extent, microscopic assessment in the laboratory.

### Sampling and preparation

Sampling and preparation alone are said to be responsible for 53–90% of all false-negative tests [11]. Possibly up to two-thirds of sampling error is due to a failure of smear-takers to harvest representative diagnostic cells from the cervix.

Depending on the sampler used, up to 90% of the cellular material scraped from the cervix may be discarded with the sampler. The amount of material transferred successfully to the glass slide ranged from 6.5% at worst to 62.5% at best [11]. Furthermore, since some spatulas have a well-recognized trapping effect and the distribution of the abnormal cells on the sampling device is not uniform, only a selected, non-random proportion of the cells is placed on the glass slide. Thus the material on the slide may not contain the most diagnostic cells removed from the cervix. Preparation and fixation of smears in the doctor's clinic setting give little control of the critical parameters required for accurate microscopic assessment – cellular morphology, clarity, density and uniformity. Smears are frequently unevenly spread and poorly fixed and many are rendered inadequate for accurate assessment. Improvements in diagnostic accuracy of the Pap test need to begin in the doctor's clinic with better-quality smear-taking, preparation and fixation.

Sampling problems are not only associated with the actual taking of the smear but are influenced by the size and site of the lesion within the cervix and its histological type. Very small lesions and lesions located mainly within endocervical crypts or high in the canal are more difficult to sample with routine spatulas. The poor sensitivity of the Pap test to detect precursors of endocervical adenocarcinoma is well recognized [12].

**Laboratory assessment**

Within the laboratory, problems have been associated with inadequate training and continuing education of technical and medical staff and with failure to provide an appropriate screening environment and equipment. It is now well accepted that quality assurance procedures are necessary to confirm the continuing competence of staff [5]. Habituation and fatigue problems are compounded where individuals are expected to screen excessive numbers of slides per day [5]. On the other hand, problems may arise from lack of regular experience, resulting from seeing too few slides or too few abnormal cases. Detection and interpretation problems are well documented. Detection is currently limited by the resolution of the light microscope and the human eye. In many cases we are not able to identify early morphological changes of neoplasia or neoplastic precursor cells. Poor fixation and preparation, particularly in the presence of inflammatory or menstrual exudate, make detection of abnormal cells difficult. This is particularly true when there are very few abnormal cells present or where the abnormal cell nuclei are small in size or hypochromatic [13].

Lack of standard terminology and, more importantly, standard criteria is the basis of interpretation problems. The presence of inflammatory or menstrual exudate makes detection and interpretation of abnormal cells difficult.

Cytological 'look-alikes' of high-grade cells such as endometrial cells, tubo-endometrial metaplasia, macrophages and follicular cervicitis may be a source of false-positive or false-negative smears. CIN infiltrating crypts may result in groups of endocervical cells with small numbers of neoplastic cells attached which may not be recognized [5,13].

Human factors are also important. Laming [14,15] describes the cyto-pathologist's tasks as the inspection of a series of rather similar slides with no immediate feedback. He constructed an experiment where subjects were asked to detect similar flashing lights and he compared the effects of immediate feedback with lack of feedback. He also noted the effect of imposing penalties for false positives. In a second experiment, he studied the interaction between successive judgements and showed that response assimilation led to accumulation of errors and judgement 'runaway'. He postulated this as the reason why some pathologists identified in some major screening scandals had failed to recognize as abnormal most of the abnormal smears referred to them by technical staff [14].

### False-negative smear patterns

In an attempt to discover why some smears were not recognized by laboratory staff as abnormal, Mitchell and Medley [16] carried out a case-control study of CIN III where false-negative smears were compared with true-positive smears. The false-negative smear profile showed that the correct diagnosis was unlikely to be made where the number of abnormal cells present in the smear was less than 50, the cells were present as single cells rather than as a combination of groups and dispersed cells, where the cell size was small and where the chromatin was normochromic with a fine chromatin pattern. Bosch *et al.* [17] showed similar findings in their study of smears preceding invasive cancers but also noted that false negatives were repeatedly missed in the routine screening situation, while often detected when cytotechnologists know they are being tested. However this was accompanied by a doubling in the screening time and a threefold increase in the false-positive rate. Robertson and Woodend [18] confirmed that false-negative smears preceding invasive cancer often had very few abnormal cells present, but noted that the abnormal cells were often present only as fragments rather than single cells. This was particularly common with adenocarcinoma (50% of cases). However, they noted that almost half the cases had moderate numbers of single cells and, in a third of cases, these were so numerous as to be detected easily on rapid review of the slide.

Robertson and Woodend [18] suggested that smears lacking an endocervical component (i.e. suggesting a poor-quality sample) were a common occurrence in negative smears preceding cervical cancer, but Mitchell and Medley [19] in their longitudinal study of 20 222 women with negative cervical smears according to endocervical status showed that the incidence of CIN was not significantly different between women whose first smear lacked endocervical cells and those whose smear included endocervical cells.

### Histological type of the invasive cervical cancer

The histological type of the invasive cancer is also important. Very frequently in women who have been adequately screened, the cancer is microinvasive or, at worst, stage 1B, i.e. at a stage where it is potentially curable. In the study of Sasieni *et al.* [4]. 26% of invasive squamous cancers were microinvasive and a further 53% were stage 1B. Is it realistic to consider these 'failures' of screening programmes? The incidence of endocervical adenocarcinoma has more than doubled in women under 35 years in the last three decades. In the study by Mitchell *et al.* [12] endocervical adenocarcinoma constituted 13% of all cervical cancers. Endocervical adenocarcinoma constitutes 22% of cervical cancers in our own area. Since cervical screening programmes are designed to detect squamous intraepithelial lesions, should adenocarcinomas be included as failures of screening? In addition, many invasive cervical cancers are mixed adenosquamous in type and it is unclear whether the natural history for these histological types is different. Among invasive cancers occurring in screened women, a higher proportion are adeno- or adenosquamous carcinoma, possibly confirming other evidence that cervical cytology has a lower sensitivity for the detection of these histological types [12,20]. It may therefore be important to separate these histological types into different categories when presenting audits of cervical screening programmes.

## The importance of specificity

No screening programme can provide 100% protection but the false-negative Pap smear may not be the biggest problem in cervical screening today. The false-positive Pap smear is far more prevalent and results in additional economic costs and emotional stress to the woman. In an attempt to lower the false-negative rate, laboratories have been increasing their false-positive rate, with resulting additional economic and emotional costs. Specificity is particularly important in screening programmes because false positives cause morbidity. Indeed, some true positives are also a problem if they identify and lead to treatment of conditions which would not have progressed to significant disease and become apparent [21]. Several studies have reported spontaneous regression rates between 6 and 60% for precursor lesions diagnosed on cervical smears. Thus both false positives and false negatives should be considered as phenomena of the Pap screening test rather than incompetence or negligence. The word 'error' should be avoided.

## Conclusion

Nationally (or, preferably, internationally) accepted standards are urgently required. Quality assurance measures are necessary to confirm that laboratory and programme standards are satisfactory. The introduction of new technologies such as thin-layer preparations should be considered in order to address some of the sampling and laboratory deficiencies of conventional screening. These new technologies lend themselves well to additional tests for other indicators of neoplasia which might improve both the sensitivity and specificity of the Pap test [22]. The role and economics of using automated pre- and post-screening devices need to be assessed in comparison to good-quality conventional screening. In the final analysis, however, the smear-taker, in collecting the sample, is the limiting factor in the whole screening process.

## References

1 Hakama M, Miller AB, Day NE. *Screening for Cancer of the Uterine Cervix*. Lyon: International Agency for Research on Cancer, 1986.
2 CRC. *Cancer of the Cervix Uteri*. Cancer Research Campaign, Factsheet 12.2, 1994.
3 Sasieni PD, Cuzick J, Lynch-Farmery E. Estimating the efficacy of screening by auditing smear histories of women with and without cervical cancer. *Br J Cancer* 1996; **73**: 1001–1005.
4 Sasieni P, Cusick J, Farmery E. Letter. *Lancet* 1995; **346**: 1566–1567.
5 Koss LG. The Papanicolaou test for cervical cancer detection, a triumph and a tragedy. *JAMA* 1989; **261**: 737–743.
6 Yobs AR, Plott AE, Hicklin MD. Retrospective evaluation of cytologic cytodiagnosis: 11. Interlaboratory reproducibility as shown in rescreening large consecutive samples of reported cases. *Acta Cytol* 1987; **31**: 900–910.
7 van der Graaf Y, Vooijs GP, Gaillard HLJ, Go DMDS. Screening errors in cervical cytologic screening. *Acta Cytol* 1987; **31**: 434–438.
8 Eddy DM. Screening for cervical cancer. *Ann Intern Med* 1990; **113**: 14–226.
9 Mitchell HS, Giles G. Cancer diagnosis after a report of negative cervical cytology. *Med J Aust* 1996; **164**: 270–273.
10 Mitchell H, Medley G, Higgins V. An audit of the women who died during 1994 from cancer of the cervix in Victoria, Australia. *Aust NZ J Obstet Gynaecol* 1996; **36**: 73–76.
11 Hutchison ML, Isenstein LM, Goodman A *et al*. Homogeneous sampling accounts for the increased diagnostic accuracy using the ThinPrep processor. *Am J Clin Pathol* 1994; **101**: 215–219.
12 Mitchell H, Medley G, Gordon I, Giles G. Cervical cytology reported as negative and risk of adenocarcinoma of the cervix: no strong evidence of benefits. *Br J Cancer* 1995; **71**: 894–897.
13 Herbert A. Achievable standards, benchmarks for reporting and criteria for evaluating cervical cytopathology. *Cytopathology* 1995; **6**: suppl 2.
14 Laming D. Screening cervical smears. *Br J Psychol* 1995; **86**: 507–516.
15 Laming D. The human element in medical screening. *J Med Screen* 1995; **2**: 52–55.
16 Mitchell H, Medley G. Differences between Papanicolaou smears with correct and incorrect diagnoses. *Cytopathology* 1995; **6**: 368–375.

17 Bosch MMC, Rietveld-Scheffers PEM, Boon ME. Characteristics of false-negative smears tested in the normal screening situation. *Acta Cytol* 1992; **36**: 711–716.

18 Robertson JH, Woodend B. Negative cytology preceding cervical cancer: causes and prevention. *J Clin Pathol* 1993; **46**: 700–702.

19 Mitchell H, Medley G. Longitudinal study of women with negative cervical smears according to endocervical status. *Lancet* 1991; **337**: 265–267.

20 Mitchell H, Medley G, Giles G. Cervical cancers diagnosed after negative results on cervical cytology: prospective in the 1980s. *BMJ* 1990; **300**: 1622–1626.

21 Robertson JH, Woodend B, Elliott H. Cytological changes preceding cervical cancer. *J Clin Pathol* 1994; **47**: 278–279.

22 McGoogan E, Reith A. Would monolayers provide more representative samples and improved preparations for cervical screening? *Acta Cytol* 1996; **40**: 107–119.

# Section 4
# Cytology Screening Programmes

# 19: Organization, Monitoring and Use of Resources for Screening Programmes

## J. Patnick

All public health systems have costs attached to them before any benefit can be gained. The financial costs must compete with many other related and unrelated priorities, whether funding is sought from the individual or public purse. Other resources used are the skills of medical, technical and nursing staff, which can be in short supply, and the time and trouble of the population coming forward for screening. It is therefore essential to be able to demonstrate that the time, effort and money are well spent.

If screening is carried out on an individual basis, then that individual may feel a benefit if reassurance is gained or a cancer found earlier than might otherwise have been the case. However, that benefit cannot be proved; for this one needs to look at screening on a population basis. Wilson and Jungner in 1968 for the World Health Organization [1] defined 10 principles against which any potential screening programme can be tested. One of these principles was that the cost of the screening programme should be balanced against the benefit provided.

Purchasers of screening will be looking for value for money, particularly when the purchasers are public health departments looking at the cost of screening an entire population. Value for money can rarely be demonstrated in a population-based screening programme which is not organized. A distinction must be made between a screening policy, which is a statement of good intent, and a screening programme, which includes making some provision for a screening policy actually to be implemented.

For a screening programme to be properly organized, a number of characteristics are needed:

1 Identification of the population to be screened.

*Correspondence*: Mrs Julietta Patnick, National Co-ordinator, NHS National Screening Programme, The Manor House, 260 Ecclesall Road South, Sheffield S11 9PS, UK.

2    Call-and-recall for screening to a planned schedule.
3    Clear screening protocols.
4    Clear referral patterns.
5    Process quality indicators.
6    Outcome quality indicators.

For cervical cancer, the population at risk is all women with a cervix, particularly those who have ever been sexually active. Women who have never had sexual intercourse may be at lower risk of squamous cell carcinoma [2], but may be at equal risk of adenocarcinoma, the incidence of which appears to be rising [3,4]. According to local patterns of incidence, the lower and upper age limits for the programme can be set, with most programmes commencing around the mid-20s and finishing around 60.

Recently it has become apparent that there is a strong relationship between certain types of human papillomavirus (HPV) and the development of cervical cancer [5]. It may be that this will enable the identification of a particularly high-risk population who should be subject to slightly different screening protocols and schedules than the general population of women.

The frequency of screening has often been debated. The International Agency for Research on Cancer (IARC) study [6] demonstrated the relative benefits of screening frequencies. These can be balanced against the resources available. To make the best use of resources and the most impact on the disease, high coverage of the identified population is essential [7]. This can most easily be achieved by personal and regular invitations to women according to a well-publicised schedule. Recruitment which is opportunistic rather than organized can be a costly method of achieving high coverage rates since this approach typically leads to overscreening of lower-risk women at the expense of those women at higher risk.

Clear screening protocols are necessary in order that all participants in the programme, the women and the professionals concerned, understand what is being offered and its limitations. Screening is a question of balance – sensitivity against specificity, advantages against disadvantages, risks against benefits. Overzealous pursuit of one area, or lack of activity in another, may disturb the balance. Women invited for cervical screening expect that their chance of benefit is greater than their chance of harm. Clear protocols ensure that the programme is kept in balance in their favour.

Where there is a multicentre screening programme, for example, a national screening programme, it is essential to have common, agreed protocols for both screening and referral in order to maintain the cohesion of the programme. This is needed if evaluation is to be attempted of the whole programme or country rather than of each individual centre within the programme. It is important, however, that these common protocols share a striving for excellence, rather than agreement on the lowest common denominator, or the overall quality of the programme could deteriorate.

There is little point in screening for abnormalities in an apparently healthy population if those abnormalities are not investigated or not treated where necessary. In the same way that protocols are needed for the initial test, then there must be agreed protocols for managing the women identified as having a cervical abnormality. Our experience in the UK has led us to the conclusion that the protocols should include not only when and how the woman is treated, but also who should treat her [8].

In order to ensure that the protocols are adhered to, and the appropriate quality maintained, process indicators must be developed and monitored. These might include the proportions of low- and high-grade lesions to be found, the positive predictive value of cytology compared with histology, the accuracy of the colposcopists' opinion and the proportion of confirmed treatment failures. These will not tell you whether the incidence of cervical cancer is falling, but all those involved in the programme – the women, the professionals and the funding bodies – can be satisfied that the programme is on target as it is operating at the current time. Outcome indicators take several years to be meaningful and if a programme is not operating correctly, it is imperative to know and take action as quickly as possible.

Outcome indicators are obviously essential for evaluation of a screening programme in the longer term. Mortality and incidence rates are the ultimate arbiters here – the measures against which value for money, time and skills can be judged. Other indicators which might be employed could include the relative proportions of women with an invasive cancer who have never been screened or ever been screened.

To conclude, the organization, monitoring and use of resources in cervical screening are inextricably linked. In order to obtain sufficient resources, a screening programme must be well organized and monitored. It must be able to demonstrate its efficacy and that it does more good than harm.

## References

1 Wilson JMG, Jungner G. *Principles and Practice of Screening for Disease*. WHO public health paper 34. Geneva: WHO, 1968.

2 Griffiths M. Nuns, virgins and spinsters. Rigoni-Stern and cervical cancer revisited. *Br J Obstet Gynaecol* 1991; **98**: 799–802.

3 Van Wijngaarden WJ, Duncan ID, Hussain KA. Screening for cervical neoplasia in Dundee and Angus, 10 years on. *Br J Obstet Gynaecol* 1995; **102**: 137–142.

4 Sigurdsson K. Quality assurance in cervical screening: the Icelandic experience 1964–1993. *Eur J Cancer* 1995; **31A**: 728–734.

5 Muñoz N, Bosch FX, Shah KV, Meheus A (eds) *The Epidemiology of HPV and Cervical Cancer*. IARC Scientific Publication no. 119. Lyon: IARC, 1992.

6 Day NE. The epidemiological basis for evaluating different screening policies. In: Hakama M, Miller AB, Day NE (eds) *Screening for Cancer of the Uterine Cervix*. IARC Scientific Publication no. 76. Lyon: IARC, 1986.

7 Chamberlain J. Reasons that some screening programmes fail to control cervical cancer: In: Hakama M, Miller AB, Day NE (eds) *Screening for Cancer of the Uterine Cervix*. IARC Scientific Publication no. 76. Lyon: IARC, 1986.

8 Luesley D (ed) *Standards and Quality in Colposcopy*. NHSCSP publication no. 2. Sheffield: NHSCSP, 1996.

# 20: Cervical Screening by General Practitioners and Nurses and Information Feedback Systems

## J. Patnick

The close relationship between women and their general practitioners is supported by evidence from the UK that most women prefer their own general practitioner to perform the cervical smear [1] and that it is advantageous if the woman's general practitioner signs the invitation letter him- or herself [2,3].

In the UK there is a National Health Service (NHS) which is free at the point of delivery. The first point of contact for an individual is with primary care. This is the family doctor, or in some contexts the community clinic. General practice in the UK has undergone major changes in the last 10 years. Most general practitioners are now working in modern health centres with several partners and practice nurses. The primary health care team and the primary-care-led NHS are the focus of current thinking.

Most smears taken in the UK are taken in the primary care setting by general practitioners and practice nurses. A national census [4] carried out in 1993 showed that 74.8% of practice nurses in England and Wales are now known to be taking cervical smears. There is some evidence to suggest that practices with a practice nurse and with a female partner have higher cervical screening coverage rates [5].

It is clearly important to report back to each practice team its coverage rate for cervical smears. In the UK the level of coverage is linked to the fees paid to the practice, with milestones at 50% and 80% coverage. In the British context, therefore, coverage rates are a vital piece of feedback.

Each individual smear-taker should also monitor his or her own inadequate and optimal smear rate. In the UK this is considered a professional matter, although from time to time where there are particular problems a laboratory may wish to discuss an individual's smear-taking technique with that person.

*Correspondence*: Mrs Julietta Patnick, National Co-ordinator, NHS National Screening Programme, The Manor House, 260 Ecclesall Road South, Sheffield S11 9PS, UK.

The laboratory will clearly report if a smear is inadequate and should be repeated, and also if, in women of reproductive age (under 50) there is evidence of transformation zone sampling. It is recommended that at least 80% of smears from women under 50 should demonstrate metaplastic and/or endocervical cells [6].

Smear-taking technique is something that has given rise to problems in the UK in the past. Scandals have hit the press and television regarding smears being taken by fingers and with tongue depressors. Therefore much emphasis is now laid on training of smear-takers and work is continuing.

The smear-taker, having invited the woman to have a smear, has the responsibility to inform the woman of the result and, if necessary, to ensure she is followed up correctly. This means that the smear-taker and cytology laboratory must be in regular communication. If referral is necessary, the smear-taker will also need to communicate with the gynaecologist regarding appropriate management and counselling of the woman concerned.

The general practitioners and nurses who undertake cervical screening are a vital part of a screening programme. The strong relationship between women and their general practitioners can be used to the benefit of the screening programme to increase uptake. The quality of the general practitioners' and nurses' input into the screening programme will be improved if they are provided with appropriate feedback on coverage, quality of smears taken, results of smears and results of referrals.

This feedback can be accomplished by paper reports, although electronic links are being increasingly used. The essential features remain considering the general practitioner and nurse as part of the screening team and building relationships between the primary care part of the team and the cytology laboratory and gynaecologists in the hospitals.

## References

1 Cullum DE, Savory JN. Patient preferences for cervical cytology. *BMJ* 1983; **287**: 329–330.
2 Eardley A, Elkind AK, Thompson R. Health Education Authority guidelines for a letter to invite women for a smear test: theory and practice. *Health Ed J* 1990; **49**: 51–56.
3 Nathoo V. Investigation of non-responders at a cervical screening clinic in Manchester. *BMJ* 1988; **296**: 1041–1042.
4 Atkin K, Lunt N, Parker G *et al*. *A National Census of Practice Nurses*. University of York: Social Policy Research Unit, 1993.
5 Majeed F, Cook D, Anderson H *et al*. Using patient and general practice characteristics to explain variations in cervical smear uptake rates. *BMJ* 1994; **308**: 1272–1276.
6 Pritchard J (ed.) Quality Assurance Guidelines for the Cervical Screening Programme. NHSCSP publication no. 3. Sheffield: NHSCSP, 1996.

# 21: Screening Programmes: Results and Expectations

## I. D. Duncan

## Introduction

The main objective of any cervical screening programme is the prevention of deaths from cervical cancer. A woman undergoing screening in the private sector may decide that excluding cervical disease is so important to her that she is willing to pay for every conceivable test to give her that reassurance. It may be that she is extremely wealthy or it may be that she considers going without other items of expenditure perfectly acceptable as long as she can be completely reassured that she does not have cervical disease. Screening programmes, however, are different. In most instances these are national and, although the private sector may be involved, it is the public purse that is the main resource. This resource is finite and there are many health issues completing for it. Public health cervical screening programmes are based, therefore, on cytology alone.

The success of these programmes depends upon several things. First, compliance – only those patients who participate in the programme can benefit  from it and the fall in national figures for cervical cancer mortality depends upon general acceptance by the population at risk. In England and Wales it is only since 1993 that this percentage has exceeded 80% and this is now reflected in a significant fall in the national mortality [1].

Identification of the population to be screened is fundamentally important. Everyone would agree that it is wasteful to screen women who are not at risk. In this respect different countries have decided upon different age groups. In addition, the screening interval should reflect what is known about the development of the disease and minimize interval cancers – the development

*Correspondence*: Dr I. D. Duncan, Department of Obstetrics and Gynaecology, Ninewells Hospital, Dundee DDI 95Y, UK.

of a cancer in a woman after a truly negative test before the next test is due. The working group of the International Agency for Research on Cancer studied screening programmes in eight different countries [2]. The data came from areas with centralized cervical cytology screening programmes where most smears pass through one laboratory; areas with a centralized programme that was responsible for only a fraction of the screening; areas where screening was not centrally organized but where all smears were evaluated by a single central laboratory; and areas where most screening was performed in private practice with several cytopathology laboratories responsible for cytological evaluation so that screening histories had to be obtained from many sources [2]. Assuming 100% compliance, they estimated figures for a percentage reduction in incidence ranging from 70% to 93%. The former figure could be expected if women aged 35–64 were screened every 5 years and the latter figure if women aged 20–64 were screened every year. The number of tests required in the former group would be six and in the latter group 45 – a huge difference in resource requirements. They concluded that screening programmes should be aimed principally at women aged 35–60 but should start some years before the age of 35 and the intervals between screening should be 3 years or less. We have recently shown that cervical intraepithelial neoplasia (CIN) typically occurs in younger women. Women over 50 with an adequate history of negative results on smear testing every 3 years are highly unlikely to develop CIN and could probably be safely discharged from further screening [3].

CIN of course is the potential progenitor of squamous cervical cancer. The latent phase is usually prolonged, allowing detection and eradication of the premalignant disease. Thus countries with well-established programmes have been able to demonstrate a reduction in mortality from squamous cervical cancer. Unfortunately, the same cannot be said for adenocarcinoma or adeno-squamous carcinomas, which now constitute a much larger proportion of cervical cancers, especially in younger women. Their aetiology may be similar. Adenocarcinoma-*in-situ*, when found, commonly coexists with CIN. The propensity for malignant transformation of adenocarcinoma-*in-situ* is not known but when it does happen the latent phase is probably much shorter than for CIN and the resulting malignancy is also more likely to spread rapidly. Two recent population studies have found no effects of cervical screening on the incidence or mortality from adenocarcinoma of the cervix [4,5].

The sensitivity and specificity of cervical screening are clearly important. In attempting to increase the sensitivity the specificity is lost and a major problem facing developed countries now is the large number of women whose smears have not been regarded as normal. Most of these women are not at risk of developing cervical cancer and do not have premalignant disease. Valuable resources, however, are used in investigating such women, probably unneces-sarily. This represents the negative side of screening programmes and almost certainly additional tests other than cytology will be necessary to help distinguish those women who are truly at risk.

False negatives will undoubtedly occur with cervical cytology. A small percentage is unavoidable but can prove expensive in medicolegal terms and disruptive to the service. Recently the issue of quality assurance in cervical screening has been addressed and the publication of guidelines and expected standards has followed in the UK [6–9].

The challenge for the developed countries as we approach the new millennium is to improve the specificity of cervical screening. In developing countries where 90% of the world's cervical cancer occurs the problem may be entirely different. Cervical screening may not be a practical proposition for the population at large and a reduction in mortality may depend upon alternative measures, including education of the population to signs and symptoms, and downstaging.

## References

1 Sasieni P, Cusick J, Farmery E. Accelerated decline in cervical cancer mortality in England and Wales. *Lancet* 1995; **346**: 1566–1567.

2 IARC Working Group on Evaluation of Cervical Cancer Screening Programme. Screening for squamous cervical cancer; duration of low risk after negative cervical cytology and its implication for screening policies. *BMJ* 1986; **293**: 659–664.

3 Van Wijngaarden WJ, Duncan ID. Rationale for stopping cervical screening in women over 50. *BMJ* 1993; **306**: 967–971.

4 Van Wijngaarden WJ, Duncan ID, Hussain KA. Screening for cervical neoplasia in Dundee and Angus: 10 years on. *Br J Obst Gynaecol* 1995; **102**: 137–142.

5 Sigurdsson K. Quality assurance in cervical cancer screening: the Icelandic experience 1964–1993; *Eur J Cancer* 1995; **31**: 728–734.

6 Duncan ID. (ed) *Guidelines for Clinical Practice and Programme Management*. Oxford: NHSCSP, 1992.

7 Herbert A. (ed) *Achievable Standards, Benchmarks for Reporting and Criteria for Evaluating Cytopathology*. Sheffield: NHSCSP, 1995.

8 Pritchard J. (ed) *Quality Assurance Guidelines for the Cervical Screening Programme*. Sheffield: NHSCSP, 1996.

9 Luesley D. (ed) *Standards and Quality in Colposcopy*. Sheffield: NHSCSP, 1996.

# 22: Screening for Cervical Cancer: Experience of the Nordic Countries

## M. Hakama

## Benefits and dangers of screening

Screening for cancer consists of the identification of preclinical disease by a relatively simple test. The objective of screening is to reduce the risk of death, i.e. mortality from cancer subjected to screening. For cervical cancer the screening test is aimed at detection of preinvasive lesions. Therefore, reduction in the incidence of invasive disease is the objective of screening for cervical cancer, and the indicator for the effect is change of incidence in time before and after application of the screening test or difference of incidence between those subjected to screening and those not subjected to screening.

Screening may have benefits other than an effect on incidence. If the treatment of disease detected at screening is less invasive, less radical or results in less morbidity than that of clinically detected disease, the quality of life of the screened population is improved. Correct negative results also have a beneficial effect in that they reassure people without the disease.

Because the aim of screening is to provide a preinvasive diagnosis of disease, there is a prolonged period of morbidity — from the time of diagnosis at screening to the hypothetical time at which a clinical diagnosis would have been made had the patient not been screened. This lead-time, while a prerequisite of effective screening, is an adverse effect because of the prolongation of anxiety and morbidity due to diagnosis and treatment of cancer.

Cases detected at screening are confirmed by standard clinical diagnostic methods. Many such cases are borderline abnormalities, some of which would progress to clinical disease and some of which would not, even if left untreated.

*Correspondence*: Dr Matti Hakama, School of Public Health, University of Tampere, Box 607, 33101 Tampere and Finnish Cancer Registry, Liisankatu 21B, 00170 Helsinki, Finland.

The diagnosis of carcinoma-*in-situ* and severe dysplasia results in an invasive treatment. A proportion of these lesions would have not progressed to clinical disease during the woman's lifespan. Any screening programme will disclose such abnormalities, which are indistinguishable from truly abnormal cases which will progress into the clinical phase in the absence of early treatment. One of the adverse effects of screening is therefore the consequent treatment of patients with such lesions. This results in anxiety and morbidity. Also false-positive screening results cause anxiety and sometimes morbidity, even if later confirmed to be benign. Conversely, a false-negative result is falsely reassuring. If it results in postponement of clinical diagnosis and worsens the outcome of treatment, screening is disadvantageous.

## Organizing a screening programme

Screening is public health policy, and the success of the whole programme must be assessed. The validity of the programme depends on the screening test used, attendance, the screening interval and the success of referral for diagnostic confirmation of cases found at screening.

An International Union against Cancer (UICC) workshop on screening for cervical cancer [1] presented statements on the organizational aspects of screening programmes which have since then resulted in several modifications. It was emphasized that, to be effective, screening should be organized according to an agreed policy. Circumstances vary in different countries, and it should not be assumed that a format suitable for one country applies to another without first testing and evaluating it with a sufficiently rigorous design. It seems, however, that many of the successful programmes have some essential elements in common:

1   The target population is identified.
2   Individuals are identifiable.
3   Measures are available to guarantee high coverage and attendance, such as a personal letter of invitation.
4   There are adequate field facilities for collecting the screen material and adequate laboratory facilities to examine it.
5   Adequate facilities exist for diagnosis and for appropriate treatment of confirmed disease or defect and for the follow-up of treated individuals.
6   There is a carefully designed and agreed-upon referral system. An agreed link exists between the patient, the laboratory, and the clinical facility for diagnosis of an abnormal screening test, for management of any abnormality found, and for providing information about normal screening tests.
7   Evaluation and monitoring of the total programme are organized in terms of incidence and mortality rates among those attending, and among those not attending, at the level of total target population.

Many of the successful programmes operate nationwide and are population-based. Individuals need to be identified to improve attendance and to evaluate the effect. Personal letters of invitation with details of time and place of screening have been used, e.g. the Finnish and Swedish screening programmes for cervical cancer. This resulted in 70–80% attendance [2]. In, Denmark, personal invitations were issued to a proportion of the population and this was shown to increase the rate of attendance considerably [3].

Much of the information on the applicability of screening for cervical cancer as a public health policy stems from the organized programmes practised in the Nordic countries since the mid-1960s [4]. Most of the Nordic countries have nationwide screening programmes for cervical cancer which fulfil the general prerequisities of an organized programme and make it possible to follow up each woman for the occurrence of cervical intraepithelial neoplasia (CIN) and for cervical cancer.

Selective screening in a community means applying the screening test to only a subpopulation in that community. The criteria for selection are based on high risk of the disease among those subjected to screening. The purpose of screening high-risk groups only is to reduce the resources required for the programme or, sometimes, to reduce the number of those at risk to the adverse effects of the screening test. A selective screening programme should detect a substantial proportion of the total number of cancer cases in the entire target population, i.e. only a few cancer cases are assumed to originate in the low-risk groups not subjected to such selective screening.

So far, selective screening based on high-risk populations defined by aetiological risk factors has failed. This is true for the approaches based on a single risk factor, as well as those based on a combination of several of them. Several attempts have used risk factors characterizing different aspects of the aetiology of a specific cancer. In such cases, programme sensitivity was low, i.e. a substantial proportion of the cancer cases diagnosed in the total target population originated in the low-risk group not subjected to screening. The present methods of selective screening for cancer based on risk factors are not likely to be sufficiently effective to be applied in public health programmes. If the efficiency and effectiveness of an established programme are to be increased, improvements are likely to come from improving the organization, attendance rate and quality of the test rather than from limiting the activities to high-risk groups only.

Improving the screening programmes by human papillomavirus (HPV) testing is a topical issue at present and is related to selective screening. Because not all the cancers are due to HPV infection and because HPV infection does not always result in occurrence of cancer, a programme based on HPV testing only will face the same problems as selective screening in general. The sensitivity will remain low. Also there may not be a reduction in cost because of the cost of the test and the need to test for HPV-positivity in all the target population.

## Effectiveness

The effectiveness of screening for cervical cancer in terms of reduced incidence has never been demonstrated in a randomized preventive trial. There is, however, non-experimental evidence of a reduction in incidence of invasive disease. Canada was the pioneer in screening for cervical cancer [5,6]. The largest of the studies on effectiveness is the collaborative study coordinated by the International Agency for Research on Cancer [7], which showed that eradication of the disease is an unrealistic goal and that maximal protection after a negative smear is about 90%, which remains roughly the same for several years after the test (Table 22.1). This conclusion is in accordance with the results of studies on the natural history of the disease, which have shown that most preinvasive lesions progress to frankly invasive cancer over several years.

In the Nordic countries there are differences in cervical cancer screening policies within the organized programmes. In Finland [4], Iceland [8] and Sweden [9], a nationwide population-based organized programme has been in operation at least since the early 1970s, whereas only a few counties in Denmark, including the most populous ones, had organized screening programmes [10,11]. The programmes are run by voluntary cancer organizations in Finland and Iceland, and by the counties in Denmark and Sweden. The recommended age groups to be covered were originally 30–55 years in Finland (later the programme was extended up to 60 years), 25–69 years in Iceland, and 30–49 years in Sweden. The screening intervals recommended are 2–3 years in Iceland, 4 years in Sweden and 5 years in Finland. In Denmark the practice varies by county, but the National Board of Health recommendation is to have a smear every 3 years from the age of 23 to 59 and every 5 years from 60 to 75. In Norway [12,13] only 5% of the population was covered by an organized programme. Cytological smears are, however, frequently taken outside the organized system, by private gynaecologists and elsewhere. Such

**Table 22.1** International Agency for Research on Cancer (IARC) collaborative study. Reduction of incidence of invasive cervical cancer after a negative smear by interval between the screens and age.

| | Screening interval | | | |
| | Reduction in incidence (%) | | Number of life-time smears | |
| Age (years) | 3 years | 5 years | 3 years | 5 years |
| --- | --- | --- | --- | --- |
| 20–64 | 91 | 84 | 15 | 9 |
| 25–64 | 90 | 82 | 13 | 8 |
| 30–64 | 85 | 77 | 12 | 7 |
| 35–64 | 78 | 70 | 10 | 6 |

Data from Day [7] and IARC working group [18].

smears are taken more often than the smears in the organized programmes in all the Nordic countries, with the exception of Iceland.

In the Nordic countries about 2500 new cases of cervical cancer were diagnosed annually before the screening programmes were initiated. Since the early 1980s the annual number of new cases has been about 1700. Denmark had a high incidence, in the early period. The age-adjusted (world standard) incidence was about 30 per $10^5$ woman-years, whereas in the other Nordic countries it was about 15, with somewhat increasing trends before the screening programmes started. In the early 1980s the rates ranged from 15 (Denmark) to 5 (Finland) [14].

There was a strong correlation between the extent of the organized screening programme and changes in the incidence of invasive cervical cancer (Table 22.2). The relative reduction in the risk was steepest in Finland and Sweden, and intermediate in Denmark. In Norway the incidence rates of cervical cancer increased up to the 1970s. During the 15-year period from 1966–1970 to 1981–1985, the incidence rates fell by 65% in Finland and 20% in Norway. The substantial decrease in incidence from the 1960s to 1970s in Iceland is partly because the prevalent microinvasive lesions were diagnosed during the first round of screening in the late 1960s more frequently than in the other Nordic countries. The rates in Iceland are subject to large random variation owing to the small population and relatively few cases of cancer.

The most substantial reduction in the risk of cervical cancer occurred in the age group 40–49 years [15], which probably came under the most intensive screening by the organized programme. Again, the reduction was highest in Finland (80%) and lowest in Norway (50%). The rates were somewhat increasing at young ages, sharply decreasing for the middle-aged and relatively stable for the elderly. The rates for women in Iceland were unstable owing to the small numbers.

**Table 22.2** Observed annual age-adjusted incidence rates (per 100 000 woman-years) of invasive cervical cancer in the Nordic countries in selected time periods.

| | Observed | | | | Predicted | |
|---|---|---|---|---|---|---|
| Country | 1956–1960 | 1966–1970 | 1976–1980 | 1983–1987 | 1998–2002 | 2008–2012 |
| Denmark | 30 | 30 | 19 | 16 | 11 | 11 |
| Finland | 14 | 14 | 6 | 4 | 2 | 2 |
| Iceland | 16 | 26 | 9 | 13 | 10 | 9 |
| Norway | 15 | 17 | 17 | 13 | 9 | 8 |
| Sweden | 18 | 18 | 10 | 9 | 7 | 7 |

Data from the Nordic Cancer Registries [14,15].

The mortality was shown to follow closely the incidence trends in the Nordic countries [2]. The estimates for deaths from cervical cancers prevented (Table 22.3) are also substantial. Compared to the hypothetical no-screening option, there was an estimate of 91% of reduction in the risk of death due to screening by year 2015 if applied as in Finland [16].

It seems that the differences in trends cannot be accounted for by the biology of the disease but the most significant determinant of risk reduction is how well the programme is organized. A comparison of the Nordic countries shows very little relation between the interval between the screening rounds and reduction of risk, or very little relation between the target age range and reduction of risk. This provides the confirmation of the estimate of the IARC Working Group [7,17,18] on the basis of several large-scale screening programmes, that the protective effect of screening is high for screening intervals up to 5 years and for lower age limits up to 30 years. Organized programmes, in contrast to opportunistic ones, promote adequate quality control [19] and high attendance (e.g. by personal letters of invitation and of response). High coverage and attendance seem to be the single most important determinant of a successful screening. Opportunistic screening has problems in catching those who would benefit the screening most from screening. Recently, Gustafsson *et al.* [20] suggested a more optimistic view of the efficiency of opportunistic screening. The conclusion was based on detection rates of carcinoma-*in-situ* in Sweden, not on the incidence of invasive disease. Such an analysis will not provide evidence for opportunistic screening. In Finland it was confirmed by a case-control study on invasive cancer at individual level, that the effectiveness was better for organized screening than for the spontaneous smear-taking activity [21].

**Table 22.3** Predicted numbers of deaths from cervical cancer in 1995 and 2015 in the Nordic countries assuming no screening (without) and the screening programme as practised in Finland (with).

| | Year | | | |
|---|---|---|---|---|
| | 1995 | | 2015 | |
| Country | Without | With | Without | With |
| Denmark | 530 | 90 | 530 | 40 |
| Finland | 290 | 70 | 310 | 30 |
| Iceland | 10 | 1 | 10 | 1 |
| Norway | 250 | 50 | 260 | 20 |
| Sweden | 470 | 100 | 480 | 40 |
| Nordic | 1550 | 310 | 1590 | 130 |

From Hristova and Hakama [16].

## Cost

In spite of coverage of the total target population, screening for cervical cancer can be relatively inexpensive: those programmes with the greatest effect have been low in cost. It seems that screening programmes, starting at the age of 25 or even at the age of 30, repeating the smears at 5-year intervals, and having the upper age limit of 60 years will practically provide maximal reduction in the risk of cervical cancer (Table 22.1). The programme assumes seven or eight smears during the woman's life-time. Such a programme favourably compares with those proposed to start at age 20 with annual smears, resulting in a total of 40 tests during the woman's lifespan.

Screening for cervical cancer is relatively inexpensive compared to the costs of screening for cancers of other primary sites. In fact, the costs of screening will be more than compensated for by savings due to more frequent treatment of early disease, compared to the treatment costs of cancers detected through normal practice without screening [22]. This is different from other screening modalities practised as a public health policy (Table 22.4).

## Equity

Equity is the third dimension, in addition to effect and cost, in the health services activities. Often there is a trade-off between effectiveness, efficiency and equity. Screening for cervical cancer is an exception. As pointed out, the effect in terms of reduction in risk is in practice inversely related to cost: programmes with a large reduction in risk are based on relatively few smears. The Finnish programme is an example of an effective programme with improvement in equity, measured by the outcome (reduction in risk) in different population groups. In the mid-1960s the risk was high in remote areas and in lower social classes. Some of the remote areas have benefited most [23] and at the same time the social class differences were reduced. In the early 1970s there was a relative risk of 2.6 between the lowest and highest social class, which was 1.7 at the

**Table 22.4** Costs of control for cervical breast and colorectal cancers in the year 2010, assuming organized screening programmes, compared to costs of control without screening in the Nordic countries.

| Primary site | Cost (US$ million) | | Difference |
|---|---|---|---|
| | With screening | Without screening | |
| Cervix | 45 | 62 | −17 |
| Breast | 154 | 88 | +66 |
| Colorectum | 211 | 156 | +62 |

From Hristova and Hakama [16].

**Table 22.5** Age-adjusted incidence rates (per 100 000 woman-years) of invasive cervical cancer among Finnish women 35–64 years old in 1971–1975 and 1981–1985 by social class (I = highest, IV = lowest).

| Period | Social class | | | |
|--------|:---:|:---:|:---:|:---:|
|        | I | II | III | IV |
| 1971–1975 | 11 | 19 | 22 | 28 |
| 1981–1985 | 8 | 8 | 9 | 14 |

From Pukkala [29].

beginning of 1980s. The differences in risk between social classes had disappeared, except in the lowest class which was still a higher risk than the others (Table 22.5).

## Conclusion

Screening for cervical cancer reduces the incidence of invasive disease and is applicable as a public health policy, but a wide variation is seen, from highly effective programmes to relatively poor ones.

While the effectiveness of screening for cervical cancer can be relatively reliably evaluated, some of the adverse effects are more problematic. First, there are lesions fulfilling histological criteria of malignancy but without the malignant potential to kill the woman during her life-time, resulting in overdiagnosis and sometimes overtreatment. The frequency of such lesions depends on the transition probabilities from dysplasia to carcinoma-*in-situ* and from carcinoma-*in-situ* to invasive disease. The transition probabilities are a reflection more of the local diagnostic practices than of any general biological phenomena. In Finland, the diagnostic standard adopted results in CIN III lesions, of which one in three would have progressed to invasive disease if left untreated [24]. In Sweden, the transition probability is substantially smaller, and in several years the annual number of carcinoma-*in-situ* lesions was about five times the number of invasive cancers before screening [25].

Second, the quality of life effects are poorly known and research is rare. Often the women who attend screening do so to be reassured [26] rather than to reduce the risk of death – the women attend because of quality-of-life reasons. Important research on anxiety caused by invitation, false- or true-positive tests and other quality-of-life aspects have been and currently are being conducted, especially in the UK [27,28].

To screen or not to screen for cervical cancer does not depend on poor information on biological effects or on organizational aspects. The decision depends on balancing the effect on the length of life (which is relatively well known and easy to establish), on the quality of life (which is poorly known and difficult to measure) and on the cost (which again, is relatively easy to measure, but relatively poorly known). It is likely that experts give greater value or weight to the length of life; women value the quality of life; while those responsible for administration are cost-conscious. Therefore, the decision to establish and continue screening programmes depends not only on the factual evidence available, but also on those whose value of the benefits, harms and costs prevail.

## References

1 Hakama M, Miller AB, Day NE. (eds) *Screening for Cancer of the Uterine Cervix*. Lyon: IARC, 1986.
2 Läärä E, Day N, Hakama M. Trends in mortality from cervical cancer in the Nordic countries: association with organized screening programmes. *Lancet* 1987; **i**: 1247–1249.
3 Lynge E. Screening for cancer of the cervix uteri. *World J Surg* 1989; **13**: 71–78.
4 Hakama M, Magnus K, Pettersson F, Storm H, Tulinius H. Effect of organized screening on the risk of cervical cancer in the Nordic countries. In: Miller A, Chamberlain J, Day N, Hakama M, Prorok P (eds) *Cancer Screening*. Cambridge: Cambridge University Press, 1991; pp 153–162.
5 Fidler HK, Boyes DA, Worth AJ. Cervix cancer detection in British Columbia. *J Obstet Gynaecol Br Commonw* 1968; **75**: 392–404.
6 Miller AB, Knight J, Narod S. The natural history of cancer of the cervix, and the implications for screening policy. In: Miller AB, Chamberlain J, Day NE, Hakama M, Prorok PC (eds) *Cancer Screening. UICC Project on Evaluation of Screening for Cancer*. Cambridge: International Union Against Cancer, 1991; pp 141–152.
7 Day NE. The epidemiological basis for evaluating different screening policies. In: Hakama M, Miller AB, Day NE (eds) *Screening for Cancer of the Uterine Cervix*. Lyon: IARC, 1986; pp 199–212.
8 Johannesson GE, Geirsson G, Day N, Tulinius H. Screening for cancer of the uterine cervix in Iceland 1965–1978. *Acta Obstet Gynecol Scand* 1982; **61**: 199–203.
9 Petterson F, Björkholm E, Näslund I. Evaluation of screening for cervical cancer in Sweden: trends in incidence and mortality 1958–1980. *Int J Epidemiol* 1985; **14**: 521–527.
10 Lynge E. Regional trends in incidence of cervical cancer in Denmark in relation to local smear-taking activity. *Int J Epidemiol* 1983; **12**: 405–413.
11 Lynge E, Madsen M, Engholm G. Effect of organized screening on incidence and mortality of cervical cancer in Denmark. *Cancer Res* 1989; **49**: 2157–2160.
12 Pedersen E, Hoeg K, Kolstad P. Mass screening for cancer of the uterine cervix in Østfold county, Norway: an experiment. Second report of the Norwegian Cancer Society. *Acta Obstet Gynecol Scand* 1971; **50**(suppl 11): 1–18.
13 Magnus K, Langmark F, Andersen A. Mass screening for cervical cancer in Østfold county of Norway 1959–1977. *Int J Cancer* 1987; **39**: 311–316.
14 Engeland A, Haldorsen T, Tretli S *et al*. Prediction of cancer incidence in the Nordic countries up to the years 2000 and 2010. *Acta Pathol Microbiol Immunol Scand* 1993; **101** (suppl 38): 1–124.
15 Hakulinen T, Andersen A, Malker B, Pukkala E, Schou G, Tulinius H. Trends in cancer incidence in the Nordic countries. *Acta Pathol Microbiol Immunol Scand Sect A* 1986; **94**: (suppl 288): 1–151.

16 Hristova L, Hakama M. Effect of screening for cancer in the Nordic countries on death costs and quality of life up to 2017. Accepted for publication as supplement for *Acta Oncologica* 1997; **36**(suppl. 9): 1–60.

17 IARC Working Group on Evaluation of Cervical Cancer Screening Programmes. Screening for squamous cervical cancer: the duration of low risk after negative result of cervical cytology and its implication for screening policies. *BMJ* 1986; **293**: 659–664.

18 IARC Working Group on Cervical Cancer Screening. Summary chapter. In: Hakama M, Miller AB, Day NE (eds) *Screening for Cancer of the Uterine Cervix*. Lyon: IARC, 1986; pp 133–142.

19 Sigurdsson K. Quality assurance in cervical cancer screening: the Icelandic experience 1964–1993. *Eur J Cancer* 1995; **31A**: 728–734.

20 Gustafsson L, Sparén P, Gustafsson M, Wilander E, Bergström R, Adami HO. Efficency of organised and opportunistic cytological screening for cancer *in situ* of the cervix. *Br J Cancer* 1995; **72**: 498–505.

21 Nieminen P, Kallio M, Hakama M. Effectiveness of the organized and spontaneous screening for cervical cancer. 1997. Submitted.

22 Hristova L. Effect of screening for cancer on mortality, costs and quality of life in Finland. Acta Univesitatis Tamperensis, ser A vol. 456, Tampere: University of Tampere 1995.

23 Hakama M, Kallio M, Pukkala E. Kohdunkaulan syövän seulonnat – vaikuttavia tai oikeudenmukaisia? *Suom Lääkäril* 1995; **50**: 2527–2533.

24 Hakama M, Räsänen-Virtanen U. Effect of a mass screening program on the risk of cervical cancer. *Am J Epidemiol* 1976; **103**: 512–517.

25 Sveriges Officiella Statistik. Gynekologisk hälsoundersökning 1967–1973. Statistiska meddelanden HS, 1, 1976.

26 Kauppinen M, Kauraniemi T, Koli T, Voipio N. Response to the written invitation in a gynaecological mass screening by cytology arranged in Helsinki in 1966. *Acta Obstet Gynaecol Scand* 1970; **49** (suppl 7): 1–20.

27 Campion MJ, Brown JR, McCance DJ *et al*. Psychosexual trauma of an abnormal cervical smear. *Br J Obstet Gynaecol* 1988; **95**: 175–181.

28 Posner T, Vessey M. *Prevention of Cervical Cancer. The Patient's View*. London: King's Fund Publishing Office, 1988.

29 Pukkala E. *Cancer Risk by Social Class and Occupation. A Survey of 109 000 Cancer Cases among Finns of Working Age*. Basel: Karger, 1995.

# 23: Screening that Failed to Work

## J. Patnick

Cervical smears were available in most parts of the UK from the mid-1960s. However, while in north-east Scotland this was well organized from the outset [1] with enviable results [2] in most of the UK smears were taken opportunistically. They were taken mainly from young women with a short interval between examinations due to their attendance for family planning and obstetric care. Older women and women in the lower socioeconomic groups were frequently missed out altogether by this sytem. These were, of course, the very women at greatest risk of developing and dying from invasive cervical cancer.

Draper [3] in 1982 showed that UK incidence had not fallen with this system. Beral and Booth [4] writing in 1986 predicted increasing incidence rates, particularly in young women, although mortality rates in older women were falling [5].

Jocelyn Chamberlain [6] identified the following as characteristics of failing cervical screening programmes in order of importance:

1   Failure to reach the women at risk.
2   Inadequate follow-up of abnormal smears.
3   Long screening interval (more than 5 years).
4   False-negative smear results.

In the early 1980s it seemed that the British screening programme suffered from all of these.

The Imperial Cancer Research Fund in 1984 [7] had called for the institution of a computerized call-and-recall system to identify and invite the wider female population as a whole. They followed this in 1986 [8] with a statement recommending further wide-ranging changes, including the estab-

*Correspondence*: Mrs Julietta Patnick, National Co-ordinator, NHS National Screening Programme, The Manor House, 260 Ecclesall Road South, Sheffield S11 9PS, UK.

lishment of a national coordination office to bring some coherence to the programme and a repeat of the call for a computerized population database.

In 1987 the Royal Colleges concerned produced a combined report on cervical screening [9] and also that year there was a major scandal involving false-negative results in a laboratory in one of our teaching hospitals. A head of steam had built up and action was taken.

Computerized call-and-recall systems were required to operate in each district by April 1988, with a recall interval of not more than 5 years. Coverage of the target population began to climb from 22% reported in 1988 to 83% by 1993 [10]. In 1990 target payments were introduced to encourage general practitioners to reach 80% coverage and financial penalties if they reached the lower 50% target or even less. This is felt to have had a major impact on coverage of the population.

The objective set in 1988 by the Department of Health was to reduce mortality [11]. Sasieni *et al.* [12] reported in 1995 that the slow decrease in mortality seen in older women had now accelerated from 1–2% per annum to around 7% per annum. In addition, the death rate in younger women was also falling. It was argued that this fall in mortality was attributable to the major increase in screening programme coverage described above.

Incidence, which is the current target [13], however, refuses to demonstrate a fall. It may be that the lead-time since the start of organized screening is as yet insufficient for a fall in incidence to be demonstrated. This may take 10 years from the start of organized screening. However, a 1992 audit [14] of smear histories of women with and without cervical cancer estimated that without the cervical screening programme the number of cases in women under the age of 70 would have been approximately 75% higher. Of those under 70 with a fully invasive cancer, 41% had no smear recorded more than 6 months before diagnosis.

There remained problems with follow-up of abnormal smears. Thirteen per cent of all patients under 70 had smear histories which indicated inadequate follow-up. Guidelines were published in 1992 [15] for clinical aspects of management of the programme and these have been followed recently by a set of quality assurance guidelines [16–18] to address continuing issues. These guidelines have been produced under the aegis of the new national coordination office for the National Health Service Cervical Screening Programme which has an ongoing remit to keep professional guidance under review.

Now the UK is moving from focusing on coverage, which is no longer the problem it was, to a focus on quality assurance. This will embrace the entire programme, from recruitment to treatment of cervical intraepithelial neoplasia and follow-up.

The computerized call-and-recall system, together with a general practitioner target payments system working on a maximum interval of 5.5 years, addresses the problem of a long screening interval. In fact, 67% of women in England aged 25–64 have had a smear within the last 3 years [19]. The problem of false-negative smears will never disappear, but with the establishment in the UK of the quality assurance initiative and national coordination, it should be minimized.

The four issues identified by Chamberlain [6] have each been addressed in turn. The UK screening programme is now working effectively. Mortality is already falling and incidence is confidently expected to follow suit shortly. The value of the application of organization and clear quality standards to the system which existed in the mid-1980s has been clearly shown.

## References

1 MacGregor JE, Baird D. Detection of cervical carcinoma in the general population. *BMJ* 1963; i: 1631–1636.
2 MacGregor JE, Moss S, Parkin DM, Day NE. Cervical cancer screening in north east Scotland. In: Hakama M, Miller AB, Day NE (eds) *Screening for Cancer of the Uterine Cervix*. IARC scientific publication no. 76. Lyon: IARC, 1986.
3 Draper G. Screening for cervical cancer: revised policy. *Health Trends* 1982; **14**: 37–40.
4 Beral V, Booth M. Predictions of cervical cancer incidence and mortality in England and Wales. *Lancet* 1986; i: 495.
5 Sasieni P. Trends in cervical smear mortality. *Lancet* 1991; **338**: 818.
6 Chamberlain J. Reasons that some screening programmes fail to control cervical cancer. In: Hakama M, Miller AB, Day NE (eds). *Screening for Cancer of the Uterine Cervix*. IARC scientific publication no. 76. Lyon: IARC, 1986.
7 ICRF. Organisation of a programme for cervical cancer screening. *BMJ* 1994; **289**: 894–895.
8 ICRF. The management of cervical screening programme: a statement. *Commun Med* 1986; **8**: 179–184.
9 Sharp F, Duncan ID, Evans DMO *et al*. Report of the intercollegiate working party on cervical cytology screening. London: Royal College of Obstetricians and Gynaecologists, 1987.
10 Farmery E, Gray JAM. Report of the first 5 years of the NHS cervical screening programme. Oxford: NCN, 1994.
11 Health Services Management. *Cervical Cancer Screening*. HC(88)1. London: Department of Health, 1988.
12 Sasieni P, Cuzick J, Farmery E. Accelerated decline in cervical cancer mortality in England and Wales. *Lancet* 1995; **346**: 1566–1567.
13 Department of Health. *Health of the Nation*. London: HMSO, 1992.
14 Sasieni P, Cuzick J, Farmery E. Estimating the efficacy of screening by auditing similar histories of women with and without cervical cancer. *Br J Cancer* 1996; **73**: 1001–1005.
15 Duncan ID. (ed) *Guidelines for Clinical Practice and Programme Management*. Oxford: NCN, 1992.
16 Herbert A, Johnson J, Patnick J *et al*. *Achievable Standards, Benchmarks for Reporting and Criteria for Evaluating Cervical Cytopathology*. Sheffield: NHSCSP, 1995.
17 Luesley D. (ed) *Standards and Quality in Colposcopy*. Sheffield: NHSCSP, 1996.
18 Pritchard J (ed.) *Quality Assurance Guidelines for the Cervical Screening Programme*. Sheffield: NHSCSP, 1996.
19 Cervical Screening Programme, England 1994–95. *Statistical Bulletin*. London: Department of Health, 1996.

# 24: Implementation and Evaluation of Cervical Cancer Screening Programmes in the European Union

## C. J. M. de Wolf

## Introduction

In most European member states, the early detection of cervical cancer is fundamental to the provision of health care and, depending on each health system, performed by the general practitioner, the gynaecologist or trained nurse. The smear-taking is often not performed within an organized and structured screening programme but performed on request. The public is highly aware of early detection methods for cervical cancer, such as Papanicolaou (Pap) smear.

If the low mortality rate of cervical cancer in Europe ($\pm 43/100\,000$ (IARC 1993) [1]) is seen as a performance parameter, this might suggest that this early detection service is adequately performed. However, a low cervical cancer mortality is not only due to early detection techniques but also to the service given within the curative health system. Moreover, a low mortality rate does not indicate that the service is efficiently performed, nor does it indicate the quality of the smear-taking, reading of the smears and adequate assessment of the patient. These performance parameters and cost-effectiveness evaluations are of prime importance for any policy decision on the implementation of a systematic cervical screening programme.

The European Commission has a task to develop acceptable and comparable quality parameters for the outcome measurement and programme evaluation of cervical cancer. In 1992, the European Commission issued a set of recommendations on cervix uteri cancer screening drafted by its committee of cancer experts. This committee recommends a set of criteria to be respected by any project intending to implement a cervical cancer screening programme. You will find these recommendations in the appendix to this chapter. These

*Correspondence*: Dr C. J. M. de Wolf, European Commission, DG V F.2 EUFO 3159, Plateau de Kirchberg, L-2920 Luxembourg.

recommendations have been followed by a document called European guidelines on quality assurance for cervical cancer screening [2], published as a supplement to the *European Journal of Cancer* in 1993.

The guidelines emphasize that no screening programme should be undertaken without clearly established goals, dedicated staff training and a proper quality assurance (QA) programme.

A QA programme for cervical cancer screening should be considered under headings relating to all elements in the programme, from the identification of the population to be screened to the evaluation and identification of screen-detected abnormalities. Ideally, a comprehensive QA programme in cervical cancer screening should also take into account an audit of treatment but, in the wide context of Europe, with all the variations involved, this is not seen as practical in the present instance.

In the first edition of the European guidelines for cervical cancer screening the following topics are addressed:

1 Organization of the screening programme, including the identification of the catchment area, definition of the target population, specification of the screening interval, integration of the screening programme into the health care system, resource implications, failsafe system, etc.

2 Screening methodologies: methods for collecting cervical smears, processing of smears and preparation of smear report.

3 Management of the patient with an abnormal cervical smear: failsafe measures, conditions for local destructive therapy, follow-up.

4 Monitoring the programme and use of resources: parameters for monitoring effectiveness and resource use in the short and long term and data-gathering requirements.

5 Training of participating personnel: smear-takers, cytotechnologists.

6 QA in the cytology laboratory: internal and external quality assurance.

The appendix gives details of tabulation of parameters and equivalent terminology used for cervical cytology reporting in the European Community.

To evaluate the effects of these guidelines, the European Commission supports in each member state a pilot project in cervical cancer screening which has adopted the European guidelines as a framework for its screening service.

These pilot projects were asked to become members of the European network of cervical cancer screening pilot projects, supporting the following aims:

1 To provide a forum for discussion of problems associated with cervical screening in individual member states and to assist with their solution by drawing on the collective experience of the members of the network.

2 To promote liaison between personnel involved in various aspects of cervical screening – smear-taking, laboratory processing, treatment, etc. and encourage exchange of ideas.

3   To provide an opportunity to introduce uniform quality standards in cervical screening throughout the European Union and to review current screening policies in the light of the European Guidelines for Quality Assurance [2].

4   To monitor quality standards in cervical cancer screening in the pilot projects.

5   To liaise with the Europe against Cancer screening committee and to make reports to them on selected aspects of cervical cancer screening pilot projects.

6   To identify those aspects of cervical cancer screening which could benefit from further research and advise the Europe against Cancer committee on them.

7   Gradually to improve the guidelines on quality assurance.

8   To disseminate the results of systematic screening on cervical cancer.

The network is at present in its initial period.

## Future possibilities and directions for cervical cancer interventions

The third action plan on cancer 1966–2000 of the European Community stated that priority would be given to support for the preparation and dissemination at a European level of a common terminology and classification in order to improve the quality of anatomical and cytopathological interpretation, particularly of suspect growths in the breast and cervix uteri, in particularly for anatomists and cytopathologists in the Community.

The priority action is one of the elements of the guidelines. Besides this terminology and classification issue, attention will be given to making cervical screening more cost-effective. This includes attendance on frequency for screening, adequate smear-taking, training of cytotechnologist, assessment procedures and follow-up to assessment and treatment. Most failures in these important areas of cervical screening are preventable.

The identified top-priority actions as well as documentation of the experiences and expertise within cervical screening settings in Europe, and the epidemiological evaluation of programme outcome based on universal collection of data and universal reporting of cervical lesions are the key to improving the quality of cervical cancer detection.

European cooperation to achieve these objectives is a clear example of Community-added value in the field of public health.

## References

1 IARC. *Facts and Figures of Cancer in the European Community*. International Agency for Research on Cancer, 1993.

2 Coleman D, Day N, Douglas G *et al.* Europe Against Cancer Programme. European guidelines for quality assurance in cervical cancer screening. *Eur J Cancer* 1993; Vol. 29A (suppl 4).

## Appendix: recommendations of the committee of cancer experts on cervix uteri cancer screening, 6 April 1992

The committee recommends that the following criteria be respected by any project intending to implement a cervical cancer screening programme.

### Effectiveness

The effectiveness of well-organized screening programmes in reducing morbidity and mortality from cervical cancer is now widely established. In successful programmes recruitment and recall to screening have been by personal invitation of women by means of population register and the quality of smear-taking, cytological examination and organization of follow-up have been monitored.

Screening by invitation should be promoted. Even where this is not available and screening is provided on the initiative of the patient or carried out opportunistically, the quality of screening should be monitored and controlled.

### Inequalities in risk and use of screening

Women of lower socioeconomic status are at higher risk of dying of cervical cancer, but make less use of screening services, especially if attendance requires individual initiative. Eforts must be directed at ensuring that all women, including those of lower socioeconomic status, are offered screening programmes.

### Target populations

Priority should be given at the start of a mass screening programme to the age group in which the incidence of invasive cervical is highest. In most populations this will be between 35 and 60 years. An optimal screening programme should aim at the population aged 25–65 years, thus aimed also at the preinvasive stages.

### Information and participation

The success of mass screening depends on achieving and maintaining a high level of participation. A high participation rate can be obtained by personal invitation. The public needs a basic understanding of the nature of this cancer, its causes and the purpose of screening. Women also need practical information about the screening service and where it is available. Back-up for a screening programme through dissemination of information by newspapers, television and leaflets in public buildings and hospitals is helpful.

## Screening text and training

Detailed information about the screening programme for health professionals, especially general practitioners, gynaecologists, pathologists and others who take smears is especially important so that they can advise patients.

The recommended method of screening is the Pap smear. The quality of smear-taking, as well as smear-reading, must be assured; organization of training programmes, proficiency testing and systems of quality control are needed. A uniform nomenclature for both cytology and histopathology between member states is recommended.

## Screening interval

In order to make best use of available screening resources, the interval between screening should be controlled. The additional benefit to be gained by screening more frequently than 3-yearly is very small. Screening every is 3–5 years is therefore generally recommended, depending on the resources available and the relative importance of the disease in the population.

## Follow-up of abnormal smears

Every screening programme should designate an individual responsible for its management. A detailed protocol for managing women with abnormal results should be drawn up for each programme. It should indicate what options are acceptable for the diagnostic investigation of screen-detected abnormalities and for their treatment follow-up. Ablative treatment should always be preceded by histological biopsy.

## Monitoring

Evaluation and appropriate adaptation of a screening programme depend on monitoring. For registration of samples and follow-up, person-based registers are of main importance. Comprehensive person-based records of invitation, screening attendance, screening results and follow-up provide the following advantages:

1  A failsafe mechanism for ensuring that abnormal smears are followed up can be incorporated.

**2**   Screening invitation can be regulated to ensure that the laboratories receive an even flow of work; too frequent screening can be discouraged and efforts concentrated on recruiting those who underutilized the service.

**3**   Cervical screenings should be evaluated as a means of reducing the incidence of invasive cancer.

**4**   False-negative smears can be reviewed; this provides a means for continuing self-education for cytology staff as well for monitoring quality.

### Exchange of information

Exchange of information between centres starting pilot projects is desirable. Areas of special interest are the success of different strategies for increasing participation in screening and assessment of cost-effectiveness. Studies of cost-effectiveness should take into account disadvantages, such as those of overtreatment, as well as the financial costs.

### Optimal use of resources

Screening of asymptomatic women every 3 years has proved to be an efficient means for reducing incidence and mortality from cervical cancer; on a population basis, the most efficient use of given resources is therefore achieved, if all women in the relevant age groups are offered screening every 3 years. Use of the public health care resources on annual screening should be avoided. To ensure that sufficient resources are available for 3-year population screening, both general practitioners and the public should be informed about the good results obtained at 3-year screening intervals for asymptomatic women.

# 25: Organization and Results of Cervical Cancer Screening in Europe Over the Past 20 Years

## C. J. M. de Wolf

Early detection of cervical cancer by the use of the Papanicolaou (Pap) smear test is common practice in all European countries. There is strong evidence that cervical cancer screening is able to reduce the incidence of and mortality from cervical cancer. The degree of this reduction is related to the organization of the provision of this service. An organized systematic screening programme offers the best possibility to achieve the reduction.

In most European countries the early detection of cervical cancer is fundamental to the provision of health care and, depending on each health system, performed by the general practitioner, the gynaecologist or trained nurse. The smear-taking is often not performed within an organized and structured screening programme.

There is a correlation between the level of organization and the reduction of cervical cancer. The organization incorporates all the screening process, from invitation to treatment and follow-up, as well integration in the existing health care system. The level of integration is determined by the limitations, legislation and restrictions of the health care system.

The experience of cervical screening of the last 20 years allows the identification of determinants and conditions for optimal organization of a (public health) screening programme. The expression of these conditions in a screening programme will determine the final result.

## Political level

1  Political support for a screening programme.
2  Long-term policy.
3  Supporting legislation.

*Correspondence*: Dr C. J. M. de Wolf, European Commission, DG V F.2 EUFO 3159, Plateau de Kirchberg, L-2920 Luxembourg.

**4** Structural financing not competing with the health care budget for cure and care.
**5** Accurate cancer and population registers.
**6** Quality-assured health care system.

## Screening level

**1** Existence of a quality assurance programme (including protocols, minimal/optimal targets, etc.).
**2** Central coordination.
**3** Call and recall system.
**4** Level of information of target population.
**5** Evaluation parameters.
**6** Audit of invasive cancer cases.

## Professional level

**1** Trained health professionals (mandatory).
**2** Accredited laboratories.
**3** Multidisciplinary follow-up of abnormalities.
The various levels of organization of the cervical screening programmes in Europe are the result of the adaptation of the organization to the existing determinants. The results vary from highly quality-assured systematic cervical screening programmes to poorly controlled voluntary screening.

## Lessons learned

The main objective of any cervical screening programme is the prevention of death from cervical cancer. A subsidiary objective is to reduce the incidence of cervical cancer:
**1** Cervical cancer screening using the Pap smear test as a screening test is able to reduce the incidence and mortality of cervical cancer.
**2** Organized, systematic screening offers the best guarantees to achieve these objectives.

### Systematic screening

**1** Systematic screening is a public health intervention and should receive political support. The organizing body of a screening programme should be held responsible throughout the programme. The delivery of a screening programme should comply with what is described in national guidelines and protocols.

2   A structural financing system for public health services separate and independent from the cure and care budget is an advantage.

3   The organization, monitoring and use of resources in cervical cancer screening are inextricably linked.

4   The keyboard for successful screening programmes is organization. The most significant determinant of risk reduction is how well the programme is organized. Therefore it seems that one of the most important conditions for a successful screening programme is the organization of the existing national health system.

5   The existence of an organized screening programme in a country will have an effect in terms of higher quality of the diagnostic procedures, treatment and follow-up in the clinical setting.

## Opportunistic screening

1   Screening without any coordination will never be successful. A central coordination is strongly advised. Screening which is not centrally coordinated is not a programme.

2   Screening should aim at the highest possible standards of quality from the medical and organizational point of view.

3   In any screening programme, the health professionals involved should be subject to quality assurance, audit and external quality control.

4   A *public health* screening programme can never be performed in an individual practice. This is opportunistic case-finding with the main objective of reassuring the women.

5   In an opportunistic screening setting, proper training of the health professional involved and a high level of quality assurance of the cytopathological performance should receive high priority.

6   On an individual basis, the cost involved in the early detection of a disease can be justified. However, in a public health setting, with limited resources, priorities in the distribution of health care services have to be identified.

7   Good screening with poor assessment is still poor prevention.

## Relevant recommendations of the Council of Europe

### Recommendation no. R (94)11 on screening as a tool of preventive medicine

#### Section 1.8

Screening is a tool which is potentially capable of improving the health of the population but it also has adverse effects. Constant care should be taken to

ensure that in any screening programme the advantages prevail over the disadvantages.

Any screening programme strikes a balance between the positive and
adverse effects. However in some countries there is a broad consensus that the
health gain is larger than the adverse effects, not only at public health level but
also for each individual participating in the screening.

### Section 4.4

Non-systematic screening or spontaneous screening results in high marginal
costs. Only systematic screening is able to provide the means to control cost.
Therefore, constant care should be taken to ensure that in any screening
programme the allocated resources are used in an optimal way.

### Section 6.3

It must be stressed that screening cannot succeed without cooperation between preventive and curative systems. Organization must be tailored to the
structures of the health system. If appropriate structures in the curative health
care system are lacking, screening should not be implemented until they are
developed (pilot programmes, for example). There are various degrees to
which screening services may be integrated with curative services or develop as
a separate specialty. The advantages and disadvantages of these should be
assessed separately in different health care systems.

## Appendix: Council of Europe, Committee of Ministers, recommendation No. R(94)11

The Committee of Ministers, Considering that the aim of the Council of
Europe is to achieve a greater unity between its members and that this aim may
be pursued, inter alia, by the adoption of common action in the public health
field;

Noting that chronic diseases are the major causes of death and a high social
and economic burden in developed countries;

Considering that screening for the early detection of some of these diseases
could, in principle, provide a method for their control;

Considering that, as yet, there is no absolute proof of the value of screening
and early treatment in most diseases;

Considering that few, if any, diseases can at the present time be regarded as

Recommendation No. R(94)11 adopted by the Committee of Ministers on 10 October
1994 at the 518th meeting of the Ministers' Deputies.

fulfilling all the desirable criteria for screening, and that the recommended evaluative procedures are not often carried out in full;

Recognising that the implementation of widespread screening programmes raises major ethical, legal, social, medical, organisational and economic problems which require initial and ongoing evaluation;

Taking into account the provisions of the European Convention on Human Rights and of the European Social Charter;

Bearing in mind the Convention for the protection of individuals with regard to automatic processing of personal data of 28 January 1981, as well as the provisions of Recommendation No. R (81) 1 on regulations for automated medical banks and Recommendation No. R (83) 10 on the protection of personal data used for purposes of scientific research and statistics.

Recommends to governments of member states that they take account in their national health planning regulations and legislation of the conclusions and recommendations set out in the appendix to this recommendation.

## Appendix to Recommendation No. R (94) 11

### 1  Introduction

1.1  For the purposes of this recommendation, screening means applying a test to a defined group of persons in order to identify an early stage, a preliminary stage, a risk factor or a combination of risk factors of a disease. In any case it is a question of detecting phenomena, which can be identified prior to the outbreak of the disease.

1.2  The object of screening as a service is to identify a certain disease or risk factor for a disease before the affected person spontaneously seeks treatment, in order to cure the disease or prevent or delay its progression or onset by (early) intervention.

1.3  The value of existing forms of screening for infectious diseases is fully acknowledged but these established methods are not considered in detail in this recommendation. Emphasis is made on screening for chronic degenerative non-communicable disorders.

1.4  Screening is only one method of controlling disease. It should be viewed in the whole context of reducing the burden of ill health to the individual and the community by, for example, socio-economic, environmental measures, health education and improvement of existing health care and disease prevention systems.

1.5  Environmental factors are recognised as important contributors to disease, but inherited factors may also play an important role. With the advent of new genetic knowledge, an increasing number of genetic diseases and genetic risk factors for disease will be identified and offer the possibility for new screening procedures. As the procedures for genetic screening are not fully established nor fully evaluated, they have not been included in this recommendation.

1.6    The present position is that the implementation of screening in European countries is fragmentary, with few national screening programmes for the total population but many screening schemes restricted to population groups.

1.7    Because there are differences in health needs and health services, as well as in ethical values and in legal norms and rules between countries, the decision to implement a particular screening programme should be taken in cooperation with the medical profession by each country. Nevertheless there are common general principles and problems which are equally relevant to all systems.

1.8    Screening is a tool which is potentially capable of improving the health of the population but it also has adverse effects. Constant care should be taken to ensure that in any screening programme the advantages prevail over the disadvantages.

1.9    The general benefits of screening are often described. It is, however, also important to be aware of the adverse effects which can be:
• stigmatisation and/or discrimination of (non) participants;
• social pressure to participate in the screening and undergo the intended treatment/intervention;
• psychological distress where there is no cure for the disease or where the treatment and/or intervention is morally unacceptable to the individual concerned;
• exposure to physical and psychological risks with limited health gains;
• creation of expectations which probably cannot be fulfilled;
• individuals who are positively screened might experience difficulties such as access to insurance, employment, etc.;
• severe side effects of invasive clinical diagnosis of false positives;
• delay in diagnosing false negatives;
• unfavourable cost-benefit relationship of a screening programme.

1.10    The various problems which are encountered in the introduction and provision of screening are interrelated. Nevertheless, a distinction may be made between those concerned with: (i) ethical and legal issues; (ii) selection of diseases (medically) suitable for screening; (iii) economic aspects and evaluation of screening; (iv) quality assurance; (v) organisation of a screening programme; (vi) scientific research.


## 2    Ethical and legal values

2.1    Effectiveness is a necessary prerequisite for the screening to be ethical. It should none the less be kept in mind that screening can be effective and still unethical.

2.2   Advantages and disadvantages of screening for the target population and the individual must be well balanced, taking into account social and economic costs, equity as well as individual rights and freedoms.

2.3   Failure to make known information on the positive and negative aspects of the screening is unethical and infringes the autonomy of the individual.

2.4   The decision to participate in a screening programme should be taken freely. The diagnoses and treatments which may follow the screening should also require a free and separate consent. No pressure should be used to lead somebody to undergo any of these procedures.

2.5   The right to privacy requires that the results of the tests as a general rule are not communicated to those who do not wish to be informed, are collected, stored, and handled confidentially, and adequately protected. It is preferable not to screen individuals who do not wish to be informed of the results of the screening.

2.6   Neonatal screening can only be justified if the intervention is of direct health benefit to the child. Otherwise screening should be postponed until the child can decide for itself.

2.7   No personal data derived from the screening should be communicated to third parties unless the data subject has given consent to it or in accordance with national law.

2.8   When a screening programme is provided as a service and conducted also for research purposes, the decision to make available personal medical data stemming from the screening programme for research purposes should be taken freely, without undue pressure.

The decision not to take part in the research should not in any way prevent the individual from participating in the screening programme.

## 3   Criteria for selecting diseases suitable for screening

3.1   The disease should be an obvious burden for the individual and/or the community in terms of death, suffering, economic or social costs.

3.2   The natural course of the disease should be well known and the disease should go through an initial latent stage or be determined by risk factors, which can be detected by appropriate tests. An appropriate test is highly sensitive and specific for the disease as well as being acceptable to the person screened.

3.3   Adequate treatment or other intervention possibilities are indispensable. Adequacy is determined both by proven medical effect and ethical and legal acceptability.

3.4   Screening followed by diagnosis and intervention in an early stage of the disease should provide a better prognosis than intervention after spontaneously sought treatment.

## 4  Economic aspects

4.1    The increasing financial burden of health care makes it necessary to assess the economic aspects of screening. However these aspects should not be the overriding consideration. In all screening programmes human consideration regarding the value and quality of life, life expectancy as well as respect for individual rights are of prime importance.

4.2    Economic assessments as necessary to enable rational decisions to be made on the priority to be given to alternative ways of using health resources.

4.3    Measurement of the economic aspects of screening is not fully mastered. Early detection and treatment may be less expensive than late treatment. However, available studies relate only to present screening costs and further work is necessary to determine possible cost control in the long term.

4.4    Non-systematic screening or spontaneous screening results in high marginal costs. Only systematic screening is able to provide means for controlling cost. Therefore, constant care should be taken to ensure that in any screening programme the allocated resources are used in an optimal way.


## 5  Quality assurance

5.1    Screening should aim at the highest possible standards of quality from the medical and organisational point of view.

5.2    Because of the expectations that screening creates as well as its adverse effects, screening should meet the highest quality assurance standards in all its aspects.

5.3    As assessment of the scientific evidence of the effectiveness of screening in the control of a disease should be made by experimental studies before introducing a screening programme as a service. The practical arrangements for a mass screening, which are directly linked to the health structures and systems, should obtain the same effectiveness as that obtained in the randomised trial.

5.4    Having implemented a screening programme, it should be subjected to continuous independent evaluation. Evaluation will facilitate adaptation of the programme, correction of deficiencies noted and verification of achievement of objectives. The adverse effects of the screening programme should not be ignored in the evaluation which should be carried out by independent public health experts.

5.5    If quality assurance standards are not met in the long term it should possible for the screening programme to be corrected, and, if this is not possible, stopped.

5.6    The programme must evaluate participation, and the percentage of people screened in the target population, the technical quality of testing and the quality of diagnosis and treatment provided as a follow-up for persons with a positive test result.

Severe side effects of false positives should be revealed and evaluated.

5.7   There is need for more teaching of medical students in epidemiology and its application to measuring the effects of screening. Similarly post-graduate education in this field is also needed to enable practising doctors to understand the principles and evaluation of screening.

5.8   Provision of screening programmes requires that training in techniques and interpretation of screening tests is included in undergraduate and post-graduate medical teaching programmes.

5.9   A screening programme requires resources in both staff and technical facilities for carrying out the screening tests. In many instances tests can be performed by non-medical staff. Provision should be made for initial and further training of the medical and technical staff who will be involved in performing the screening tests and interpreting their results. Technical methods, including automated techniques, are useful in screening for some diseases. Quality of screening methods should be monitored.

## 6   Organisation

6.1   The organising body of a screening programme should be held responsible throughout the programme. The organisation of a screening programme should comply with what is described in national guidelines and protocols.

6.2   Within the organisational framework the target population should be defined (by age or otherwise) as well as the frequency of screening tests and the general and specific objectives and quality assurance guidelines.

6.3   It must be stressed that screening cannot succeed without co-operation between preventive and curative systems. Organisation must be tailored to the structure of the health system. If appropriate structures in the curative health care system are lacking, screening should not be implemented until they are developed (pilot programmes, for example). There are various degrees to which screening services may be integrated with curative services or develop as a separate speciality. The advantages and disadvantages of these should be assessed separately in different health care systems.

6.4   Provisions should be made for the financing of the programme, the cost of organising and evaluating the structure, the cost of testing, the cost of quality assessment and monitoring, and the cost of the follow-up care of those people who screen positively.

6.5   Process and outcome indicators should be constantly evaluated.

6.6   Systematic collection of data is required in screening programmes to serve the needs of the individual and of the health service. To that end, data should be collected on the target population, on persons screened (with dates and the results of the test carried out), and on the results of eventual diagnostic examinations. Access to a morbidity register considerably facilitates evaluation.

6.7  Adequate protection of all data collected by means of a screening programme should be guaranteed.

6.8  Participation of the public in screening programmes is determined by personal factors (for example attitudes, motivation and anxiety) and by situational factors (waiting time and efficient organisation, for example). These can be influenced for instance by health education and by good organisation of the screening procedure.

6.9  In order to ensure optimal participation by the target population, the best possible information should be widely provided and awareness-raising and education programmes should be organised for both the target population and the health professionals.

6.10  Invitations should be accompanied by written information on the purposes and effectiveness of the programme, on the test, on potential advantages and disadvantages, on the voluntary nature of participation and on how data will be protected. An address should be provided for those who require further information.

6.11  Participants should be informed on how, when and where their test results will be available or will be communicated to them.

6.12  The positive results found at screening should always be confirmed by subsequent diagnostic tests before commencing a treatment/intervention, unless the screening test is a diagnostic test. It is absolutely essential that adequate diagnostic facilities are available to confirm or reject the screening finding as soon as possible. Similarly, treatment facilities must be available and easily accessible to the confirmed cases. The work load placed on the health services by screening can be very large, especially since most screening programmes also lead to incidental pathological findings unrelated to the disease at which the programme is aimed.

6.13  Combining screening for several diseases into a multiple screening procedure may seem to be convenient to the individual and economic to the programme, but such a 'package deal' may negatively influence the extent to which most of the criteria for screening including age limit and frequency would be met.

## 7  *Research*

7.1  Research into new, more effective, screening tests must be encouraged and the long-term effects of the various methods of treatment and provision for positive subjects studied. Research must be further developed to answer the numerous social, ethical, legal, medical, organisational and economic questions as well as psychological problems raised by screening, on which evidence is incomplete.

7.2 Quality assurance concerning research programmes should be conducted into the effectiveness of the various screening tests, the practical arrangements for screening, the measures to increase participation, the means of improving test efficiency, follow-up to and provisions for those screened positive, an assessment process and all the economic aspects.

7.3 Information gathered during screening should be available for the purpose of scientific research, for the improvement of health services, and for the benefit of future screening, taking into account full respect of autonomy and confidentiality and the protection of personal privacy.

## 8 General remarks

8.1 It is particularly important that political decision-makers and target groups should be kept informed of the current state of knowledge about the value of screening for particular diseases. Improved communication should be encouraged.

8.2 Governments should promote the research and evaluation necessary for assessing the value of both new and existing programmes. This form of research necessarily means large-scale research which, in some instances, may be designed as international collaborative studies. Scientific evaluation is the only way in which the positive and negative effects of screening can be assessed in order that a rational decision can be taken on whether a screening programme should be implemented and what resources should be allocated.

### Quality assurance (as defined by World Health Organization)

'All those planned and systematic actions necessary to provide adequate confidence that a structure, system or component will perform satisfactorily in service (ISO 6215-1980). Satisfactory performance in service implies the optimum quality of the entire diagnostic process, i.e. the consistent production of adequate diagnostic information with minimum exposure of both patients and personnel.'

### Quality control (as defined by World Health Organization)

'The set of operations (programming, co-ordinating, carrying out) intended to maintain or to improve ... (ISO 3534-1977). As applied to a diagnostic procedure, it covers monitoring, evaluation and maintenance at optimum levels of all characteristics of performance that can be defined, measured, and controlled.'

# 26: Spontaneous Screening: Benefits and Limitations

## J. Monsonego

Cancer of the uterine cervix is a common gynaecological cancer which occurs worldwide. It is a major cause of death, especially in Third World countries, where screening is often not routinely performed. Papanicolaou (Pap) smear screening is designed to detect precursor lesions which may antedate the development of invasive cancer by several years. For this reason, the Pap test should be a central part of a strategy to prevent the development of invasive cancer.

Evidence of the effectiveness of Pap smear screening is largely derived from retrospective analyses of the incidence of cervical cancer and associated mortality. In at least three cases of northern countries where a screening programme has been introduced (Finland, British Columbia and Iceland), a considerable reduction (50–85%) in incidence and mortality has been shown over the last 30 years [1]. Despite the lack of randomized trials, the data provide compelling evidence for the effectiveness of Pap smear screening in the prevention of cervical cancer [2].

Nevertheless, although the smear test is a satisfactory means of mass screening, its imperfections have meant that the disease has not been eradicated in any of the populations studied to date.

Recent analysis of data concerning national screening programmes set up at a later date (UK, Norway, Denmark, etc.) shows that the results of these organized programmes, recommending a smear test every 3–5 years, are far from those which could have been expected [3–7].

In many developed countries the incidence of cervical cancer has remained the same. In Europe, 22 000 new cases of invasive cancer are diagnosed each year and 8000 women die as a result of the disease [8]. At the same time, the

*Correspondence*: J. Monsonego, Head of Cyto-Colposcopic Screening Unit, Institut Alfred Fournier, 25 Boulevard St Jacques, 75014 Paris, France.

incidence of premalignant lesions is on the increase. Although the global incidence of cervical cancer does appear to have stabilized, this can be explained by a decrease in cases in older women, whereas figures tend to be increasing amongst younger women [8,9]. In many developed countries, screening for cervical cancer remains voluntary. As a result, in most of them, the incidence rate of the disease has remained the same over the last 20 years [10].

In France, 5000–6000 new cases are registered every year; of these patients, 2000 die from the disease. The ineffectiveness of voluntary screening has been reported and can give rise to the same effects as the inappropriate organized programmes [5, 7, 11–14]. The lack of coverage of the target population, the absence of quality control and the non-evaluation of the system are some of the reasons for this failure.

## Factors necessary for the success of organized screening

The success of organized screening programmes requires specific conditions. Ten years ago, experts met at the International Agency for Research on Cancer (IARC) in Lyon and, after assessing numerous screening systems of the 1970s, came to the conclusion that an organized programme carried out among a target population, using the smear test as the means of detection every 3 years after two initial negative smears, is an effective way of reducing the incidence of, and mortality from, cervical cancer [2].

Analysis of the data from organized programmes of the 1970s leads to these comments:

**1**  Relative protection decreases with increasing screening interval, whatever the programme. Protection decreases strongly after the 3–5-yearly screening test.

**2**  The relative protection is lower with one previous negative smear than after two or more negative smears. Two first negative smears give more marked protection than the initial first negative smear. The best protection is given with two initial negative smears and a screening interval of 1–2 years.

**3**  Whatever the screening interval, the protection varies strongly between centres. This protection is lower when the screening programme is random, compared to centres with organized programmes.

It was suggested that drawing any conclusions from studies performed in a number of countries with widely different approaches and conducted with contrasting study designs was clearly hazardous. However, the disparate nature of the sources of the information strengthened any convergence towards a common interpretation. Therefore, maximum protection is observed with an annual smear but the protection is broadly acceptable with a 2-year interval and begins to reduce after 3- and 5-year intervals (Table 26.1).

**Table 26.1** Summary of relative protections, geometric mean values over the centres.

| Time since last negative smear (months) | Relative protection (no. of cases in brackets) | 95% confidence intervals |
|---|---|---|
| 0–11 | 15.3 (25) | 10.0–22.6 |
| 12–23 | 11.9 (23) | 7.5–18.3 |
| 24–35 | 8.0 (25) | 5.2–11.8 |
| 36–47 | 5.3 (30) | 3.6–7.6 |
| 48–59 | 2.8 (30) | 1.9–4.0 |
| 60–71 | 3.6 (16) | 2.1–5.9 |
| 72–119 | 1.6 (6) | 0.6–3.5 |
| 120+ | 0.8* (7) | 0.3–1.6 |
| Never screened | 1.0 | |

* Based on figures from Aberdeen and Iceland only.

Bearing in mind these results, the IARC group has suggested that organized programmes using a smear test every 3 years after two initial negative smears gives significant protection compared to annual screening (Table 26.2).

The following conclusions were drawn by the IARC working group on the sensitivity of cytological screening:

1  Risk factors have little effect.
2  There was no differentiation between younger and older women as regards fast-growing tumours.
3  Most invasive tumours were asymptomatic.
4  In the first 2 years, after at least two negative smears, the risk of cervical cancer is less than 10%.
5  At 3–5 years, after two negative tests, the risk of cervical cancer rises slowly (9% to 15%).
6  The false-negative rates vary widely, from 40% to 10%.
7  The lowest false-negative rates are seen in results from centrally organized programmes.

**Table 26.2** Percentage reduction in the cumulative rate of invasive cervical cancer over the age range 35–65, with different frequencies of screening.

| Screening frequency | Reduction in the cumulative rate (%)* | No. of tests |
|---|---|---|
| 1 year | 93.3 | 30 |
| 2 years | 92.5 | 15 |
| 3 years | 91.4 | 10 |
| 5 years | 83.9 | 6 |
| 10 years | 64.2 | 3 |

* Assuming screening takes place at age 35, and that a previous screen has been performed.

**8** Three-year screening intervals give a significant risk reduction of cervical cancer. However, the group has pointed out: 'It must be remembered that this reduction is brought about only if the policy is adhered to, and that bringing all women into a screening programme will be a main factor in its success' [2].

## Failure of cervical cancer screening in developed countries

Despite the success of screening programmes, cervical cancer in developed countries remains a reality. Various explanations can be proposed for such differences, but prominent among them are the absence of organized programmes (voluntary screening) and differences in the organization and implementation of the screening services. The main factors for failure are the lack of coverage of the target population and false-negative smears due to inadequate samples or lack of interpretation. The minor factors are error of management of abnormal smears and rapidly growing cancers.

### Lack of coverage

Evidence from Nordic countries shows that coverage is a critical factor in successful screening programmes. Although clinicians throughout Europe support the concept of cervical screening as a method of preventing cervical cancer, national screening programmes have been introduced in relatively few countries. These include Iceland, Finland, Denmark, Sweden, Norway, the Netherlands and the UK. If we examine the screening programmes in these countries it can be seen that, although the programmes were launched at about the same time in the mid 1960s, each country had adopted a very different policy towards screening, with regards the selection of women, screening intervals and the methods of invitation. In the UK, for example, the national policy was to take a cervical smear every 5 years from women aged 35 or over, although no call-and-recall system was in place to ensure that this happened. In Iceland, on the other hand, women between the ages of 25 and 69 were regularly screened at 3-year intervals [2].

Although the national screening programmes in the Nordic countries have been in place for over 20 years, their effectiveness as determined by a reduction in incidence and mortality from cervical cancer has varied from country to country and even within a single country. Review of the effectiveness of screening in the UK in the 1980s revealed that in the Grampian region of Scotland there was a significant reduction in the mortality and incidence of invasive cervical disease – a finding that contrasted significantly with the results in the rest of the UK. A comparative review of the effectiveness of screening in the Nordic countries showed a similar contrast between mortality rates in Iceland and Finland compared with Sweden, Norway and Denmark [1].

**Table 26.3** Variations (%) in mortality from cervical cancer between 1963–67 and 1978–82 in the Nordic countries and by age group.

| Country | Age group (years) | Patients covered by nationally organized mass screening (%) | Variations of mortality (%) by age group | | | |
|---|---|---|---|---|---|---|
| | | | 30–39 | 40–49 | 50–59 | 60–69 |
| Iceland | 25–69 | 80 | −100 | −77 | −66 | −66 |
| Finland | 30–55 | 75 | −172 | −77 | −66 | −66 |
| Sweden | 30–49 | 70 | −59 | −63 | −40 | +7 |
| Denmark | 30–50 | 35 | −61 | −53 | −26 | +1 |
| Norway | 25–60 | 3 | −48 | −23 | −2 | +14 |

Europe against Cancer, 1993.

Table 26.3 illustrates the fall in mortality rates in the Nordic countries over the last 20 years by age group [8]. It shows that the decline in mortality from cervical cancer is directly related to the percentage of the female population which has been screened. Thus, in Finland and Iceland, where the fall in mortality has been the greatest, 75–80% of women at risk have had a cervical smear. A similar observation has been made from statistics released from the UK. In the Grampian region of Scotland, 95% of women at risk of cervical cancer have had a cervical smear, compared with 40% of women in the rest of the UK.

In Table 26.4, the effect of screening programmes on different proportions of the population at different frequencies is shown [15]. It is clear that it is more cost-effective to recruit a high proportion of the population and screen them infrequently than to recruit a low proportion and screen them at regular intervals. These findings serve to emphasize the importance of comprehensive coverage of the population at risk if cervical screening programmes are to be effective.

**Table 26.4** Reduction in the cumulative incidence of cervical cancer according to the proportion of the population covered by screening programmes and according to the interval between smear tests (age group between 35 and 64 years).

| Frequency of smear tests | Proportion of population screened (%) | Reduction in cumulative incidence (%) | No. of tests* |
|---|---|---|---|
| 1 year | 20 | 19 | 6 |
| 2 years | 30 | 28 | 4.5 |
| 3 years | 40 | 37 | 4 |
| 5 years | 50 | 42 | 3 |
| 10 years | 80 | 51 | 2.4 |

* Per female patients in the entire population.

In many European countries where screening is offered on a voluntary basis, coverage of the population is poor. Women who are most at risk – older women, women who are promiscuous, women from lower social groups – may not have even one smear test during their life-time, whereas women who are least at risk may have annual smears. Although nearly 5 000 000 smears were taken annually in France (enough to screen the population at risk every 3 years), fewer than half of women aged between 25 and 65 have had a cervical smear. The consequence of this neglect was demonstrated in a retrospective review of women who died from cervical cancer [16].

Unscreened women are the main problem in countries where screening programmes are not organized. In countries where the screening is opportunistic, the rate of coverage is around 20–40%, compared to organized programmes, where it is of the order of 80–90%.

## Lack of sensitivity of cytology: problems of false negative smears

False-negative cytology may be partly responsible for the failure to diagnose cervical cancer, and it is estimated that between 13 and 31% of cervical malignancies have been associated with negative smears in the 3 years preceding the diagnosis [17–19]. When cases of cervical intraepithelial neoplasia (CIN) are examined for false-negative cytology, rates of between 16 and 36% are quoted for CIN cases that had negative cytology in smears taken at the time of the biopsy [20–24].

Various reasons for these false-negative results have been suggested. These include inadequate sampling, which may arise due to errors made by the sample-taker, differences between the effectiveness of the sampling devices, and physical properties of the lesions which make effective sampling less likely due to diminished cellular exfoliation. The absence of endocervical cells also contributes. In a recent study by Beeby et al. [25] it was pointed out that a number of other factors contributed to the production of false-negative smears; these included the young age of the patient, fewer pregnancies, less severe grades of referring smears, the absence of endocervical smears, no visible lesion at colposcopy and lesion size.

Lesion size is significantly associated with cytological status [26–29]. Jones et al. [28] have shown that small-volume high-grade lesions (CIN III) exist in the presence of the minor-grade cytological smears in some 12% of cases who at one time had an abnormal smear, which was subsequently followed by a negative smear. Hartmann et al. [29] have also shown in a morphometric study of CIN in cone biopsy specimens that false-negative cytology exists in association with small surface lesions. This would seem to suggest that a small volume of CIN is closely associated with false-negative cytology. It has also been suggested that the site of the lesion is most important. Beeby et al. [25] in their study showed that 8% of brush smears taken in patients with false-negative cytology showed no abnormality, suggesting that these particular lesions may lie in a position that is inaccessible to sampling by spatula. They suggested that the severity of the lesion may also be an important factor, since the cases with false-negative cytology tended to have a less severe grade of CIN than those with abnormal cytology. A more likely explanation is that less severe and possibly smaller lesions may be less likely to exfoliate. It is suggested that small-volume high-grade disease has minimal malignant potential [28].

Another important factor is the quality of Pap smear interpretation by the laboratories as a result of lack of training, poor quality control or scanner exhaustion. Indeed, an analysis of false-negative cytology at the Mayo Clinic over a 4-year period showed errors in 63 cases. Sample error accounted for 39 (62%) of these errors, screening failure for 10 (16%) and interpretation error for 15 (22%) [30]. Human error has been blamed for many failures in smear analysis. Often a small cell lesion did not trigger the appropriate reaction in the screener, mostly because of inattention or fatigue [4].

Higher false-negative rate are seen in results from non-organized programmes [2–13] compared to national screening programmes [2–6].

Problems of false negatives are not only a reality of voluntary screening but are also observed in some inadequately organized programmes [2–13]. The study of Raffle conducted in the Bristol, UK area [3] shows that, despite the introduction of a 5-yearly test programme since 1970, in terms of mortality rate from cervical cancer there is no difference before and after the screening programme despite the increasing coverage and introducing quality control of the smears in the laboratories.

In France, a recent survey among gynaecologists concerning invasive cervical cancers observed since the last negative smear showed that 45% of cases had a normal smear 1 year before the diagnosis [31].

### Minor factors of failure

The minor factors of failure of cervical cancer screening are errors in the management of abnormal smears and rapidly growing cases. Fewer than 15% of invasive cervical cancers are due to these circumstances [2,11,32].

## Spontaneous screening experience in France

### Cervical cancer incidence

De Vathaire and colleagues [33] have provided an assessment of the incidence of cervical cancer from the incidence data of eight registers of the Francim network between 1983 and 1987 and the mortality data for the whole country between 1985 and 1989.

The annual incidence varies according to the age group, as we know (Fig. 26.1; Table 26.5). The incidence rate is low in young women, increases after the age of 60 and decreases after the age of 70. There is a wide variation between areas. The incidence rate may vary by a factor of 10, mostly in young women.

The mortality rate indicates a low rate in young women and a higher rate in older women but again, the standardized incidence rate shows a variation between the different registers.

Figure 26.1 shows annual incidence according to age between 1983 and 1987. Analysis of this figure shows a low incidence in young women but increasing cases until the age of 45, suggesting the failure of screening or the particular characteristics of the disease in this period. The high incidence between the ages 50 and 65 is probably due to the drop in attendance of these women in this period. The annual incidence is the same as in the UK, lower than in Denmark but much higher than in southern countries of Europe.

Points to note from these observed French data are:

1  Number of cases per year: 4325.
2  Gross annual incidence rate: 15.3/100 000.
3  Annual incidence rate standardized against the world population: 12.1/100 000.
4  Cumulated incidence rate between the ages of 0 and 64: 0.92%.
5  Cumulated incidence rate between the ages of 0 and 74: 1.24%.

## Recent survey results

In France, there is no nationally organized screening programme. Most patients see their own private gynaecologist spontaneously to have smears

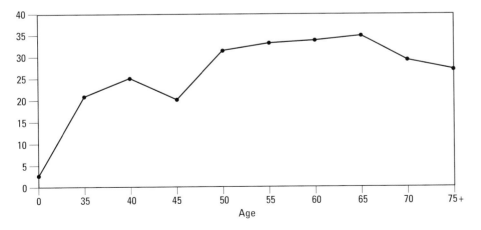

**Fig. 26.1** Cervical cancer in France: estimated incidence (per 100 000 women) between 1983 and 1987.

**Table 26.5** Cervical cancer in France: (a) observed annual incidence and (b) estimated incidence (per 100 000) during the period 1983–1987.

| AC | Area | Age (years) | | | | | | | | | | Gross | Standardized | Rate per year |
|---|---|---|---|---|---|---|---|---|---|---|---|---|---|---|
| | | 0–34 | 35–39 | 40–44 | 45–49 | 50–54 | 55–59 | 60–64 | 65–69 | 70–74 | 75+ | | | |
| (a) | | | | | | | | | | | | | | |
| 14 | Calvados | 2.3 | 28.1 | 35.5 | 31.7 | 54.1 | 43.6 | 38.6 | 43.7 | 34.6 | 31.5 | 18.5 | 20.2 | 57 |
| 21 | Côte d'Or | 1.4 | 14.5 | 20.1 | 23.1 | 25.2 | 42.1 | 42.9 | 39.1 | 28.6 | 31.4 | 14.4 | 14.8 | 36 |
| 25 | Doubs | 2.0 | 4.5 | 21.2 | 12.7 | 31.0 | 31.2 | 27.4 | 27.3 | 41.8 | 25.1 | 11.4 | 12.4 | 28 |
| 34 | Hérault | 6.7 | 48.5 | 38.0 | 47.5 | 36.4 | 35.4 | 27.7 | 26.3 | 35.3 | 31.5 | 22.4 | 22.2 | 89 |
| 38 | Isere | 2.6 | 15.2 | 22.6 | 15.6 | 22.6 | 26.7 | 33.0 | 29.7 | 29.1 | 20.2 | 12.1 | 12.8 | 59 |
| 67 | Bas Rhin | 2.5 | 23.1 | 20.8 | 15.4 | 22.0 | 28.4 | 40.8 | 41.4 | 29.6 | 27.7 | 14.0 | 14.4 | 67 |
| 80 | Somme | 4.9 | 30.9 | 59.4 | 41.0 | 40.5 | 41.5 | 39.6 | 46.0 | 37.8 | 29.4 | 21.1 | 23.1 | 59 |
| 81 | Tarn | 2.6 | 10.2 | 15.6 | 15.1 | 20.4 | 20.6 | 19.6 | 14.3 | 30.1 | 28.5 | 12.5 | 10.4 | 22 |
| (b) | | | | | | | | | | | | | | |
| | Women | 2.8 | 20.7 | 25.0 | 20.2 | 31.6 | 33.1 | 33.8 | 35.2 | 29.1 | 26.9 | 15.3 | 15.3 | 4325 |

From De Vathaire [33] with permission. AC, area codes.

taken. Although screening has existed for many years, cervical cancer is still the most commonly encountered form of gynaecological cancer and the incidence rate has not changed significantly.

The results of the survey as regards smear testing by general practitioners cause us to observe that the situation in France needs careful attention [34]. The survey, carried out on a national scale, amongst a representative sample of general practitioners in April 1994, reveals that approximately 70% of general practitioners conduct screening by smear tests. There seems to be a discrepancy between this high figure and the reality of cervical cancer in France. However, when these physicians were questioned about their training as regards taking a smear test, 50% replied that they were either insufficiently or not at all trained. In reality, over a third of these practitioners do not react when faced with an abnormal smear. These results indicate therefore that if general practitioners are to take part in cervical cancer screening, priority must be given to ensuring adequate training and to motivating them to perform this examination. They will then be in a position to understand why they should move from opportunistic screening to systematic screening.

A survey carried out among gynaecologists following a questionnaire which appeared in the press [31] reveals certain worrying – even alarming – preliminary results. We carried out this appraisal so that the medical history of the cervical smears of women who went on to develop cervical cancer could be assessed. In order to evaluate the factors associated with the development of cervical cancer, within a population undergoing spontaneous screening, a confidential survey was carried out following publication in a medical journal. We focused the questions on the period of time, the grade of previous smears and the characteristics of cancer developing after recent normal smears. A total of 550 cases have been analysed to date. It appears that 92% of physicians are against smear tests being conducted only once every 3 years; 91% feel sure they will observe an increase in cases of cervical carcinoma-*in-situ* and invasive carcinoma. Finally, 79.7% have already been confronted with cervical carcinoma (*in-situ* or invasive) in patients whose last smear test, carried out during the previous 36 months, was normal. Examination of the replies (Table 26.6) to the detailed questionnaire regarding the profile of the diagnosis in women

**Table 26.6** Observed cases of cervical cancer.

| Diagnosis | Number | % | |
|---|---|---|---|
| Carcinoma-*in-situ* | 413 | 75 | |
| Microinvasive squamous carcinoma | 49 | 9 | |
| Invasive squamous carcinoma | 66 | 12 | 137 (25%) |
| Adenocarcinoma | 22 | 4 | |
| Total | 550 | 100% | |

**Table 26.7** Assessment of cervical cancer since last negative smear.

|  | +5 years | 3–5 years | 2–3 years | 1 year | < 1 year | No response |
|---|---|---|---|---|---|---|
| Carcinoma-*in-situ* (*n* = 413) | 7 (1.5%) | 16 (3.9%) | 138 (33.4%) | 204 (49.4%) | 34 (8.2%) | 15 (3.6%) |
| Invasive carcinoma (*n* = 137) | 1 (0.7%) | 7 (5.1%) | 45 (32.8%) | 43 (31.5%) | 35 (25.5%) | 6 (4.4%) |
| Total | 7 (1.3%) | 23 (4.2%) | 183 (33.3%) | 247 (44.9%) | 69 (12.5%) | 21 (3.8%) |

presenting with invasive cancer after a normal smear test during the previous 3 years reveals that about 75% (413/550) of these lesions were carcinoma-*in-situ* and 25% (137/500) invasive carcinoma. In the majority of cases, the diagnosis was confirmed by biopsy or conization.

It is important to note (Table 26.7) that, in 78% of cases, the smears were normal during the 3 years beforehand (33% had normal smears 2–3 years before; 45% had normal smears 1 year before). The distribution is more or less equal for carcinoma-*in-situ* and invasive cancer. It is also worth noting that in 27.5% of cases (151/550) the slides of normal smears were reread; in 75.5% of cases (114/151), the diagnosis was confirmed as normal, and in 21.2% (32/114) the diagnosis was revised as abnormal. Finally, it must be specified that in 74% of cases, the patient consulted on a regular basis.

The outcome in relation to mortality was available in 20% (109/550) of cases. Among them, 15 (13.8%) died. Table 26.8 shows the mortality rate according to time since last negative smear. The mean age of the patient at death is low (38 years).

Again, in this survey, the mortality rate since last negative smear is greater in cases of short time interval since the smear (1 year). There is a correlation between the interval between smears and the prognosis of the disease.

It can nevertheless be pointed out that if the sample of participating practitioners can be said to be representative, then around 30% of cases of invasive cancer reported in women who are regularly screened occur in those

**Table 26.8** Mortality rate and time since last normal smear.

| Time since last normal smear | 2–3 years | < 1–2 years | 1 year |
|---|---|---|---|
| Mortality rate | 1/15* | 4/15† | 10/15‡ |
| Mean age (years) | 34 | 40 | 35 |

* One previously diagnosed microinvasive carcinoma.
† Two previously diagnosed carcinoma-*in-situ* and two invasive carcinomas.
‡ Seven invasive carcinomas and three adenocarcinomas.

who have had normal smears during the previous 2–3 years. Based on this survey, it is possible to state that cervical cancer in France is of course observed in unscreened women, but it also remains a reality among those who undergo regular voluntary screening. This statement gives rise to questions about the natural history of the disease, the quality of samples taken, the quality of the interpretation of the smear tests and the urgency with which a reliable, centralized system of quality assurance must be set up.

## Spontaneous screening: the dilemma of smear interval

Efforts to control cervical cancer can be traced back many years to when gynaecologists first encouraged the early reporting of symptoms. The development of cytology as an effective tool for cancer screening, an increasing emphasis on prenatal care, the changes in contraceptive care and an increasing prevalence of sexually transmitted disease ensured that the concept of the cervical examination was well accepted in preventive care. Currently, the scientific community advocates annual examination, including cervical cytology.

The most cost-effective interval for Pap smear screening is unknown. The American College of Obstetricians and Gynecologists and the American Cancer Society recommend that annual screening should commence when women become sexually active or reach the age of 18 years [35,36]. If three or more consecutive annual examinations have been normal, Pap tests may be performed less frequently at the physician's discretion in women at low risk of cervical cancer.

After the publication of the IARC working group report in 1986 [2] on the subject of the effectiveness of 3-yearly screening, some countries with no organized programmes have adopted these specific conclusions, chiefly for economic reasons and without applying the prerequisite conditions to these recommendations [37].

In voluntary screening, several aspects must be considered before increasing the interval between screening tests.

### *Avoid mixing organized screening and spontaneous screening*

Cervical cancer screening aims to protect women from a potentially fatal disease: invasive cancer. The justification for cytological screening once every 3 years following two negative smears is based on mass screening programmes in place, for example, in northern Europe and in British Columbia, where programmes were set up during the 1960s. In these countries, where the organization of screening programmes ensures ideal coordination of sample-taking, where the smear test reporting is carried out by national laboratories of a high standard, where quality control can be ensured without difficulty and where women are recalled on a regular basis, these systems have proved their effectiveness with smear tests once every 3 years leading to a reduction in cervical cancer figures in the region of 91% [1–2]. None of these conditions exist in the voluntary screening sector where the majority of the screening system is performed on a voluntary basis by independent physicians and independent laboratories and where access to medical information is limited by confidentiality. As a result, cytological false negatives can reach 15–35% and interobserver variations are high [6,13,17–20,24]. These false-negative results include, of course, misinterpretations resulting from samples of poor quality. Information intended for the pathologist is sometimes missing from the physician's notes, although it is necessary to encourage the cytologist to do a systematic rereading. The sample-taking technique is not always simple and requires careful and painstaking practice. Individual efforts have been made within some laboratories with regards to rereading slides so as to guarantee some form of quality control, but on a national scale this remains insufficient. Sometimes smear test screening errors include undercalling and, at other times, inadequate interpretations, particularly as regards small cell endocervical lesions, which do not reveal enough to instigate an appropriate reaction from the person reading the slide. These disorders are naturally all dealt with and more often than not corrected within centralized and organized screening programmes. They escape any form of assessment or control in countries without organized screening programmes.

### Bear in mind recent developments

The incidence of premalignant lesions has been steadily increasing over the past few years and at the same time it has been observed that women are affected by carcinoma-*in-situ* or even invasive cancer at a far younger age [3]. The concept of slow evolution (in the region of 10 years, on average) from dysplasia to cancer is not always certain. Although this is a generally accepted fact, there have nevertheless been many reports concerning lesions which were severe from the onset [7–12]. Several studies have concerned the evolution of lesions; these should be criticized since they rely solely upon cytological follow-up or on a diagnosis made following biopsies, which are known to be capable of modifying the natural history of the lesions [38]. Furthermore, rapidly evolving cancer, particularly in young women, is on the increase and testifies to the epidemiological development of this disease [6,13,39]. The increasing incidence of adenocarcinoma is proof of this. In the UK, although a decrease of approximately 32% was noted in mortality from cervical cancer between 1979 and 1992, mortality before the age of 40 showed a marked increase, justifying urgent measures and careful attention [3].

*Note that cervical cancer is still found in*
*regularly screened women*

It has been somewhat overstated that in spontaneous screening, cervical cancer is observed in the unscreened population whereas the fact that it remains a reality among women who undergo regular check-ups is not to be ignored. These observations are reported in studies analysing the results of screening programmes introduced more recently, about 20 years ago [3,5,6,39,40]. It is possible to demonstrate in France that at least one-third of cases of invasive cervical cancer are observed in women who undergo regular examination and screening. Among these women who have undergone regular screening and yet now present invasive cancer, 37% underwent a smear test but were not followed up (due to lack of information, change of residence, etc.) and 20% were incorrectly treated.

*Consider the risk factors*

The risk factors could help establish the interval of individual screening. In April 1994, under the patronage of the World Health Organization and the European Union, European Research Organization on Genital Infection and Neoplasia (EUROGIN) invited international experts to United Nations Educational, Scientific and Cultural Organization (UNESCO) in Paris. Screening carried out in the countries where it is well organized was clearly distinguished from that performed in other countries on a voluntary basis and where the notion of risk factors and quality assurance ought to encourage physicians to take the responsibility for assessing the frequency of smear-testing [37].

Nowadays, it is widely accepted that certain types of papillomavirus are involved in the onset of cervical cancer. A large number of studies, both epidemiological and biological, have demonstrated the transformation effect of these viruses, their integration into the host genome, their genetic activity within neoplastic cells, the expression of certain viral genes (E6, E7) in order to maintain the malignant phenotype of neoplastic cells and the specific interaction of the viral proteins E6 and E7 with the tumour suppressor gene proteins p53 and pRb. The latest high-performance polymerase chain reaction (PCR) techniques have shown that human papillomavirus (HPV) 16 and 18 are reliable markers of prediction and progression of dysplasic. Therefore, HPV 16 or 18 infection [41–43] or human immunodeficiency virus (HIV) seropositivity [44] increases the risk of cervical neoplasia in women. The risks brought on by smoking, sexually transmitted diseases, multiple pregnancies and low socioeconomic conditions are well demonstrated.

*Keep up-to-date with the literature*

The most recent publications should encourage careful analysis of the situation. The history of screening based on smear tests can be divided into three main periods. The first goes back to the 1950s when the Papanicolaou test was initiated and was responsible for an enormous success since both the incidence and mortality of cervical cancer dropped significantly as a result of a relatively simple test. In the absence of systematic screening, this test also led to the detection of early invasive cancer and therefore to a reduction of mortality from this disease.

In the 1960s, a few countries or provinces set the example by organizing mass screening (Finland, British Columbia, Iceland) and showing particularly satisfactory results with a smear test once every 3–5 years, justified by irreproachable organization of the screening programme.

Recent reports on the organized screening which was set up in the 1970s and 1980s have shown that the results obtained are far from what could be hoped for, to the extent that some of them may even attempt to blame the failure on organized screening and the carrying-out of smear tests every 3 or 5 years, claiming that this would not significantly alter the incidence or mortality rates of cervical cancer, compared to previous times when there was no screening [3,5,6,13,40]. Although this information must be accepted with some reservations, we can only express surprise that they coincide with the increased mortality from cervical cancer in the under-40s, such as has been reported since the 1970s, and therefore that there must recently have been an epidemiological upheaval as regards this disease.

Finally, certain studies pertaining to the performance of cytological testing should be subjected to critical analysis [45].

## Voluntary screening: what are the priorities?

Examination of the dynamics of cervical cancer prevention shows that the two most important factors which determine the success or failure of cervical cancer screening are coverage of the population at risk and quality standards in the collection, processing and interpretation of cervical smears. Clinicians and public health authorities who are currently offering a cervical screening service should ensure that their programme meets the requirements set out above in order to justify the human and financial resources committed to the screening programme.

Laboratory performance is an important factor in determining the success or failure of cervical screening and it is essential that laboratories operate to a high standard at all times. A key determinant of laboratory standards is the quality of the staff employed on the screening programme. Only staff who have demonstrated their proficiency in the interpretation of cervical smears in nationally recognized examinations should be permitted to undertake the analysis of cervical smears.

Many laboratories have introduced internal quality assurance measures to monitor laboratory performance on a day-to-day basis. These include selected rescreening of negative smears, review of previous cytology and histological/cytological correlation of abnormal cases. The introduction of external quality assurance measures in the form of regular proficiency testing may be helpful, for example. Each member of the laboratory may be asked to report on 10% of cervical smears; failure to recognize an abnormal smear may result in suspension from screening.

Improvements in cervical cytology screening must come from the development of population-based information systems that are incorporated into screening programmes, such as the call-and-recall systems that exist in Nordic countries and the UK, and the introduction of compulsory quality control systems in cytological laboratories. Call-and-recall systems have been introduced in a number of countries in an attempt to increase the efficiency of an existing screening programme. In the UK, from 1987–1988 a system employing general practitioners or family physicians has been underway and the latest indications are that well over 85% of the targeted population have been screened. These encouraging statistics have been achieved because of the use of computerization and advanced information technology, which allows the governing health authority (the Family Health Service Authority) to present to the family practitioner a programme with which he or she can call and recall patients.

Cervical cancer screening is a failure in some developed countries. Over the past 20 years, the number of cases of invasive cancer has remained stable, even though it is widely agreed that 98% of these could have been avoided. It cannot be denied that in these countries, where the system of screening is not an organized practice, the smear test is far from flawless, for the reasons previously outlined and also because it is not a reliable reflection of cervical lesions. Nevertheless, this method does achieve its purpose when carried out at reasonable intervals.

A beneficial approach would have been to improve and extend the concept of quality control, to encourage the involvement of general practitioners, particularly in rural areas, training them and giving full support to their participation in this action. At the same time, all women, including those in underprivileged areas, who manage to elude this system, should have easier access to information and somehow be motivated to participate. Cervical cancer screening lacks cohesions in some developed countries. It hardly lends itself to regulation by administrative orders. It is quite clear that the whole situation requires a new starting point.

**Table 26.9** Spontaneous screening in developed countries.

| Situation | Actions | Perspectives |
|---|---|---|
| Heterogeneous in Europe. ~ 22 000 cases of cervical cancer every year | Ensure adequate quality control of smears | Improvement of smear test screening by using: <ul><li>Adequate sampling material (brush)</li><li>Liquid-based cytology</li><li>Automation</li><li>HPV testing as primary or secondary screening</li><li>Polar probe</li></ul> |
| Cases of invasive cervical cancer are observed in both screened and non-screened women | Implicate and motivate GPs<br><br>Extend coverage through education of target population | |
| This is the consequence of: <ul><li>the absence of any official quality control of smear test</li><li>high rates of false negatives (5–30%)</li><li>— due to laboratory errors (~ 50%)</li><li>— due to indequate samples (~ 50%)</li><li>low coverage of target population</li><li>rapid evolution of certain tumours (< 10%)</li></ul> | Ensure appropriate treatment and follow-up of CIN<br><br>Screening interval should not be imposed before application of these conditions | We are still awaiting complete evaluation of each of these systems |

GPs, General practitioners; CIN, cervical intraepithelial neoplasia; HPV, human papillomavirus.

Nowadays, cervical cancer is observed as often among closely monitored women as among those who are not screened. Extending screening to those women who are presently not covered has to be a political decision and depends upon the resources and the means that those in charge will deem necessary in order to ensure the widest possible coverage of the population. This is the main proviso for the success of screening. The present-day problems raised by cervical cancer in regularly monitored women constitute a medical responsibility. The medical profession must find the most appropriate measures for improving the system.

Tables 26.9–26.11 present the various screening strategies used in various countries.

## Conclusions

If organized programmes cannot be introduced in developed countries, the following comments should be taken into consideration:

**Table 26.10** Organized screening programme in developed countries.

| Situation | Actions |
|---|---|
| It has been proved that organized programmes imposing smear tests every 3 years are an effective way of reducing mortality and morbidity from cervical cancer (about 91%)<br>There are:<br>• adequate programmes<br>• inadequate programmes | Spread screening evenly across a wide age range<br>Ensure a high rate of participation among the target population<br>Repeat the test at a suitable interval, not exceeding 3 years<br>Ensure adequate facilities and quality control for both taking and interpreting smears<br>Ensure prompt follow-up and appropriate treatment<br>Call-and-recall must be effective |

**1** The amalgamation between organized screening and spontaneous screening must not be exacerbated.

**2** The most important aspect, increasing the coverage of the target population, remains the responsibility of health authorities.

**3** Invasive cervical cancer occurs in regularly screened women ($\sim 30\%$) and remains the responsibility of the practitioner.

**4** Before deciding on any particular frequency between smear tests, an evaluation should be made of the implications of the following points:

(a) False-negative smears.

(b) Quality control of smears.

(c) Rapidly developing cancers.

(d) Impact of the disease in young women.

(e) Impact of risk factors on the interval between smears.

(f) Cost-effectiveness of spontaneous screening compared to organized programmes.

(g) Defensive medicine.

**Table 26.11** Absence of screening in developing countries.

| Situation | Actions | Perspectives |
|---|---|---|
| Three-quarters of the cases of cervical cancer throughout the world (around 500 000 cases per year)<br>Lack of resources<br>Lack of competence | Downstaging<br><br>Treatment of early cervical cancer (brachytherapy) | Polar probe<br><br>HPV vaccines |

HPV, Human papillomavirus.

The short-term goals will be to gain additional experience with the new technologies including monolayer systems, HPV testing and automation as methods for improving the sensitivity of the smear test. In fact, the screening interval could be appropriately defined. The future goals will be to protect women from papillomavirus infection through the use of effective vaccines.

## References

1 Hakama M, Louhivvori K. A screening programme for cervical cancer that worked. *Cancer Surv* 1988; 7: 403–416.
2 IARC working group on Cervical Cancer Screening. Conclusions. In: Hakama M, Miller AB, Day N (eds). *Screening for Cancer of the Uterine Cervix*. Lyon, France: International Agency of Research on Cancer, 1986, pp 133–142.
3 Raffle AE, Alden B, Mackenzie EFD. Detection rates for abnormal smears: what are we screening for? *Lancet* 1995; **345**: 1469–1473.
4 Koss LG. The Papanicolaou test for cervical cancer detection. A triumph and a tragedy. *JAMA* 1989; **261**: 737–743.
5 Forsmo S, Buhaug H, Stalsberg H. Use of Pap smears in a population without a mass screening program. *Acta Obstet Gynecol Scand* 1994; **73**: 824–828.
6 Slater DN. Multifactorial audit of invasive cervical cancer: key lessons for the national screening programme. *J Clin Pathol* 1995; **48**: 405–407.
7 Boyce JG, Fruchter RG, Romanzi I *et al*. The fallacy of the screening interval for cervical smears. *Obstet Gynecol* 1990; **76**: 627–632.
8 European Guidelines for Quality Assurance in Cervical Cancer Screening. *Eur J Cancer* 1993; **4**: S2.
9 Austoker J. Screening for cervical cancer. *Br Med J* 1994; **309**: 241–248.
10 Muir C, Watherhouse J, Mack T, Powell J, Whelan S. Cancer incidence in five continents. *IARC Sci Publ* 1987; **V**: 88.
11 Chamberlain J. Reasons that some screening programmes fail to control cervical cancer. In: Hakama M, Miller AB, Day N (eds) *Screening for Cancer of the Uterine Cervix*. Lyon: IARC Scientific Publications, 1986, pp 161–168.
12 Peters RK *et al*. Invasive squamous cell carcinoma of the cervix after recent negative cytologic test results. A distinct subgroup? *J Obstet Gynecol* 1988; **158**: 926–935.
13 Janerich DT *et al*. The screening histories of women with invasive cervical cancer, Connecticut [see comments]. *Am J Public Health* 1995; **85**: 791–794.
14 Monsonego J. Dépistage spontané du cancer du col: faits et arguments. *Réf Gynécol Obstet* 1995; **3**: 147–162.
15 Miller AB. *Cervical Cancer Screening Programmes Managerial Guidelines*. Geneva: World Health Organization, 1992; p 23.
16 Wilson SH, Johnson J. An audit of cervical cancer deaths in Nottingham. *Cytopathology* 1992; **3**: 79–83.
17 Morell ND, Tyler JR, Snyder RN. False negative cytology rate in patients in whom invasive cervical cancer subsequently developed. *Obstet Gynecol* 1982; **60**: 41–45.
18 Mitchell H, Medleu G, Giles G. Cervical cancers diagnosed after negative results on cervical cytology; perspectives for the 1980s. *BMJ* 1990; **300**: 1622–1626.
19 Kristensen GB. Skyggebjerg KD, Holund B *et al*. Analysis of cervical smears obtained within three years of a diagnosis of invasive cervical cancer. *Acta Cytol* 1991; **35**: 47–50.
20 Smith HK, Bostron SG, Galey WT. Correlation between cervical cytology and biopsy in an airforce colposcopy clinic. *J Repro Med* 1985, **30**: 681–684.

21  Wetrich DW. An analysis of factors involved in the colposcopic evaluation of 2194 patients with abnormal Papanicolaou smears. *Am J Obstet Gynecol* 1986; **154**: 1339–1349.

22  Walker EM, Dodgson J, Duncan ID. Does mild atypia on a cervical smear warrant further investigation? *Lancet* 1986; **ii**: 672–673.

23  Giles JA, Deery A, Crow J, Walker P. The accuracy of repeat cytology in women with mildly dyskaryotic smears. *Br J Obstet Gynaecol* 1989; **96**: 1067–1070.

24  Wheelock JM, Kaminsky PF. Value of repeat cytology at the time of the colposcopy for the evaluation of cervical intraepithelial neoplasia on Papanicolaou smears. *J Reprod Med* 1989; **34**: 815–817.

25  Beeby AR, Wadehra V, Keating P, Wagstaff T. A retrospective analysis of 94 patients with CIN and false negative smears taken at colposcopy. *Cytopathology* 1993; **4**: 331–337.

26  Jarmulowicz MR, Jenkins D, Barton SE, Singer A. Cytological status of lesion size; a further dimension in cervical intraepithelial neoplasia. *Br J Obstet Gynaecol* 1989; **96**: 1061–1066.

27  Tidbury P, Singer A. CIN 3. The role of lesion size in invasion. *Br J Obstet Gynaecol* 1992; **99**: 583–587.

28  Jones MH, Jenkins D, Cusick J *et al*. Mild cervical dyskaryosis; safety of cytological surveillance. *Lancet* 1992; **339**: 1442–1443.

29  Hartmann B, Kaplan B, Boone D. Morphometrics analysis of dysplasia and carcinoma *in situ* in cone biopsy specimens in cases with false-negative cytology. *Obstet Gynecol* 1986; **68**: 832–837.

30  Gay JD, Donaldson LD, Goellner JR. False negative cytology rates. *Acta Cytol* 1985; **29**: 1043.

31  Enquête sur le Dépistage du cancer du col auprès des gynécologues. *Gynécol Obstét Pratique* 1996; **81**: 1–5.

32  Anderson MC. Invasive carcinoma of the cervix following local destructive treatment for cervical intraepithelial neoplasia. *Br J Obstet Gynaecol* 1993; **100**: 657–663.

33  De Vathaire F et réseau Francim. *Cancer du Col de l'Utérus: Estimation de l'incidence du cancer du col en France entre 1983 et 1987*. Editions de l'INSERM, 1997 (in press).

34  Enquête sur le Dépistage du cancer du col auprès des Médecins Généralistes. *Impact Médecin Hebdo* 1994; **231**: 24–26.

35  American Cancer Society. Guidelines for the cancer-related checkup: recommendations and rationale. *CA* 1980; **30**: 195–230.

36  American College of Obstetricians and Gynecologists. *The Frequency with which a Cervical-vaginal Smear should be Performed in Gynecologic Practice*. ACOG technical bulletin n° 29. Washington; DC: American College of Obstetricians and Gynecologists, 1975.

37  Monsonego J. Opportunistic screening of cervical cancer. In: Monsonego J (ed) *Screening for Cervical Neoplasia: For Whom, Why and How?* Paris: EUROGIN Scientific Publications, 1995.

38  Monsonego J. Quelle est l'evolution naturelle des dysplasies du col? *Gyn Obs* 1992; **284**: 1–5.

39  Robertson J, Woodend B. Letter to the editor: Cervical screening: what is the point? *Lancet* 1995; **346**: 245.

40  Bjorge T, Gunbjorud AB, Langmark F *et al*. Cervical mass screening in Norway – 510 000 smears a year. *Cancer Detect Prev* 1994; **18**: 463–470.

41  Cuzik J, Szarewski A, Terry G *et al*. Human papillomavirus testing in primary cervical screening. *Lancet* 1995; **345**: 1533–1536.

42  Koutsky LA, Holmes KK, Critchlow CW *et al*. Cohort study of risk of cervical

intraepithelial neoplasia grade 2 or 3 associated with cervical papillomavirus infection. *N Engl J Med* 1992; **327**: 1272–1279.

43 Cuzik J, Terry G, Ho L *et al*. Human papillomavirus type 16 in cervical smears as a predictor of high grade cervical intraepithelial neoplasia. *Lancet* 1992; **339**: 959–960.

44 Fruchler RG, Maiman M, Sillman FH *et al*. Characteristics of cervical intraepithelial neoplasia in women infected with HIV. *Am J Obstet Gynecol* 1994; **171**: 531–537.

45 Fahey MT, Irwig L, Macaskill P. Metaanalysis of Pap test accuracy. *Am J Epidemiol* 1995; **141**: 680–689.

# 27: Is Cervical Cancer Cytological Screening Valuable in Developing Countries?

R. Herrero,[1] M. H. Schiffman,[2] A. Hildesheim,[2] C. Bratti,[3]
A. C. Rodriguez,[4] M. E. Sherman[2] & J. Morales[5]

## Summary

Cytological screening is considered a valuable tool for reducing the incidence and mortality from cancer of the cervix. However, several developing countries have established programmes that have been in operation for a number of years with very limited or no impact at all in the corresponding indicators. For example, in Costa Rica, the age-adjusted incidence of cervical cancer has remained around 24 per 100 000 women during the last 12 years, without evidence of a decreasing trend for any specific age group. Incidences twice as high are reported from the less developed areas in the country.

We present a preliminary analysis of results from a survey and screening of a random sample of 10 049 women in Guanacaste, a high-risk province of Costa Rica. A vast majority of the women report having had a Papanicolaou (Pap) test at least once (87%), and almost 70% report having had one in the previous 3 years. In addition, almost 75% report having had more than one examination. Screening is more common among women between 25 and 54 years of age and is also correlated with higher education, higher socioeconomic level and a history of having used oral contraceptives. Women with invasive cancer and high-grade cervical intraepithelial neoplasia have been screened almost as frequently as women without disease, indicating that the screening programme operates ineffectively. These results suggest that in this area,

*Correspondence*: Dr Rolando Herrero, Unit of Field and Intervention Studies, International Agency for Research on Cancer, 150 Cours Albert Thomas, F-69372 Lyon Cédex 08, France.
[1]Unit of Field and Intervention Studies, International Agency for Research on Cancer, 150, Cours Albert Thomas, F-69372 Lyon Cédex 08, France; [2]Environmental Epidemiology Branch, National Cancer Institute, Bethesda, MD, USA; [3]Guanacaste Project, FU-CODOCSA, Caja Costarricense de Seguro Social, Costa Rica; [4]National Tumor Registry, Ministry of Health, Costa Rica; [5]Caja Costarricense de Seguro Social, Costa Rica.

despite the relatively high participation of the population in the screening, the disease remains largely uncontrolled. A reorganization is proposed, including the centralization of laboratories and treatment facilities and the establishment of a country-wide information system. The results of screening in this area could be improved by optimization of the use of resources already available.

## Introduction

Despite recognized limitations, cervical cancer screening is considered a successful public health intervention that is at least partially responsible for the significant decline in incidence and mortality observed in the last few decades in several developed countries [1].

However, the incidence and mortality from cervical cancer remain very high in most developing countries, particularly in Latin America, Africa and South-East Asia, where it is often the leading cancer among women [2]. In most countries in those regions, the availability of incidence data is limited, but in the majority of those where such data are available, the declines in incidence from cervical cancer are very limited or non-existent. This is so despite the fact that, in some of these areas, important amounts of resources are devoted to cytological screening, and programmes of varying intensity and organizational level have been in place for a number of years.

In Costa Rica, for example, a small country in Central America with 3.5 million inhabitants and a national health system, screening activities have been available for at least 20 years, but very limited impact on the incidence has been observed. In this report we present incidence data from Costa Rica and use preliminary results from a recent population-based survey and screening to analyse screening behaviour in this population in relation to prevalent cervical disease.

## Materials and methods

Age-specific rates of invasive cervical cancer are presented, based on data from the National Tumor Registry of Costa Rica. The Registry has been in operation since 1977, achieving national coverage by 1980. It receives mandatory reports of all cases o cancer occurring within the universal health system that exists in the country. All pathology and health statistics departments, either public or private, submit reports of any cancer diagnosed to the Tumor Registry, which is a dependency of the Ministry of Health. The Registry verifies and codes the reports and keeps a computerized database for the preparation of cancer statistics, which are included in the last two editions of *Cancer Incidence in Five Continents* [3].

Age-specific rates are calculated by dividing the number of cases in a specific age group by the population in that sex/age group. Age-standardized rates are calculated by applying age-specific rates to the age structure of the world population. We restrict the analysis to the period 1982–1993, because the quality of the registration process is considered more reliable from there on. For the year 1981, slightly higher rates were observed, but this is thought to be related to the inclusion of prevalent cases when the registry started.

We also present results of the Guanacaste project, a population-based survey of 10 049 randomly selected women conducted in Guanacaste, a province of Costa Rica with a high incidence of cervical cancer. Methodological aspects of the study are presented elsewhere [4]. Briefly, a random sample of approximately 20% of the sensus segments in the province was selected, and enumeration of adult women residing in those segments was performed by staff of the Costa Rican Ministry of Health. The 11 742 women in the sample were invited to participate by personal letters to the nearest local government clinics, where study staff performed the corresponding procedures between June 1993 and December 1994. Eligible women (after exclusion of the pregnant and mentally or physically ill) signed informed consent and were interviewed on demographic and socioeconomic characteristics, cervical cancer risk factors and screening histories. On those reporting previous sexual activity, a pelvic examination was performed and cervical cells for cytological analysis were collected. The analysis of the smears was done blindly and independently using the Bethesda system, based on three different methods: conventional smear read as usual, conventional smear read with the aid of computer analysis (Neuromedical Systems Inc., Suffern, NY) and monolayer cytology (Cytyc, Marlborough, MA). In addition, a cervigram (magnified photograph of the cervix) was performed after application of acetic acid and interpreted by an expert colposcopist. Any cytological or cervicographic abnormality prompted referral to colpobiopsy, complete diagnostic work-up and treatment of significant lesions. Final diagnoses were defined after review of all available materials for each subject.

A total of 10 738 women were eligible for interview and of those, 10 049 were interviewed (93.6%). After exclusion of women without prior sexual activity, 9466 were considered eligible for a pelvic exam, and such an exam was performed on 9175 women (96.9%). Twelve women in the sample were diagnosed with invasive cervical cancer, corresponding to a prevalence of 0.14% (excluding hysterectomized women from the denominator). Another 128 were diagnosed with high-grade cervical intraepithelial neoplasia (CIN) giving a prevalence of 1.5%, and 189 were diagnosed with low-grade CIN for a prevalence of 2.2%. The rest were either equivocal or normal diagnoses.

In this report, we present descriptive data on the screening histories of the population in the study. Cross-tabulations of the screening variables with questionnaire data and with the final diagnosis are presented.

**Table 27.1** Incidence of invasive cervical cancer in Costa Rica, 1982–1993.

| Year | Cases* | Crude rate |
|------|--------|------------|
| 1982 | 209 | 17.4 |
| 1983 | 222 | 18.0 |
| 1984 | 221 | 17.4 |
| 1985 | 233 | 17.8 |
| 1986 | 240 | 17.9 |
| 1987 | 263 | 19.1 |
| 1988 | 273 | 19.3 |
| 1989 | 259 | 17.8 |
| 1990 | 262 | 17.6 |
| 1991 | 273 | 17.9 |
| 1992 | 261 | 16.7 |
| 1993 | 290 | 18.1 |

Data from National Tumor Registry, Ministry of Health, Costa Rica.
*Excludes 44 cases reported as 'death certificate only' (DCO).

## Results

Table 27.1 presents the number of cases and crude rates per 100 000 women for the whole country from 1982 to 1993. The rates during the period have remained very stable, at around 18 per 100 000 women (corresponding to an age-adjusted rate of 24 per 100 000). However, as expected given stable rates, the number of cases has increased over time, with the consequent additional burden to the health services.

Figure 27.1 presents age-specific incidence rates per 100 000 women in

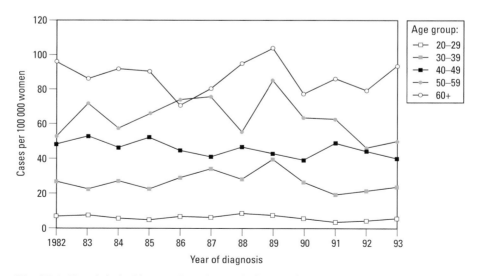

**Fig. 27.1** Trends in incidence of invasive cervical cancer in Costa Rica by age group, 1982–1993. Data from National Tumor Registry, Costa Rica, with permission.

**Table 27.2** Average annual incidence of invasive cervical cancer in Costa Rica, 1982–1993, by province.

| Province | Cases in period* | Crude rate | ASR |
|---|---|---|---|
| San José | 1192 | 24.0 | 29.3 |
| Alajuela | 385 | 17.3 | 23.9 |
| Cartago | 255 | 17.1 | 23.5 |
| Heredia | 205 | 17.6 | 21.6 |
| Guanacaste | 285 | 31.2 | 42.7 |
| Puntarenas | 388 | 28.2 | 47.0 |
| Limón | 272 | 28.8 | 45.4 |

ASR, Age-standardized rates, adjusted for the world propulation.
Data from National Tumor Registry, Ministry of Health, Costa Rica.
*Cases of unknown residence excluded.

different age groups for the years 1982–1993. The rates are increasingly higher for each 10-year age group, but are remarkably stable over the 12-year period within all age groups.

Table 27.2 presents incidence rates by province in Costa Rica. The three coastal provinces (Limón, Guanacaste and Puntarenas) present the highest incidence rates in the period, almost reaching an age-adjusted incidence of 50 per 100 000 women, which doubles the national rate and is among the highest reported in the world. The population survey described below was conducted in Guanacaste and will be used as an example of the screening situation in the country.

The population of Guanacaste, as shown in the survey is relatively young, with a median age of 37 years. It is characterized by low educational levels, with only 32% having gone beyond elementary school, and low income, with a vast majority of women reporting an estimated family income under US$ 4100 per year. Regarding sexual behaviour, 54% report having had only one life-time sexual partner, and only 12% report four or more. The population is also characterized by high parity, with almost 40% reporting more than five pregnancies. Smoking is uncommon (11% ever) and 60% of the women have used oral contraceptives. In addition, 6.8% of the participants reported having had a hysterectomy.

Table 27.3 presents cervical cytological screening histories of the women in the sample. A total of 87% reported ever having been screened at least once. Sixty per cent of the participants reported having had a Pap smear in the last 2 years, according to the local medical recommendation, and 70% reported having had one in the last 3 years. More than 50% of these women reported having had at least four examinations in their life-time and about 75% reported at least two.

Table 27.4 presents screening histories in different age groups. The proportion of women who have never been screened is naturally higher among the

**Table 27.3** Screening histories* of women in Guanacaste.

|  | Number | (%) |
|---|---|---|
| *Ever had a Pap?* |  |  |
| Yes | 8208 | 86.8 |
| No | 1242 | 13.2 |
| *Interval since last Pap (months)* |  |  |
| 0–12 | 3814 | 40.7 |
| 13–24 | 1805 | 19.2 |
| 25–36 | 905 | 9.6 |
| 37–48 | 477 | 5.1 |
| 49–60 | 283 | 3.0 |
| 61+ | 855 | 9.1 |
| Never | 1242 | 13.2 |
| *Number of Paps in life-time* |  |  |
| 0 | 1242 | 13.2 |
| 1 | 1176 | 12.4 |
| 2 | 1078 | 11.4 |
| 3 | 1164 | 12.3 |
| 4 | 1054 | 11.2 |
| 5–6 | 1420 | 15.0 |
| 7+ | 2316 | 24.5 |

* Restricted to women reporting previous sexual activity.
Pap, Papanicolaou test.

**Table 27.4** Screening histories* by age, Guanacaste.

| Age (years) | *n* | Never Pap | No recent Pap† | Recent Pap‡ |
|---|---|---|---|---|
| 18–19 | 241 | 45.6 | 1.2 | 53.1 |
| 20–24 | 938 | 22.7 | 7.5 | 69.8 |
| 25–29 | 1321 | 8.7 | 12.8 | 78.5 |
| 30–34 | 1373 | 6.3 | 13.9 | 79.8 |
| 35–39 | 1183 | 4.6 | 16.9 | 78.5 |
| 40–44 | 979 | 4.7 | 17.5 | 77.8 |
| 45–49 | 791 | 6.2 | 18.8 | 75.0 |
| 50–54 | 593 | 8.0 | 25.3 | 66.0 |
| 55–59 | 525 | 13.7 | 26.1 | 60.2 |
| 60–64 | 453 | 18.8 | 29.4 | 52.0 |
| 65–69 | 370 | 25.7 | 24.6 | 49.7 |
| 70–75 | 297 | 34.3 | 25.3 | 40.4 |
| 75+ | 317 | 51.4 | 24.0 | 24.6 |

* Restricted to women with previous sexual activity.
† No Pap in the last 36 months.
‡ Pap in the last 36 months.

young until age 24, but from that age to age 54, only about 5% of the women report never having been screened. However, after age 55, the percentage of women who have never been screened increases consistently up to more than 50% among those 75 or older. The proportion of women who have not had a Pap in the last 36 months increases after age 50 but remains constant at around 25% until advanced ages. Thus, almost 80% of women between 25 and 49 years of age report having had a Pap in the previous 36 months, this proportion decreasing steadily afterwards to a low of 25% for the group of 75 years or older. Furthermore, in the group of women aged 25–49, more than 85% have had at least two Paps, and more than 75% have had three or more examinations (data not shown). Other positive correlates of screening, education and income, were increasing as well as previous use of oral contraceptives.

Table 27.5 presents the intervals since last examination by final diagnosis. The intervals since last examination are similar for all the diagnoses, with the exception of women with invasive cancer, among whom the proportion without a Pap in the last 5 years was twice that of the other groups. It must be noted, however, that there is only a small number of invasive cancers in this series.

All the 12 women with cancer reported having had a Pap smear before, 4 (33%) of them within 1 year before our diagnoses (2 in the previous 3 months and 2 at least 7 months before diagnosis). However, of those having had a Pap in the last 12 months, only 2 had been told that they ever had an abnormal Pap (not necessarily the last one). Nine (75%) of the invasive cervical cancer cases had had a Pap in the previous 5 years.

Of the women with high-grade CIN, 83.4% reported having had a Pap in their life, 34.6% within 1 year and 65% within 3 years. Twenty-four per cent of the women diagnosed with high-grade CIN reported having been told that they had an abnormal Pap in the past. When interpreting these findings, it

**Table 27.5** Interval since last Papanicolaou test (Pap) by final diagnosis (per cent in each category).

| Interval (months) | Cancer ($n = 11$) | High-grade CIN* ($n = 127$) | Low-grade CIN† ($n = 188$) | Normal/other ($n = 8162$) |
|---|---|---|---|---|
| 0–12 | 36.4 | 34.6 | 42.0 | 41.7 |
| 13–24 | 27.3 | 20.5 | 19.2 | 19.9 |
| 25–36 | 9.1 | 11.0 | 10.1 | 9.6 |
| 37–60 | 9.1 | 8.7 | 5.9 | 8.0 |
| 61+ | 18.2 | 8.7 | 6.9 | 8.3 |
| Never | 0.0 | 16.5 | 16.0 | 12.5 |

Excludes hysterectomized women, women without a pelvic exam and unknowns.
HSIL, High-grade squamous intraepithelial lesion; LSIL, low-grade squamous intraepithelial lesion.
* Includes CIN 2 and CIN 3.
† Includes CIN 1 and koilocytotic atypia.

should be kept in mind that the screening examinations that lead to the diagnosis in the study were done after administering the interview; thus, possible bias was minimized.

## Discussion

Screening has been available through a national health care system in Costa Rica during at least the last 20 years. Mortality from cervical cancer has decreased to some extent in Costa Rica during the last 35 years [5], probably as a result of reductions in parity and other risk factors, better access to treatment and detection at earlier clinical stages. However, incidence remains at high levels since adequate registry data are available, particularly in certain areas of the country. Most countries where screening programmes are in operation describe reductions in incidence mainly among the younger groups, which are more likely to participate in such programmes. In the case of Costa Rica there is no apparent continuing beneficial effect of screening for any age group, at least during the last 12 years examined.

We present preliminary data from a recently completed survey and screening conducted in Guanacaste, one of the provinces with the highest incidence of cervical cancer in the country, to investigate the patterns of utilization of screening. It is clear that the majority of women participate with a relatively high frequency both in terms of intervals and number of Paps reported. Women in the younger age groups and those with better education and socioeconomic conditions, as well as those who have used oral contraceptives, are more frequently screened.

Interestingly, 80% of the women in the 25–49 age group report having been screened in the last 3 years and most of them also report having had multiple examinations. If this pattern, or one with even higher participation, is present in the country as a whole (which is likely, given that Guanacaste is one of the poorest provinces), we would expect some impact on the incidence of the disease, at least in the age groups that appear to be covered. However, such an impact is not observed in the country, suggesting that screening as currently practised is ineffective. Alternatively the current level of activity of the programme might be keeping under control what would otherwise have been a recent increase in incidence.

With the exception of invasive cancers, that were more likely to have an extended period since their last examination than women with CIN or normal diagnoses, the percentages of women having had an exam and the intervals since the last examination were very similar for the different diagnostic groups. In a previous case-control study of screening in four Latin American countries, we described some protective effect of screening against invasive cancer [6]. In that study, risk associated with lack of screening was highest for women who had never had a Pap (relative risk = 3.0, confidence interval = 2.3–4.0). However, we also noted that an important proportion of the cases (32%) had relatively recent histories of screening (12–47 months), even when excluding diagnostic Paps.

The fact that around 70% of the cancers and high-grade CINs in the study report a Pap in the last 3 years is worrisome because, theoretically, an important proportion of those women already had disease when examined, and should have been detected and treated. Screening programmes require high coverage of the population, smears that are appropriately taken and read, and further diagnosis and treatment of neoplastic lesions [1]. We do not have data at this moment to determine at what levels the failure of the system occurred, but it is clear that it was not related to a lack of participation of the patients. The high participation rates in the Guanacaste project (93.6%) also demonstrate the potential compliance of this population.

We have in the past described the possible reasons for the lack of impact of the screening programme in Costa Rica [7] and proposed a reorganization based on the establishment of a central coordinating unit, the centralization of the many small laboratories that operate without quality control in the country, the creation of a national information system to monitor the activities of the programme and the establishment of a colposcopy and treatment network. Less intensive screening of improved quality may be cost-effective in this setting and major improvements could be made by better use of available resources.

## Acknowledgement

This study was supported by contracts N01-CP-21081 and N01-CP-31061 of the National Cancer Institute, National Institutes of Health, USA.

## References

1 Pontén J, Adami H-O, Bergström R et al. Strategies for global control of cervical cancer. *Int J Cancer* 1995; **60**: 1–26.
2 Parkin DM, Pisani P, Ferlay J. Estimates of the worldwide incidence of 18 major cancers in 1985. *Int J Cancer* 1992; **54**: 594–606.
3 IARC, World Health Organization. *Cancer Incidence in Five Continents.* vol. VI. IARC Scientific Publications no. 120. Lyon: International Agency for Research on Cancer, 1992.
4 Herrero R, Schiffman MH, Bratti C et al. Design and methods of a population-based natural history study of cervical neoplasia in a rural province of Costa Rica: the Guanacaste project. *Bull PAHO* (in press).
5 IARC, World Health Organization, UICC. *Trends in Cancer Incidence and Mortality.* IARC Scientific Publication no. 121. Lyon: International Agency for Research on Cancer, 1993.
6 Herrero R, Brinton LA, Reeves WC. Screening for cervical cancer in Latin America: a case-control study. *Int J Epidemiol* 1992; **21**: 1050–1056.
7 Caja Costarricense de Seguro Social. *Programa Nacional de Deteccion y Control de Cancer de Cuello del Utero.* Costa Rica: CCSS, 1992.

# 28: Screening in Cervical Cancer Prevention in Porto Alegre, Brazil: The Experience of a Programme in a Developing Country

P. Naud,[1-4] M. C. Bozzetti,[2,4] J. C. Prolla,[2,3,5] E. Becker, Jr,[2,4]
A. Camozzato,[2,4] R. Siegle,[2-4] T. P. Duarte,[2-4] P. P. Zanatta Filho,[2-4]
G. B. Lima,[2-4] J. Cavagnolli,[2,4] J. C. Mattos,[2,4] A. R. Timm[2,4] & C. I. Filho[4,6]

## Summary

Cervical cancer is a major worldwide public health problem, corresponding to 15% of all cancer diagnosed in women. About 80% are among women in developing countries.

Since cervical cancer is a potentially preventable disease, cytological mass screening and effective health educational programmes to detect and to reduce all cervical cancer precursor lesions would have an effect in reducing the risk of developing cervical cancer among the population at risk. Also, adequate treatment of sexually transmissible diseases would have an impact in reducing the incidence of this type of cancer due to its strong relationship with sexual activity.

The current national situation indicates cervical cancer in Brazil as a strong public health problem. Morbidity and mortality data vary among regions within the country, mostly because of under-registration. According to available official information, cervical cancer ranks first among all cancers in women, corresponding to 23.6%, skin cancer ranks second (22.5%) and breast cancer is third – 15.1% of all cancers diagnosed in women in Brazil.

Human papillomavirus (HPV) infection is highly associated with the development of precursor lesions and cancer of the cervix. A previous study coordinated by the Department of Gynecology at the Federal University of Rio Grande Sul, which enrolled 190 women with clinical evidence of HPV infection, indicated that in 85% the location of the lesion was the uterine

*Correspondence*: Dr Paulo Naud, Av. Soledade, 234, Porto Alegre, RS, Brazil.
[1]Department of Gynecology; [2]Hospital de Clinicas de Porto Alegre; [3]Federal University of Rio Grande do Sul; [4]EUROGIN/BRAZIL; [5]Citology Department; [6]State Health Department.

cervix alone; and in 15% the lesions were located in the cervix and/or vagina and/or vulva.

As cervical cancer is a preventable disease, the need for a national information system with a regular update and quality control to understand the real situation in Brazil would help to evaluate the impact of screening mass programmes and health education programmes on reducing and even eliminating this disease, which is a major public health problem.

## Introduction

Cervical cancer accounts for approximately 15% of all cancer diagnosed in women in the world. About 80% of these cases occur in developing countries, where cancer of the cervix is consistently the leading cancer among women [1]. It ranks fifth when all cancer sites for both sexes are combined, accounting for 7.3% of all human cancers [2].

The importance of cervical cancer as a public health problem, particularly in developing countries, makes the knowledge of its incidence and its variation in distinct regions of the world one of the first tasks in understanding the problem. An adequate system of epidemiological investigation is essential to further the development of efficient programmes to prevent and control progress of the disease [3].

Cervical cancer is a potentially preventable disease. The well-established benefit from screening and the existence of an effective treatment contribute to the reduction of incidence and mortality of the disease. Health education programmes focused on reducing sexually transmissible diseases would also have an effect in reducing the incidence of cervical cancer due to its strong relationship to sexual activity. Considering the extent of the problem in developing countries, various measures could be taken to approach the problem. Among them are taking Papanicolaou (Pap) smears of all population at risk of developing cancer of the cervix, performing colposcopy in women with abnormal exams and collecting biopsy specimens of the lesion in reference centres for adequate treatment.

The present study aims to evaluate different approaches to further the development of screening programmes, adequately identify the population at risk of developing cancer of the cervix and therefore reduce the disease incidence and mortality.

## The current national situation

A rational programme is only possible with an adequate registry system. Within Brazil, the reliability of specific morbidity and mortality data varies between regions, and the major contributory factor is under-registration. Such

**Table 28.1** Age-specific incidence rates of *in situ* and invasive carcinoma of the uterus (Brazil: 1976–1980).

| Age (years) | Carcinoma-*in-situ* n (%) | Invasive carcinoma n (%) | Total n (%) |
|---|---|---|---|
| 15–19 | 28 (58.3) | 20 (41.7) | 48 (100.0) |
| 20–24 | 313 (61.7) | 194 (38.3) | 504 (100.0) |
| 25–29 | 1025 (56.1) | 802 (43.9) | 1827 (100.0) |
| 30–34 | 1531 (46.9) | 1734 (53.1) | 3265 (100.0) |
| 35–39 | 1737 (36.8) | 2977 (63.2) | 4714 (100.0) |
| 40–44 | 1634 (30.5) | 3728 (69.5) | 5362 (100.0) |
| 45–49 | 1400 (25.7) | 4037 (74.3) | 5437 (100.0) |
| 50–54 | 809 (17.7) | 3156 (82.3) | 4565 (100.0) |
| 55–59 | 482 (14.0) | 2955 (86.0) | 3437 (100.0) |
| 60–64 | 298 (11.2) | 2369 (88.8) | 2667 (100.0) |
| Total | 9257 (29.1) | 22572 (70.9) | 31829 (100.0) |

factors directly affect the statistical analysis of morbidity and mortality data throughout the country [4,5].

Table 28.1 describes the age-specific incidence of carcinoma-*in-situ* and invasive carcinoma diagnoses in the same time period. The age-specific incidence rates of carcinoma-*in-situ* are higher among younger women and the age-specific incidence rates of invasive carcinoma are higher among older women.

Incidence rates of the disease for the City of Porto Alegre, located in southern Brazil, are presented in Table 28.2. The data show no difference in incidence rates for the two periods. Such figures reach about 46.5 and 35.1 per 100 000 women in Fortaleza and São Paulo, respectively [1].

In 1986, 73 897 people died due to cancer [4] in Brazil. Cancer ranks second among all causes of mortality in women accounting for 13.4% of all deaths. Mortality data for Rio Grande do Sul are shown in Table 28.3.

Comparing data from Table 28.3 with Table 28.2; it may be suggested that, even though there was no apparent changes in incidence rates over the period, mortality rates have increased, indicating a possible failure or inadequacy in a secondary level of prevention such as treatment of precursor lesions.

The available data presented here reinforce the importance of cervical

**Table 28.2** Incidence rates of cervical cancer for the city of Porto Alegre, State of Rio Grande do Sul (1979–1982 and 1990).

| Time period | Incidence (per 100 000 women) |
|---|---|
| 1979–1982 | 23.7 |
| 1990 | 23.8 |

**Table 28.3** Age-standardized rates on mortality data for the city of Porto Alegre and the State of Rio Grande do Sul, Brazil (1970–1992).

| Year | Mortality (per 100 000 women) | |
|------|-------------|------------------|
|      | Porto Alegre | Rio Grande do Sul |
| 1970 | 4.95 | 2.18 |
| 1980 | 7.23 | 4.41 |
| 1990 | 6.30 | 5.22 |
| 1991 | 5.64 | 5.82 |
| 1992 | 7.78 | 5.85 |

cancer as a public health problem. Its prevention through early detection and treatment would certainly have an impact on its morbidity and mortality, and would alter the present figures on cost–benefit of such an important disease.

## Cytological screening

In Brazil, the Ministry of Health recommends that all women aged 25 years or older who are sexually active should have a smear taken annually and repeated triannually after two consecutive normal smears taken in the recommended interval, even though some believe that, due to the high prevalence of sexually transmissible diseases, the early age at first intercourse and the low socioeconomic status of the Brazilian population, women aged 15 years and up who are sexually active should also be recommended for prevention programmes. However, a careful evaluation of the effect of such an approach on programme cost–benefits, which are well described elsewhere [6], should be considered before introducing such a recommendation into screening programmes. It is the proposal of the present protocol to initiate the screening programme with women 35 years and older and in future to extend it to younger women (25 years and older).

Even though there are federal recommendations, the feasibility of such prevention programmes varies greatly within the country. Each state coordinates its own actions in public health and the differences, including financial and staffing resources, create important limitations for an adequate development of such programmes.

In the state of Rio Grande do Sul, the state's Secretary of Health is responsible for planning and implementing the state cervical cancer screening programme; however, it does not consider a significant number of exams taken in hospitals and in private clinics which may follow a different scheme for screening women at risk. In addition, even though recommendations exist, smears are not taken on a regular basis. The state has its own laboratories for reading smears, which may differ from other private and public services. In

1993, 146 308 exams were performed, where the most frequent abnormality reported was cervical intraepithelial neoplasia (CIN) grade I (29% of abnormal exams), followed by CIN grade II (17%), CIN grade III (17%), carcinoma epidermoid (7%) and adenocarcinoma (2%). These are official results from the state Secretary of Health data bank and include women of all ages.

## Epidemiological predictors of high risk

Prevention and treatment of the precursor lesions are the key to avoiding cervical cancer, so the Bethesda classification, which indicates low-grade (CIN I) and high-grade CIN (CIN II and III), is of prognostic and therapeutic significance, considering that the relative risk of a lesion to progress either carcinoma-*in-situ* or a cytological abnormality depends on its grade and/or its correlation with histological abnormalities. The relative risks in relation to cervical cancer are shown in Table 28.4 [6].

Several epidemiological studies have studied and established the risk factors for cervical neoplasia [7–14]. The major and most important factor for deciding on the target population to allow us to obtain an optimal cost–benefit relationship is age. Therefore we should include patients within the age group at risk of developing the disease. However, sexual activity is also strongly associated with cervical cancer, therefore, we believe that even though incidence rates of cervical cancer are higher among women over 35 years of age [6], and based on official data which show that a considerable number of cases are younger than 35 years of age, it should be a further aim of the programme to screen younger women to detect and treat precursor lesions which may be either premalignant lesions of sexually transmissible diseases (particularly HPV infections) affecting younger women.

## Implementation of a screening programme

Some considerations have to be established for the implementation of a screening programme to detect and avoid cancer of the cervix:
1  Epidemiological evidence that cervical cancer is a public health problem.
2  Ethics and behavioural characteristics of the population.

Table 28.4 Relative risks of initial diagnosis in relation to cervical cancer.

| Initial diagnosis | Relative risk |
| --- | --- |
| Control | 1.0 |
| CIN I | 4.0 |
| CIN II | 14.5 |
| CIN III | 46.5 |

From Miller [6] with permission. CIN, Cervical intraepithelial neoplasia.

3   Establishing a target population.
4   Appropriate health system.
5   Technical conditions in taking, reading and interpreting smears.
6   Adequate conditions for diagnosis, follow-up and treatment.
7   Adequate information system.

For those patients whose smear shows any abnormality, adequate treatment and follow-up are important. In Brazil, school hospitals are among the institutions that can offer specific and specialized care to the at-risk population. In addition, national and regional public health policies related to prevention programmes, including cervical cancer, change their guidelines with each new government.

## Screening modalities for cervical cancer: a review

### Cytology (cervical smear)

Screening by cytology using Papanicolaou smear is a well-established method. Several studies have shown the impact on the incidence of cervical cancer and mortality of cytological screening programmes. This method has, however, some pitfalls. For instance, it may not be cost-effective if the majority of screened women are at low risk. Mostly as a result of scarce financial and staffing resources, many developing countries have failed to establish good screening programmes at a national level and any such country would probably benefit more by adopting selective screening of women that can be identified at high risk of developing cervical cancer. Even though this corresponds to reality, it is also true that, at present, the majority of cases are likely to be found among normal and low-risk women. Therefore, by not limiting the screening population to those at higher-risk, we may have a higher impact upon the population.

### Cervicography

This technique involves the preparation of the cervix in a similar way as for colposcopy. The cervix is visualized in a self-retaining speculum. A specifically designed hand-held camera (cerviscope) is used. An electronic data bank permits accurate identification of the slides (cervigrams) of each patient. Its sensitivity and specificity in relation to cytological screening have yet not been established.

### Cervical inspection

Cervical inspection has always been part of cervical cytology screening; however, its contribution to screening programmes has not been established.

Demonstration of the effectiveness of such an approach would probably have an important impact on screening costs, assuming that only women with suspected findings at cervical inspection would be selected for cytological screening. This would be particularly helpful for the introduction and development of screening programmes in developing countries where financial and staffing resources have been the greatest inhibitors to furthering the development of such programmes.

Cervical visualization requires good light and an examination table, preferably with stirrups, swabs and a vaginal speculum. Approaches to visualization include unaided visual inspection of the untreated cervix (aimed at detecting early cancer) and aided visual inspection of the acetic acid-treated cervix (aimed at detecting CIN III).

During the examination, lesion and/or cervical abnormalities seen on inspection, through the Schiller test, will also be referred for further investigation.

## Aims of screening

### General goals

The general goals of screening are to further the development of strategies, in our setting; to screen adequately the population at risk of developing cancer of the cervix; and to reduce disease incidence and mortality.

### Objectives

1   To screen women at risk of developing cancer of the cervix.
2   To evaluate the required strategies to maintain an adequate participation rate and follow-up of subjects.
3   To determine the prevalence of premalignant lesions among women considered at high risk of developing cervical neoplasm.
4   To treat adequately all cervical lesions that may progress to cervical cancer.
5   To evaluate the impact of the programme on morbidity and mortality of cervical cancer.
6   To determine the cost-effectiveness of a screening programme based on unaided visualization compared to cervical cytology.
7   To evaluate the effect of the screening programme on hospital costs in the treatment of cervical cancer (surgery and all other therapeutic approaches).
8   To make recommendations for a national policy on cervical cancer screening based on the pilot study results.
9   To promote and diffuse cervical cancer screening programmes not only to the general population but also to health professionals (gynaecologists, family

doctors, nurses and other related professionals) who have contact or work with the population at risk of developing the disease of interest.

## Methodology

### Selection of the screening centre

The gynaecology department at the Hospital de Clinicas de Porto Alegre (HCPA) was chosen as the setting for the pilot study as it had the qualified staff and the infrastructure to conduct the study in order to reach its aims.

### Study design

This is a pilot study which has been planned to evaluate different approaches for cervical cancer screening in a cohort of women age 35–64 years attending the gynaecology outpatient clinic at the HCPA. The main outcome measures will be the rates of detection of preinvasive lesions (CIN I–III) and invasive carcinoma of the cervix.

### Screening population

All women attending the gynaecology department at the HCPA will be taught about preventive measures directed to preventing and/or avoiding exposure to known risk factors. They will also be informed about the importance of early disease detection and invited to participate in the screening programme. All sexually active women aged 35–64 will be eligible for screening. A later aim of the present study is to extend the screening to younger women (aged 25 and over).

### Selection of the study groups

Eligible women will be distributed at random to two screening groups. One group will be invited to attend for a visual inspection and cervical cytology. In the other group the screen will consist of visual inspection alone. All women with abnormalities on visual inspection will be referred for further investigation to the outpatient clinic where resources are available to carry out such an evaluation.

Twenty per cent (at random) of women selected (in both groups) will have an additional endocervical exam to consider the possibility of missed lesions in that area. Such a procedure will help the investigators to measure the size of such a loss. To overcome the possibility that women who have been assigned to the inspection group will not receive the best method for mass cervical cancer screening currently known, the random sample will also include cytology of the ectocervix and an interim analysis will be performed to compare the results of inspection and cytology in this group.

### Frequency of screening

After the first screen (on entry), women will have the second screen within a year. If the second examination results are negative, women will be screened every 3 years. The follow-up period for the study is 5 years.

Women with abnormalities will be treated if they have cervical lesions, which will be determined by colposcopy. The follow-up of those women will consist in a smear taken within 3 months of treatment, and a year after that. If at this time the findings are normal, the woman returns for regular follow-up if results are negative.

### Method of treatment

Treatment measures will be applied following the Bethesda system for all those women who will present with abnormalities. The measures are as follows:
1   Low-grade lesions: observation and a new smear taken after 3 months, with the exception of all exophytic lesions, which will be removed.
2   High-grade lesions: removal of the lesion and free margins according to the lesion's size and extent.

### Sample size considerations

Data on frequency of women seen at the gynaecology department at the HCPA in 1993 show a total of 27 970; these numbers have been stable during the last few years. About 40% of all women would be eligible to participate in the screening programme (approximately 12 000 women). The pilot study aims to screen 1000 women in each arm of the study to achieve the main goal of the study.

### Coding and data entry

All data will be coded and entered into computer files. Ongoing monitoring of the accumulating data will be carried out.

### Analysis

Data analysis will be performed using either the Statistical Analysis System (SAS) or Statistical Package for Social Sciences (SPSS).

## Preliminary results

From 1 November to August 1, 150 women enrolled in the Early Detection and Prevention Programme for Cervical Cancer in Porto Alegre, Brazil.

The mean age of the study population was $41.2 \pm 13.5$ years. Most women were married (65%); 35% were unmarried. Thirty-eight per cent were smokers and the daily average consumption was $11.5 \pm 8$ cigarettes; the average length of tobacco exposure was $17.1 \pm 9.8$ years. Caucasians were predominant among the study group (85.3%). The mean age at first intercourse was $19.6 \pm 4.7$ years and the life-time prevalence of sexually transmitted disease (STD) corresponds to 15.1% of the population. Women had on average $3 \pm 2$ life sexual partners (Tables 28.5 and 28.6).

Information on contraceptive methods was also explored. Approximately 75% reported ever having used contraceptive methods. Amongst these women, 49.3% have been using oral contraceptives.

Univariate analysis was performed to compare some of the variables studied. Age at first intercourse (using 19 years as the cut-off point) and previous STD were significantly related, with a $P$ value of 0.003. Also, the relationship between the results of the acetic acid test and Schiller test was statistically significant ($P < 0.00$). In all those women who tested negative for acetic acid and for Schiller, cytology was also negative.

## Discussion

The main objective of this report is to present local data relating characteristics known to be associated to cervical cancer. Cervical cancer incidence rates are higher among women over 35 years of age. The population attending HCPA has a mean age within the ages of higher risk for the disease.

Marital status does not appear to be a factor associated with outcome. Beuret *et al.* [15] however, have found a significant relationship between marital status and HPV infection; unmarried women are at higher risk. In this study, marital status was not related to previous STD.

**Table 28.5** Characteristics of the study population.

| Characteristic | Mean $\pm$ SD | Median |
| --- | --- | --- |
| Age (years) | $41.2 \pm 13.5$ | 41 |
| Age at first intercourse (years) | $19.6 \pm 4.7$ | 18 |
| Number of partners | $3 \pm 2$ | 2 |
| Number of cigarettes/day | $11.5 \pm 8$ | 10 |
| Smoking exposure (years) | $17.1 \pm 9.8$ | 15 |

SD, Standard deviation.

**Table 28.6** Prevalence of other factors among the study population.

| Factors | HCPA prevalence (%) | Local literature data (%) |
|---|---|---|
| *Contraceptive method* | | |
| No | 25.3 | 27 |
| Yes | 74.7 | 73 |
| *Oral contraceptive use* | | |
| No | 50.7 | 60 |
| Yes | 49.3 | 40 |
| *Smoking habit* | | |
| No | 62 | 67 |
| Yes | 38 | 33 |
| *Previous STD* | | |
| No | 74.9 | NA |
| Yes | 15.1 | NA |

HCPA, Hospital de Clínicas de Porto Alegre; STD, sexually transmitted disease; NA, not available.

Tobacco is described as an independent risk factor for the development of cervical neoplasia [16,17]. Prevalence rates of smoking consumption among women in Porto Alegre, Rio Grande do Sul, was 33% in 1987, and 51% among males during the same period. Regarding smoking status, the results of this study (37.8%) are in agreement with such findings, and this could be a small indication that may be the study population represents to some extent the original population.

The study protocol was unable to detect ethnic variations among the population, creating limitations for the analysis of such a variable.

Age at first intercourse seemed to be related to previous STD, taking age as a variable with the cut-off point at the age of 19, which is the mean age of the population studied. Such findings are in agreement with the findings in the literature [18]. The life-time STD prevalence was 18.4%. In a given population, incidence and prevalence rates depend on adequate registration and communication of cases; under-registration is a common occurrence. Therefore, such data must be carefully interpreted.

The prevalence rate of contraceptive methods, including condom, intrauterine device, sterilization, oral contraceptives, diaphragm and spermicide was 73% in southern Brazil in 1986. Oral contraceptives alone corresponded to 40%. The study results were very similar to such findings. This is another factor that may indicate that the original population is adequately represented, as far as oral contraceptive use is concerned.

The Schiller test and acetic acid test were significantly associated. For all those patients who tested negative for both Schiller and acetic acid tests, the cytology was negative, perhaps denoting that the clinical tests were sensitive.

The preliminary results suggest that a better knowledge of the variables relating to increased risk of STD infection and cervical cancer are of great relevance. Data related to STD and demographic features vary from region to region; local studies are necessary to learn the local profile of such disease. The ability of primary health care in detecting and preventing cervical cancer can be increased with adequate information about the risk factors and screening methods, like automated reading Pap smear machines, of early signs of such neoplasms.

## References

1 Muñoz N, Bosh FX. *Epidemiology of Cervical Cancer*. Lyon: International Agency for Research on Cancer, 1989, pp 9–39.

2 Parkin DM, Laara E, Muir CS. Estimates of the worldwide frequency of 16 major cancers in 1980. *Int J Cancer* 1988; **41**: 184–197.

3 Brumini R. (ed) *Cancer no Brasil: Dados Histopatologicos – Cancer in Brazil: Histopathologic Data 1976–1980*. Rio de Janeiro: Ministerio da Saude, Campanha Nacional de Combate ao Cancer, 1982, p 480.

4 Gadelha MIP *et al*. Cancer: Um Problema de Saude Publica no Brasil. *JBM* 1992; **63**: 38–46.

5 Ministerio da Saude. *INCA/Pro Onco Cancer no Brasil: Dados dos Registros de Base Populacional*. Rio de Janeiro: Ministry of Health, 1991, p 35.

6 Miller AB. *Cervical Cancer Screening Programmes. Managerial Guidelines*. Geneva: World Health Organization, 1992.

7 Harris RWC, Brinton LA, Cowdell RH *et al*. Characteristics of women with dysplasia or carcinoma *in situ* of the cervix uteri. *Br J Cancer* 1980; **42**: 359–369.

8 Reeves WC, Brinton LA, Brenes MM *et al*. Case-control study of cervical cancer in Herrera province, Republic of Panama. *Int J Cancer* 1985; **36**: 55–60.

9 Clarke EA, Hatcher J, Mckeown-Eyssen GE, Lickrish GM. Cervical dysplasia: association with sexual behavior, smoking, and oral contraceptive use? *Am J Obstet Gynecol* 1985; **151**: 612–616.

10 Brinton LA, Hamman RF, Huggins GR *et al*. Sexual and reproductive risk factors for invasive squamous cell cervical cancer. *J Natl Cancer Inst* 1987; **79**: 23–30.

11 Greenberg ER, Vessey M, McPherson K, Yates D. Cigarette smoking and cancer of the uterine cervix. *Br J Cancer* 1985; **51**: 139–141.

12 Brinton LA, Schairer C, Haenzel W *et al*. Cigarette smoking and invasive cervical cancer. *JAMA* 1986; **255**: 3265–3269.

13 Peters RK, Thomas D, Hagan DG *et al*. Risk factors for invasive cervical cancer among latinas and non-latinas in Los Angeles county. *J Natl Cancer Inst* 1986; **77**: 1063–1077.

14 Schiffman MH, Haley NJ, Felton JS *et al*. Biochemical epidemiology of cervical neoplasia: measuring cigarette smoking constituents in the cervix. *Cancer Res* 1987; **47**: 3886–3888.

15 Beuret TH, Sadoul G, Farj A, Ionesco M, De Brux J. Étude epidemiologique comparative enter 120 patientes atteintes de lesion condylomateuse et 120 patientes temoins. *J Ginecol Obstet Biol Rep* 1987; **16**: 555–564.

16 Villa LL, Franco ELF. Epidemiologic correlates of cervical neoplasia and risk of human

papillomavirus infection in asymptomatic women in Brazil. *J Natl Cancer Inst* 1989; **81**: 332–340.

17 Brinton LA, Fraumeni JF Jr. Epidemiology of uterine cervical cancer. *J Chronic Dis* 1986; **39**: 1051–1065.

18 Naud P, Bozko L, Catalan F *et al*. Human papillomavirus and precursor lesions of uterine cervical cancer. In: *Papillomavirus in Human Pathology*. Ares Serono Symposia, 1995; p. 261.

# Section 5
# Automation in Cytology

# 29: Automation and Cervical Cytopathology: An Overview

## E. McGoogan

## Summary

The main thrust of automation development has focused on the laboratory. The three main areas targeted include thin-layer technologies, 'helper computers' and automated scanning devices for primary screening or quality control. Thin-layer technologies offer the opportunity to improve sample content and presentation and decrease the time required for microscopic assessment; helper computers may assist in training technical and medical staff and in quality assurance; and automated scanning devices may be used for quality control or for primary screening to reduce the numbers of samples requiring assessment by conventional microscopy. In addition, the recent advances in telepathology need to be assessed before it is introduced widely into laboratory practice. If automation is to be cost-effective, it must address some of the deficiencies in the current screening programme, improve the overall sensitivity of conventional screening and thereby provide less expensive health care.

## Introduction

In this era of advancing technology, it is not surprising that automated devices are being introduced into health care and screening programmes. Conventional cervical screening programmes are generally poorly funded and any changes to the conventional methods must be shown to be cost-effective. If automation is to be cost-effective, it will require to improve the sensitivity of the overall conventional screening programme, thus providing less expensive care for the whole population at risk. In particular, it would not be reasonable

*Correspondence*: Dr Euphemia McGoogan, Department of Pathology, University of Edinburgh Medical School, Teviot Place, Edinburgh EH8 9AG, UK.

to improve sensitivity at the expense of specificity since this would have unacceptable emotional and economic costs.

Cervical cancer screening programmes fail to achieve their full potential for a variety of reasons, including patient-related factors such as sections of the population remaining unscreened, difficulties in persuading women to attend regularly for routine smears, deficient follow-up processes for women identified with abnormalities and failures of treatment to cure women with pre-invasive disease [1–6] as well as specimen-related factors such as inadequate sampling during smear-taking and inadequate transfer of the sample on to the glass slide and, only to a lesser extent, deficiencies in the microscopic assessment of the slide [1,2,4,5,7–15]. In view of this it is unlikely that improving the microscopic assessment of the conventional cervical smear alone would significantly alter the overall sensitivity of the programme.

The development of automation has been focused on the laboratory. Laboratory tasks can be divided into several areas: clerical; cytopreparation; microscopic assessment; diagnosis and prognosis; quality assurance; continuing education and training. Automation has something to offer each of these areas.

## Clerical and computer tasks

Sophisticated computer links and databases have been developed which allow transfer of appropriate information from laboratories to central data registries for progamme monitoring, audit and patient follow-up purposes. In the clerical area of the laboratory, optical character recognition (OCR) for 'reading' request forms is being introduced to avoid transcription errors in recording patient and specimen information; bar codes are being used to identify not only the specimen but also sender information; paper records are being replaced by electronic filing systems and voice recognition is beginning to be used to dictate reports directly into laboratory computers. The majority of reports are now computer-generated.

## Cytopreparation and microscopic assessment

There are three main areas of development which should be considered under the heading of automation in the preparation and screening areas of cyto-pathology laboratories:

1    Thin-layer technologies either for conventional microscopy or automated scanning which may also permit adjuvant testing of cervical scrape material.
2    Helper computers attached to conventional microscopes to assist the human observer in more accurate assessment of the slide.
3    Automated scanning devices for primary screening and/or quality control.

## Thin-layer technologies

In the cytopreparation laboratory, computer-controlled robotic devices are commonly used for many tasks, including staining, cover-slipping and cyto-centrifugation. The requirement of the early quantitative analysis systems for a single cell preparation has led to the development of the thin-layer technology [16–25]. Thin-layer preparations offer the advantage that the sample removed from the cervix is rinsed from the sampler into a transport fluid so that all the cellular material is sent to the laboratory and is preserved in an optimal state [10,13,26]. In the laboratory, the samples can be batched and prepared by skilled technical staff using robotic preparation devices such as ThinPrep (Cytyc Corp.), CytoRich (Roche Image Analysis Systems) or Megafunnel (Shandon) [27–29]. Excess blood, inflammatory exudate and debris can be removed before representative randomized sampling of cells on to a small area of the slide. The result is that any abnormal cells present in the sample are not obscured or diluted out by normal cells. The belief is that thin-layer preparations could reduce the number of inadequate tests, can be screened more easily, quickly and efficiently than conventional smears and would facilitate increased detection of abnormal cells in the cervical scrape samples [13,26,30–35]. Another important advantage is that multiple parallel thin layers can be produced, or the residual cell suspension used, for additional adjunctive investigations (e.g. human papillomavirus (HPV) typing and testing) [36].

## Helper computers

A generation of helper computers attached to microscopes is being marketed (CompuCyte: Pathfinder, AccuMed: AcCell 2000 and Zeiss: HOME) which allow mapping of the area of the slide which has been screened and electronic tagging and labelling of any suspect cells or objects [37–39]. Thus the individual screener can check that all the cellular material on the slide has been assessed and can quickly review any suspect area before passing or signing out the slide. These devices also keep records of the work performed by each screener, facilitating the maintenance of quality control records for laboratories.

## Automated scanning devices

There have been many attempts to develop machines to assist the cytotechnologist in the microscopic assessment of cervical scrape samples over the last 40 years [15,40–55]. There were many false starts and no dramatic breakthroughs. Nevertheless, patient and persistent efforts on the part of engineers and clinicians directly involved in the field and the spectacular and continuing advances of the underlying electronic and computer technologies have resulted in a generation of machines which appear to be technically adequate. The key questions facing automation in the laboratory are: Will it improve the false-negative rate? Can this be done without a significant increase in the false-positive rate? Can this be achieved in a cost-effective and timely manner?

The general requirements for an automated prescreening device include:

1   A sensitivity better than or at least equal to conventional methods.
2   A specificity sufficiently high to assure cost-effectiveness.
3   Ability to detect inadequate samples.
4   Ability to detect all abnormal specimens.
5   Ideally, the facility to show the human observer a suspect cell or cells.
6   The time taken to assess each sample should not be excessive.
7   The system should not be more expensive than conventional methods.

The final decision whether an automated system is acceptable will depend on accuracy, reliability, practicality and economic efficiency. Most commercial companies have concentrated their efforts in North America because of the enormous potential market for automated cervical screening systems in that part of the world.

Two automated scanning systems are currently being marketed in the USA for assistance with cervical cytopathology quality control (NSI: Papnet and Neopath: AutoPap 300QC). Both of these have been approved by the Food and Drugs Administration but specifically limited for use in quality control [56,57]. They have not been approved for primary screening and are not to replace the mandatory 10% manual rescreening for quality control. The use of automated systems simply for quality control purposes additional to conventional microscopy would increase the cost of each Papanicolaou (Pap) test and probably be unacceptable outside the USA. However, both of these systems could be adapted for primary screening purposes. Two other systems are being developed specifically as primary screening devices: Roche Image Analysis Systems Autocyte and Xillix Cyto-savant [58,59]. AutoCyte is currently being evaluated in Edinburgh University Department of Pathology. The AutoPap 300QC and Papnet are designed for Pap-stained conventional smears. Cyto-savant is designed for Feulgen-stained conventional smears while the AutoCyte requires Pap-stained thin-layer preparations. It is accepted that those systems designed for routine conventional smears are likely to perform better with thin-layer preparations. Automated systems have a problem deciding whether some objects on the slide are actual cells and this may require a human decision. Some systems will ask for human confirmation for objects that it has assessed as abnormal cells. This interaction is usually done on screen using digitized images but some systems also provide the possibility of relocating the cell in question on the glass slide down the microscope. The Papnet and AutoCyte scanning systems have such an interactive phase.

Each system is expected to be able to handle large numbers of samples but they will be costly and smaller laboratories may have to amalgamate if this technology is introduced. Past experience with devices introduced into clinical chemistry and haematology laboratories suggests that prior evaluation is essential to identify the advantages and disadvantages and, more importantly, the cost-effectiveness of each system before decisions are made about purchasing machines.

The process towards automation is being driven largely by three factors: the quality of the service, human resources and cost-effectiveness. If automated is to be successful it must affect each of these positively.

## Can automation address the deficiencies in conventional screening?

The quality of service (measured by the false-negative rate) is affected by sampling, interpretational and detection problems. It is difficult to see how automated scanning devices can influence sampling (unless the new thin-layer technology is used). As far as interpretation is concerned, automated scanning devices do not suffer from habituation or fatigue and can work 24 h a day without suffering deterioration in performance. Detection of abnormality is normally limited by the resolution of the light microscope and the human eye. We are unable to recognize molecular biological changes in the DNA of cells before they result in gross macroscopic nuclear changes. Automated scanning devices should be able to provide a more objective and quantitative evaluation of DNA and nuclear structure which might allow us to recognize neoplasia precursors at an earlier stage. The philosophy is that the skilled human plus a computer working together can achieve better results.

There is a worldwide shortage of trained cytotechnologists and cytopathologists. The situation has been exacerbated by the limit on the number of smears which an individual is allowed to assess each day Clinical Laboratory Improvement Amendment 1988 (CLIA 88) and British Society for Clinical Cytology Recommended Code of Practice 1986 (BSCC). It takes at least 2 years to train a cytotechnologist to the level of competence required and there are a limited number of training courses being provided worldwide. The situation is likely to worsen, as workloads appear to be increasing even in those countries with well-established screening programmes. If automated scanning devices were used as prescreening devices, it should reduce the number of slides which require manual conventional microscopy and cytotechnologists would only look at those slides in which alarms had been raised. In addition, if the new thin-layer technologies were utilized, this should result in better slide preparation and staining, a smaller area to assess and increased accuracy of interpretation of any abnormalities in cells.

Interactive automated scanning devices have major implications for laboratory staff. Assessing digitized images on a computer monitor is a very different task from assessing three-dimensional real images down a microscope and laboratory staff would require extensive training in order to achieve accuracy in this new technique. Automated scanning devices could replace the primary screener in the laboratory, thereby promoting cytotechnologists to checkers or reviewers. Here cytotechnologists will quality control the machines instead of machines quality controlling the cytotechnologists.

Automated computerized systems are being investigated with a view to providing more accurate diagnostic and prognostic information. Image and DNA analysis systems and cytogenetics systems are commonly used to provide additional information in the field of diagnosis and treatment for other cancers. Molecular biological techniques could be performed on the residual cell suspension to identify high-risk HPV subtypes. Fluorescent *in situ* hybridization, hybrid capture assay and polymerase chain reaction (PCR) techniques are now well-developed and are being automated and may provide additional prognostic information.

## Conclusion

In summary, we can expect automation to:

1   Improve the quality of a cervical screening programme by decreasing the false-negative rate, increasing the precursor recognition and decreasing the unsatisfactory smear rate without an increase in the false-positive rate.

2   Improve the human resource issue by decreasing the workload per cytotechnologist and allowing an increased throughput of laboratory work in a timely manner.

3   Be cost-effective, allowing cost containment for quality screening or possibly a decrease in the cost per test.

Finally, the recent advances in telepathology offer much to improving diagnosis by making second opinions more easily accessible and permitting quick access to experts. More importantly, telepathology opens up a whole new way of bringing experts together for consensus diagnosis; it could be used to overcome some of the problems of external quality assurance in cervical cytopathology by making relevant images available to large numbers of individuals simultaneously, recording their opinions and providing feedback immediately; teleconferencing linked to telepathology could be used for regular training seminars for junior pathologists or cytology screeners; and similarly, seminars with experts could be provided for continuing medical education and continuing professional development. In this era of limited resources for travel and locums, telepathology offers a good alternative to attending every meeting in person.

# References

1 Coppleson LW, Brown B. Estimation of the screening error rate from the observed detection rates in repeated cervical cytology. *Am J Obstet Gynecol* 1974; **119**: 953–958.

2 Creasman WT, Rutledge F. Carcinoma *in situ* of the cervix. An analysis of 861 patients. *Obstet Gynecol* 1972; **39**: 373–380.

3 Day NE. Screening for cancer of the cervix. *J Epidemiol Commun Health* 1989; **43**: 103–106.

4 Koss LG. The Papanicolaou test for cervical cancer detection: a triumph and tragedy. *JAMA* 1989; **261**: 737–743.

5 Morell ND, Taylor JR, Snyder RN, Ziel HK, Salz A, Willie S. False negative cytology rates in patients in whom invasive cervical cancer subsequently developed. *Obstet Gynecol* 1982; **60**: 41–45.

6 Schwabw HW, Unz F (eds) *Automation der zytologischen Diagnostik: Beitrage zur Entwicklungsstand neuer Technologian*. Cologne: Verlag TUV Rheinland, 1984.

7 Bogdanich W. The Pap test misses much cancer through labs' errors. *Wall St J* November 2 1987.

8 Gay JD, Donaldson LD, Goetliner JR. False negative results in cervical cytologic studies. *Acta Cytol* 1985; **29**: 1043–1046.

9 Hughes RG, Colquhoun M, Haddad NG *et al*. The cytological detection of persistent cervical intraepithelial neoplasia after local ablative treatment: a comparison of sampling devices. *Br J Obstet Gynaecol* 1992; **99**: 498–502.

10 Hutchinson ML, Isenstein LM, Goodman A *et al*. Homogeneous sampling accounts for the increased diagnostic accuracy using the ThinPrep processor. *Am J Clin Pathol* 1994; **101**: 215–219.

11 McGoogan E. *Report of the Inquiry into Cervical Cytopathology at Inverclyde Royal Hospital, Greenock*. London: HMSO, 1993.

12 McGoogan E. *Comparative Evaluation of Thin Layer Devices for Cervical Cytopathology. Report for the Advisory Panel on Evaluation of Medical and Scientific Equipment and Health Service Supplies 1994* (unpublished).

13 McGoogan E, Reith A. Would monolayers provide more representative samples and improved preparations for cervical screening? Overview and evaluation of systems available. *Acta Cytol* 1996; **40**: 107–119.

14 Rubio CA. The false negative smear. II. The trapping effect of collection instruments. *Obstet Gynecol* 1977; **49**: 576–580.

15 Wheeless LL, Robinson RD, Berkan TK, Brooks CL, Reeder JE. A statistical analysis of rescreening alarms in a population of normal and abnormal specimens. *Cytometry* 1986; **7**: 205–211.

16 Bahr GF, Bibbo M, Oehme M, Puls JH, Reale FR, Wied GL. An automated device for the production of cell preparations suitable for automatic assessment. *Acta Cytol* 1978; **22**: 243–249.

17 Barrett DL, King EB. Comparison of cellular recovery rates and morphologic details obtained using membrane filter and cytocentrifuge techniques. *Acta Cytol* 1976; **20**: 174–180.

18 Husain OAN, Watts KC. Preparatory methods for DNA hydrolysis, cytochemistry, immunocytochemistry and ploidy analysis: their application to routine diagnostic cytopathology. *Anal Quant Cytol Histol* 1987; **9**: 218–224.

19 Oud PS, Zahniser DJ, Haag DJ *et al*. A new disaggregation device for cytology specimens. *Cytometry* 1984; **5**: 509–514.

20 Oud PS, Zahniser DJ, Harbers-Hendriks R, van Boekel MCG, Raaijmakers MCT, Vooijs

GP. The development of a cervical smear preparation procedure for the bioPEPR image analysis system. *Anal Quant Cytometry* 1981; **3**: 73–80.

21 Rosenthal DL, Stern E, McLatchie C *et al*. A simple method for producing a monolayer of cervical cells for digital image processing. *Anal Quant Cytol* 1979; **1**: 84–240.

22 Rosenthal DL, Manjakian V. Techniques in the preparation of a monolayer of gynecologic cells for automated cytology. *Anal Quant Cytol Histol* 1987; **9**: 55–59.

23 Tanaka N, Ikeda H, Ueno T, Okomoto Y, Hosoi S. CYBEST-CDMS: automated cell dispersion and monolayer smearing device for CYBEST. *Anal Quant Cytol* 1981; **3**: 96–102.

24 Van Driel Kulker ANJ, Ploem-Zaaijer JJ, Van der Zwan M, Tanke HJ. A preparation technique for exfoliated and aspirated cells allowing different staining procedures. *Anal Quant Cytol* 1980; **2**: 243–246.

25 Grohs HK, Zahniser DJ, Geyer JW. Standardization of specimen preparation through mono/thin-layer technology. In: Grohs HK, Husain OAN (eds) *Automated Cervical Cancer Screening*, vol. 11. New York: Igaku-Shoin, 1994, pp 176–185.

26 Laverty CR, Farnsworth A, Thurloe JK, Bowditch RC. The importance of the cell sample in cervical cytology: a controlled trial of a new sampling device. *Med J Aust* 1989; **150**: 432–436.

27 Hutchinson ML, Agarwal P, Denault T, Berger B, Cibas ES. A new look at cervical cytology: ThinPrep multicenter trial results. *Acta Cytol* 1992; **36**: 499–504.

28 Knesel EA, Geyer JW, Gahm T, Nguyen T, Fischer J, Dörrer R. The Roche cytology systems: Cyto-Rich and Autocyte. In: Grohs HK, Husain OAN (eds) *Automated Cervical Cancer Screening*, vol 11. New York: Igaku-Shoin, 1994; pp 294–303.

29 Zahniser DJ, Sullivan PJ. CYTYC Corporation. *Acta Cytol* 1996; **40**: 37–44.

30 Hutchinson ML, Cassin CM, Ball HG. The efficacy of an automated preparation device for cervical cytology. *Am J Clin Pathol* 1991; **96**: 300–305.

31 Linder J. The coming era of cytologic automation. *Am J Clin Pathol* 1991; **96**: 293–294.

32 Papillo JL, Lee KR, Manna EA. Clinical evaluation of the ThinPrep method for the preparation of nongynecologic material. *Acta Cytol* 1992; **36**: 651.

33 Schumann JL. Standardization of specimen acquisition for automated Pap smear screening. In: Grohs HK, Husain OAN (eds) *Automated Cervical Cancer Screening*, vol. 11. New York: Igaku-Shoin, 1994; pp 165–175.

34 Vassilakos P, Cossali D, Albe X, Alonso L, Hohener R, Puget E. Efficacy of monolayer preparation for cervical cytology. Emphasis on suboptimal specimen. *Acta Cytol* 1995; **39**: 368.

35 Wilbur DC, Cibas ES, Merritt S, James P, Berger BM, Bonfiglio TA. ThinPrep processor clinical trials demonstrate an increased detection rate of abnormal cervical cytologic specimens. *Am J Clin Pathol* 1994; **101**: 209–214.

36 Hall S, Wu T-C, Fields AL, Sherman M, Erozan Y. Suitability of ThinPrep specimens for immunocytochemistry and gene amplification by polymerase chain reaction. *Acta Cytol* 1992; **36**: 585.

37 Berger BM. Statistical quality assurance in cytology. The use of the pathfinder to continuously assess screener process control in real time. *Acta Cytol* 1996; **40**: 97–106.

38 Grohs DH, Gombrich PP, Domanik RA. Meeting the challenges in cervical screening: the AcCell series 2000 automated slide handling and data management system. *Acta Cytol* 1996; **40**: 26–36.

39 Kamentsky LA, Gershman RJ, Kamentsky LD, Pomeroy BM, Weissman ML. Compu-Cyte Corporation Pathfinder system: computerising the microscope to improve cytology quality assurance. *Acta Cytol* 1996; **40**: 31–36.

40 Bloss WH, Greiner W, Kringler W, Schlipf W, Schwarzman P, Straub B. Fazytan-IPS-

prescreening system. In: Burger G, Ploem JS, Goertler K (eds) *Clinical Cytometry and Histometry*. London: Academic Press, 1987; pp 18–23.

41 Carothers A, McGoogan E, Vooijs P *et al*. A collaborative trial of a semi-automatic system for slide preparation and screening in cervical cytopathology. *Anal Cell Pathol* 1994; 7: 261–274.

42 Husain OAN, Henderson MJ. Observations on the use of the Quantimet image analysing computer in automatic scanning for malignant cells. In: Evans DMD (ed) *Cytology Automation*. Edinburgh and London: E & S Livingstone, 1970.

43 Husain OAN, Allen E, Hawkins J, Taylor JB. The Quantimet Cytoscreen and the interactive approach to cancer screening. *Histochem Cytochem* 1974; **22**: 678–684.

44 Jakobsen A, Kristensen PB, Poulsen HK. Flow cytometric classification of biopsy specimens from cervical inter-epithelial neoplasia *Cytometry* 1983; **4**: 166–169.

45 Millett JA, Husain OAN. Analysis of chromatin on carcinoma *in situ*. In: Pattison JR, Bitensky L, Chayen J, (eds) *Quantitative Cytochemistry and its Application*. London: Academic Press, 1979.

46 Naujoks H, Sprenger E. Planung, Durchfuhrung und Ergebnisse einer automatisierten vaginalzytologischen Diagnostik. *Gynäkologe* 1990; **23**: 322–327.

47 Ploem JS, van Driel-Kuller AMJ, Goyarts-Veldstra L, Ploem-Zaaijer JJ, Verwoerd NP, van der Zwan M. Image analysis combined with quantitative cytochemistry – results and instrumental developments for cancer diagnosis. *Histochemistry* 1986; **84**: 549–555.

48 Stenkvist B, Bergstrom R, Brinne U *et al*. Automatic analysis of Papanicolaou smears by digital image processing. *Gynecol Oncol* 1987; **27**: 1–14.

49 Tanaka N, Ikeda H, Ueno T *et al*. Automated cytologic screening system (CYBEST model 4): an integrated image cytometry system. *Appl Optics* 1987; **26**: 3301–3307.

50 Tucker JH, Husain OAN, Watts KC, Farrow ASJ, Bayley RJH, Stark M. Automated densitometry of cell populations in a continuous motion cell scanner. *Appl Optics* 1987; **26**: 3315–3324.

51 Tucker JH, Burger G, Husain OAN *et al*. Measuring the accuracy of automated cervical cytology pre-screening systems based on image analysis. *Report EUR 11451 EN*. Luxembourg: Commission of the European Communities, 1988.

52 Tucker JH, Stenkvist B. Whatever happened to cervical cytology automation? *Anal Cell Pathol* 1990; **2**: 259–266.

53 van Driel Kulker AMJ, Ploem-Zaaijer JJ. Image cytometry in automated cervical screening. *Anal Cell Pathol* 1989; **1**: 63–78.

54 Wheeless LL, Patten SF, Berkan TK *et al*. Multi-dimensional slit-scan prescreening system: preliminary results of a single blind clinical study. *Cytometry* 1984; **5**: 1–8.

55 Zahniser DJ, Oud PS, Raaijmakers MCT, Vooijs GP, van de Walle RT. Field tests results using the BioPEPR cervical smear prescreening system. *Cytometry* 1980; **1**: 200–203.

56 Patten SF, Lee JSJ, Nelson AC. Neopath, Inc: Neopath AutoPap 300 Automatic Pap screening system. *Acta Cytol* 1996; **40**: 45–52.

57 Mango LJ. Neuromedical systems Inc. *Acta Cytol* 1996; **40**: 53–59.

58 Knesel EA Jr. Roche Image Analysis Systems, inc. *Acta Cytol* 1996; **40**: 60–66.

59 Palcic B, Garner D, MacAuley CE, Matisic J, Anderson GH. Oncometrics Imaging Corporation and Xillix Technologies Corporation: use of the Cyto-savant in quantitative cytology. *Acta Cytol* 1996; **40**: 67–72.

# 30: Automation in Cervicovaginal Cytology: System Requirements and Benefits

## L. G. Koss

## Summary

The requirements of automated screening systems for cervicovaginal cytology are listed and the applications discussed in three categories – system performance, system reliability and cost. The reasons for future widespread applications of such systems to primary screening are presented, based on personal experience with one of them.

## Introduction

Screening of cervicovaginal smears is a very monotonous, time-consuming and taxing occupation that poses great demands on trained cytotechnologists or other screening personnel. To perform this task well, on the average about 5 min per smear is required, with some smears easier and some more difficult to interpret. At the onset of population screening by *vaginal smears*, as initially advocated by Papanicolaou and Traut, the task of finding abnormal cells was much more difficult than in the cervical and endocervical samples, as currently practised. None the less, even today the finding of a few abnormal cells in a smear composed of anywhere from 50 000 to 300 000 cells or more is still a formidable task. It is therefore not surprising that, ever since, the onset of mass screening efforts have been made to automate the function of screening. The first apparatus constructed for this purpose was the Cytoanalyser, a relatively simple machine by today's standards [1].

The studies performed with the Cytoanalyser brought into focus a number of fundamental problems with automation of cervicovaginal cytology. It

*Correspondence*: Dr L. G. Koss, Department of Pathology, Montefiore Medical Center, Albert Einstein College of Medicine, Bronx, New York 10467, USA.

became quite evident that simple measurements of the size of the cell and its nucleus, and of the nucleocytoplasmic ratio were insufficient to separate benign cells from malignant cells. The reason for this failure was the *similarities* between benign and malignant cells which are much greater than the differences, a problem that must be considered even today. Further, the machine was unable to differentiate cell clusters from malignant cells.

Similar problems occurred with much more sophisticated computerized systems, based on image analysis. The most elaborate was the system proposed by Wied and colleagues [2], known as TICAS, for taxonomic intracellular analysis system. TICAS was capable of a rather sophisticated analysis of cell types in cervical smears, using not only cell measurements but also a number of mathematical algorithms, derived from histograms of cells. The system provided some important basic information in reference to analysis of cells and was applied not only to cervical smears but also to a number of other cytological targets [3]. However, none of the applications of TICAS and related systems proved to be of practical value, for reasons that were similar to the experience with the Cytoanalyser: the TICAS-based machines in an automated or semiautomated mode were not only too slow to perform but also failed in the differentiation between cell clusters and other artefacts and cancer cells. Several variations on the theme were suggested by other investigators, none of them any more successful than TICAS and its variants (see summary [4–6]).

## Principles of application

Still, this period of automation allowed the formulation of certain principles that are applicable to all automated systems. These can be summarized as follows:

1 The performance of the machine in the identification of abnormal cells should be equal to or, preferably, superior to that of a trained human screener.

2 It should be easy to maintain and reliable to use.

3 It should be cost-effective.

Other requirements that were formulated in a number of international forums were of secondary significance. For example, one of the expressed preferences was for the machine to identify infectious agents in a cervical smear, clearly not one of the most important goals of automation of cervical cancer detection. I will address the three important issues sequentially.

## Performance of the machine

A screening instrument operates on a totally different principle from the human eye–brain axis. Even the most sophisticated computer systems are still only elaborate calculating machines that perform certain tasks better than humans but lack the tremendous power of the human eye–brain axis to adapt a very rapidly changing scene. A cervical smear is a constantly changing scene. Further, the computers are still very far from having the power of human memory and of very rapid associations to reach diagnostic conclusion on visual targets, as a trained person can do. Therefore the computer-based devices cannot analyse the entire scene but must select among objects those targets that are most likely to give the most reliable practical results. There are two automated systems currently approved for quality control of cervical smear screening in the USA [7]. I am familiar with one of them, the PAPNET system.

The PAPNET system (Neuromedical Systems, Inc., Suffern, NY) utilizes two-stage analysis of the smears: a conventional image analysis technology as the first stage of cell selection and a trained neural network technology to select individual cells for display on the high-resolution screens. The technical details of the proprietary software and hardware were published [8,9]. The decision to rescreen or not to rescreen is based entirely on the judgement of a trained human observer. Further, the cells seen on the screen can be identified on the smear using a coordinated microscope stage. A permanent record of cell displays can be easily generated for the patient's file. The system was tested on known abnormal smears; the displays of abnormal cells were obtained in 97% in one trial and in 97.2% in the second trial [8]. In many of these cases the diagnosis of a malignant lesion and its type could be established on the cells displayed on the screen [8]. As a quality control instrument, the machine recognized 30% of false-negative smears in 228 women who subsequently developed a high-grade lesion or invasive cancer of the uterine cervix (unpublished data; see Hematology and Pathology Devices Panel [7]).

This figure is comparable with the results of manual rescreening in similar cases from a large number of participating laboratories, recently published by Jones [10]. The PAPNET system is highly reproducible, as documented by 10-fold rescreening of the same abnormal smears in our laboratories (unpublished data; paper in preparation).

The crucial task for an automated system is the identification of targets of the rescreening: not all the errors are significant for the patients. The finding of atypical cells of unknown significance or even of low-grade lesions (mild dysplasia, cervical intraepithelial neoplasia (CIN) I, flat condyloma) is less important than the discovery of precancerous lesions composed of small cells and located in the endocervical canal. These are the abnormalities that are most difficult to identify and are the most frequent cause of invasive cancer. In our experience with such cases the PAPNET was capable of discovering such cells, singly and in clusters in false-negative smears.

## Ease and reliability of use

A comparison in the performance of automated instruments is difficult. The Autopap® 300QC system is installed in individual laboratories, whereas the PAPNET system has created a system of scanning centres wherein the machines are maintained by trained technicians. Time will tell which system is easier to use and maintain.

## Cost-effectiveness of the automated systems

Without any doubt the use of the automated instruments as tools in quality control is initially going to increase the cost of screening of cervical smears. The cost has to be measured against the cost of screening errors, some of which may lead to invasive cancers that may be the cause of enormous suffering and lives lost. The human cost of such errors vastly exceeds the significance of costly legal proceedings which may result from such cases, at least in the USA. The cost of treatment of invasive cervical cancer must also be compared with the cost of treatment of precancerous lesions.

More importantly, however, a consensus is slowly emerging that cervical smears should be screened twice, either by technologists or by machines. Hutchinson recently wrote about this issue and tentatively calculated the cost of discovery of missed lesions [11]. Although her figures were highly preliminary and based in part on incomplete data, the basic concept of dual screening was clearly discussed.

The manufacturers of automated screening machines currently on the market are eager to address this question. Preliminary data on the use of PAPNET as a screening instrument are available [12] and they suggest that the performance of this machine as a screening tool was superior to the performance of trained cytotechnologists. There is little doubt that this is the future of automated instruments. Their use will probably lead to some savings in the cost of screening personnel but I do not envision a fully automated future in which the verdict will be rendered by machine alone. The need for trained personnel will remain but the results of screening may prove to be superior to the current system.

## References

1 Tolles WB, Bostrom RC. Automated screening of cytological smears for cancer: the instrumentation. *Ann NY Acad Sci* 1956; **63**: 1211–1218.
2 Wied GL, Bartels PH, Bahr GF, Oldfield DG. Taxonomic intracellular analytic system (TICAS) for cell identification. *Acta Cytol* 1968; **12**: 180–204.
3 Koss LG. *Diagnostic Cytology and its Histopathologic Bases*, 4th edn. Philadelphia: J.B. Lippincott, 1992.

4 Koss LG. Analytical and quantitative cytology: a historical perspective. *Anal Quant Cytol Histol* 1982; **4**: 251–256.

5 Koss LG. Automated cytology and histology: a historical perspective. *Anal Quant Cytol Histol* 1987; **9**: 369–374.

6 Husain OAN, Henderson MJ. Observations on the use of the Quantimet image analysing computer in automated scanning for malignant cells. In: Evans DMD (ed) *Cytology Automation*. Edinburgh: E&S Livingstone, 1970.

7 Hematology and Pathology Devices Panel of the Medical Devices Advisory Committee to the FDA. Federal Department of Health and Human Services. Transcript of Proceedings, Rockville, MD, August 7–8, 1995.

8 Koss LG, Lin E, Schreiber K, Elgert P, Mango L. Evaluation of the PAPNET cytologic screening system for quality control of cervical smears. *Am J Clin Pathol* 1994; **101**: 220–229.

9 Mango LJ. Computer-assisted cervical cancer screening using neural network. *Cancer Lett* 1994; 77: 155–162.

10 Jones BA. Rescreening in gynecologic cytology. Rescreening of 3762 previous cases for current high-grade squamous intraepithelial lesions and carcinoma – a College of American Pathologists Q-Probes study of 312 institutions. *Arch Pathol Lab Med* 1995; **119**: 1097–1103.

11 Hutchinson ML. Assessing the costs and benefits of alternative rescreening strategies (editorial). *Acta Cytol* 1996; **40**: 4–8.

12 Ouwerkerk-Noordam E, Boon ME, Beck S. Computer-assisted primary screening of cervical smears using the PAPNET method: comparison with conventional screening and evaluation of the role of the cytologist. *Cytopathology* 1994; **5**: 211–218.

# 31: Automated Screening Using the AutoPap® 300 Device

R. M. Richart,[1] S. F. Patten, Jr[2] & L. J. S. J. Lee[2]

## Introduction

We have previously described the use of the AutoPap® 300 QC Papanicolaou smear screener system as an adjunctive tool for the quality control of Pap smears during the routine screening process [1]. In that study, it was shown that the AutoPap® QC device could provide up to a fivefold improvement over a 10% random selection method in the detection of false negative slides. Subsequent to that study, there have been a number of improvements in the algorithms, and the device has been trained on a larger set of slides than was used for the device in the quality control mode.

The present study was designed to evaluate the AutoPap® device in the primary screening mode using the improved algorithms and the training enhancements. An anomaly score algorithm was designed to detect slides with epithelial cell abnormalities. The performance of the anomaly score algorithm was evaluated in this study.

## The AutoPap® 300 automatic pap screener system

The AutoPap® device is an automated cervical cytology screening system [2,3,4] with which images are obtained using a high resolution scanner through a high-speed video microscope. These images are digitized, and the data passed through image interpretation software. Specially-designed algorithms are used to recognize, analyze, and classify both individual cells and slides using a conventionally-prepared Papanicolaou smear preserved under glass coverslips. In use, each slide is labelled using a barcode. After being loaded in a slide tray

[1]Departments of Pathology and Obstetrics & Gynecology, Columbia University College of Physicians & Surgeons; [2]NeoPath, Inc.

and placed in the AutoPap® device, the process is automatic and provides a print-out for the laboratory at the conclusion of the AutoPap® screen.

## Materials and methods

A ninefold cross-validation method was applied to the training slides to test the anomaly score algorithm. The data set included 4922 slides (2115 randomly-selected normal slides and 2807 abnormal slides) acquired from 14 laboratories. In addition, an independent data set was used to test the algorithm for further performance validation. The independent data set included 2353 slides (1235 randomly-selected normal slides and 1118 abnormal slides) acquired from 10 laboratories. All slides were processed on two AutoPap® systems. Normal specificities and abnormal sensitivities were evaluated using the data from both systems.

## Results

The results, based on the ninefold cross-validation method are listed in Table 31.1.

**Table 31.1** Detection sensitivities by manually-screened fraction.

| Normal specificity (%) | LSIL sensitivity (%) | HSIL sensitivity (%) | Sq-Ca sensitivity (%) | AIS sensitivity (%) | Ec-Adca sensitivity (%) | Em-Adca sensitivity (%) |
|---|---|---|---|---|---|---|
| 10.7 | 98.7 | 99.7 | 100.0 | 96.7 | 100.0 | 97.5 |
| 20.1 | 97.3 | 99.3 | 100.0 | 96.7 | 100.0 | 94.4 |
| 30.3 | 95.8 | 98.3 | 100.0 | 94.5 | 98.7 | 93.1 |
| 40.1 | 93.5 | 97.6 | 100.0 | 92.6 | 98.7 | 90.0 |
| 50.2 | 89.3 | 96.7 | 100.0 | 92.6 | 98.7 | 86.9 |

LSIL, low-grade squamous intraepithelial lesion, HSIL, high-grade squamous intraepithelial lesion.

The independent test results (not shown in the table) showed that at a specificity of 50% the sensitivities are 88.4% for LSIL slides, 95.1% for HSIL slides, 96.4% for squamous cell carcinoma slides (Sq-Ca), 100% for endocervical adenocarcinoma slides (Ec-Adca), 100% for adenocarcinoma-*in-situ* slides (AIS), and 88.2% for endometrial adenocarcinoma slides (Em-Adca).

The cross-validation and the independent test results were similar. At 50% specificity, the AutoPap® 300 screener algorithm yielded above 95% sensitivities for significant squamous and endocervical lesions. The sensitivities for LSIL, HSIL, and endometrial and extra-uterine adenocarcinoma slides are all within the range of manual cyotechnologist's screening sensitivities.

## Discussion

There has been little change in the screening of Papanicolaou smears since they were introduced into clinical medicine over 40 years ago. The cytotechnologist, then and now, manually screens physician-prepared smears which are stained by a standard method. Any abnormalities which are detected by the cytotechnologist are flagged by ink dots, and the dotted slide is sent to and reviewed by a cytopathologist who makes the final diagnosis. Smears interpreted as negative by the screening cytotechnologist are generally not reviewed by another person unless they are part of a so-called directed rescreening programme or chosen for the mandated (in the USA) 10% random rescreening which is observed by most laboratories.

This manual screening process is highly labour intensive and requires the services of specially-trained technologists who, because of their high skill level, are generally relatively scarce and relatively well paid. Because both Europe and North America introduced Papanicolaou screening at an early phase of its development and because both are relatively affluent continents, cervical cancer screening programmes are widely available and widely used in both these settings. However, the screening process is still expensive, even in affluent societies, and in recent years (particularly in the USA) a shortage of trained cytotechnologists occurred following the imposition of workload limitations by regulatory authorities. In addition, the quality and skill level of cytotechnologists varies substantially, false negative rates vary widely from laboratory to laboratory, and it has been impossible to achieve a 'standard product' with a high degree of sensitivity and specificity. Further, cervical cancer is the leading cause of death from cancer among women in developing countries and the leading cause of death from any cause in the 35–45 year old cohort. Due to the rigours required for cytotechnologist training, to the cost and complexity of establishing screening laboratories, and the high cost of manual screening, it is unlikely that widespread screening in developing countries using a manual approach will be possible to achieve in the near future.

Many attempts have been made to automate the screening process [5] and most have ended in failure. It is clear, retrospectively, that much of this failure was due to a lack of understanding of the rigour needed for automated device-based screening and that the technology was too primitive to be up to the task. It was only after the development of high resolution scanning devices and sophisticated computer programs that it became possible, realistically, to expect to be able to automate the cytology screening process. The two devices which have been approved by the United States Food and Drugs Administration are currently only approved for adjunctive screening and, in the case of the AutoPap® 300 QC system, to replace the mandated 10% rescreening required in the USA. It would be highly desirable if a device could be used for primary screening as well, as that goal would potentially enable screening to become less expensive, more reproducible, and achieve a higher level of sensitivity and specificity than is currently achieved in most screening laboratories. Such a development would also potentially enable screening devices to be placed widely in developing countries, to increase substantially their ability to screen much of their populations for cervical cancer and its precursors, and to reduce substantially the extraordinarily high death rate which occurs from this disease.

The AutoPap® QC device is becoming widely used in North America and in other industrialized countries. In the laboratories in which it has been used, it has increased the detection of abnormal cells falsely interpreted as being negative by the screening cytotechnologist. In the present study, using a device which has been improved substantially over that originally reported, it has been found that the AutoPap® device, when used in a screening mode, is capable of detecting between 96% and 100% of the high-grade CIN lesions and invasive cancers — both squamous and glandular. To achieve these detection rates, the device is used at a 'sort rate' of 50%. The device hierarchically orders abnormal slides, and the laboratory screens the upper 50% of the hierarchically-ordered queue. The lower 50% are archived unscreened. Using a 50% sort rate the ASCUS, AGUS, and LoSIL categories have a lower detection rate than the high-grade CINs and invasive cancers. To achieve a higher detection rate of these abnormalities using the system in its present configuration would require that the sort rate be decreased and that a larger proportion of slides be screened manually. Clearly, with this configuration there is a trade-off between sort rate and detection rate, and this will result in a trade-off between detection rate and monetary expenditure.

It is generally conceded that the detection of ASCUS, AGUS, and LoSIL lesions is less important than that of high-grade CINs and invasive cancers. As can be seen from Table 31.1 even in a scenario in which only 50% of the smears are manually rescreened after having been examined by the AutoPap® device, a very high proportion of significant lesions are detected. This approach may be particularly useful in developing country settings where there is an enormous premium placed upon the detection of significant lesions and upon increasing the availability of cervical cancer screening. Even in developed country settings, the AutoPap® device, at a 50% sort rate, will achieve detection sensitivities equal to or superior to those achieved by cytotechnologists in most screening laboratories. Thus it would appear that the goal of augmenting or largely replacing manual screening is likely to be achieved as automated devices are more extensively trained, as the algorithms become more sophisticated, and as hardware enhancements continue to be made. It is likely that such devices will become the standard for screening and that manual examination of smears will take place after device screening has taken place.

# References

1 Richart RM, Patten SF Jr, Lee JSJ. Prospects for automated cytology. In: Lorincz A & Reid R (eds) *Obstetrics & Gynecology Clinics of North America*. Philadelphia: WB Saunders. In press.

2 Lee JSJ, Bannister W, Kuan LC, Bartels PH, Nelson A. A processing strategy for automated Papanicolaou smear screening. *Anal Quant Cytol Histol* 1992; **14**: 415–425.

3 Anderson TL. Automatic screening of conventional Papanicolaou smears: the AutoPap® 300 and AutoPap® 300 QC systems. In: *The Computerized Cytology and Histology Laboratory*. Chicago: Tutorials of Cytology, 1994, pp 306–311.

4 Patten SF Jr, Lee JSJ. Detection of true false negative slides by the NeoPath AutoPap® 300 QC system: comparison with random rescreen. In: *Compendium on Quality Assurance, Proficiency Testing and Workload Limitations in Clinical Cytology*. Chicago: Tutorials of Cytology, 1995, pp 167–169.

5 Husain OAN. The history of automated cell scanners. In: Grohs HK, Hussain OAN (eds). *Automated Cervical Cancer Screening*. New York: Igaku-Shoin, 1994, pp 3–15.

# 32: Liquid-based Cytology: Comparison of ThinPrep 2000 with Conventionally Prepared Pap Smears

J. Linder

## Summary

To evaluate the performance of the ThinPrep 2000 system, a liquid-based alternative for the conventional method of Papanicolaou (Pap) smear preparation, a prospective multicentre clinical study was conducted. The objective of the ThinPrep clinical study was to determine if gynaecological specimens prepared using the ThinPrep 2000 system were as effective as or more effective than conventional methods for the detection of atypical cells and cervical cancer or its precursor lesions. The clinical study protocol was a blinded split-sample matched-pair study for which a conventional Pap smear was prepared first, and the remainder of the sample (the material that would normally be discarded) was immersed and rinsed into a vial of PreservCyt solution.

At the laboratory the ThinPrep 2000 system was used to prepare a standardized thin layer of cells. ThinPrep and conventional Pap smear slides were examined and diagnosed independently by cytotechnologists. For low-grade squamous intraepithelial lesions (LSIL) or more severe lesions the ThinPrep method was statistically favoured over the conventional Pap smear. At screening centres, the improved rate of detecting LSIL or more severe diagnoses was up to 73%, with an average improvement of 65%, as compared to conventional Pap smears. For specimen adequacy, the ThinPrep method was statistically favoured over the conventional cytology method at four study sites, reducing the Bethesda system of classification of 'satisfactory but limited by . . .' by up to 58%, with an average reduction of 29%.

When compared to the corresponding conventional smears the ThinPrep method showed equivalent detection of benign cellular changes. These im-

*Correspondence*: Professor James Linder, Department of Pathology and Microbiology, University of Nebraska Medical Center, 600 South 42nd Street, Omaha, Nebraska 68198, USA.

provements in disease detection were confirmed by an independent patholo-gist review demonstrating that there was no loss in specificity with the ThinPrep method.

This multicentre clinical trial demonstrates that the ThinPrep Pap Test is more effective than the conventional Pap smear for the detection of atypical cells, cervical cancer and its precursor lesions. In addition, the collection of cells in a liquid-based medium offers the opportunity to improve the Pap test by adjunctive testing for human papillomavirus or other tests. This may permit the opportunity for better triage and management of patients with cervical abnormalities.

## Introduction

The cervical Pap test is the most widely used cancer screening test. In this role it has been remarkably effective in reducing the incidence of cervical cancer. For example, in the USA over the past 50 years there has been a 70% reduction in cervical cancer deaths. Remarkably, the manner that the Pap smear is collected, processed and interpreted is substantially similar to the way it was performed at the time of its introduction by Dr Papanicolaou 50 years ago. Despite the success of reducing cervical cancer deaths, there are several limitations to the conventional Pap smear. These include the potential for inadequate sampling of the uterine cervix, incomplete transfer of the sample from the sampling device to the glass slide, and the potential for compromised morphological presentation due to thick smears, or the obscuring of diagnostic cells by blood, mucus, inflammation or epithelial elements. Combined, the difficulties related to sampling, smear preparation and screening contribute to a Pap smear false-negative rate that may average 25%* [1,2].

In the USA concern regarding the false-negative rate and deaths that have been attributed to cytology screening errors has created a crisis in the public's confidence in the Pap smear. This has led to increased federal regulation, principally through the Clinical Laboratory Improvement Amendments of 1988 [3], and an effort by industry to improve the Pap smear, principally through the development of computer-based rescreening devices [4]. These instruments, two of which have received Food and Drugs Administration approval for adjunctive or rescreening purposes, essentially serve as proof-readers, examining glass slides screened as negative by cytotechnologists. The instruments suggest images or cases to the cytotechnologist that may require

---

*Here, false-negative is described according to terminology proposed by Naryshkin and Davey [1] where a 25% false-negative rate would imply that one in four women who had disease would not be detected. It does not imply that 25% of all women receiving Pap smears have an erroneous diagnosis.

rescreening, but in their present implementation, these devices do not classify the abnormality. While these devices may overcome some inferior morphological presentations of cells inherent on a smear, they cannot, however, visualize cells which have not been sampled, not been transferred to the glass slide, or are totally obscured on the smear.

An alternative approach to improve the Pap test has been to make a relatively simple change in the manner of specimen collection. Instead of smearing the patient sample on to a glass slide, the sample is immersed and rinsed into a vial of preservative solution [5]. This approach has principally been advocated by Cytyc Corporation (Boxborough, MA). The results of the most recent clinical trials evaluating the ThinPrep 2000 system will be the subject of the study.

## Methods

A prospective multicentre clinical study was conducted to evaluate the performance of the ThinPrep 2000 system and compare it to the conventional Pap smear. The clinical study protocol was a blinded, split-sample matched-pair study for which a conventional Pap smear was prepared first using the Papett sampling device. The sampling device was then immersed and rinsed into a vial of PreservCyt solution, a buffered methanol solution specifically formulated for the ThinPrep 2000 system. Thus, ThinPrep slides were made from cells that otherwise would have been discarded. At the cytology laboratory the PreservCyt sample vial was placed into a ThinPrep 2000 processor along with a disposable filter cylinder. Using the ThinPrep 2000 processor, a thin layer of cells were prepared, then transferred to a glass slide in a 20 mm circle for subsequent fixation and Pap staining.

There were 7360 patients enrolled in the study at six sites. The sites included three cytology screening centres with prevalence of LSIL or more severe abnormalities ranging from 2.3 to 3.8%, and three high-risk sites serving a high proportion of patients having previously abnormal smears (18.2–40.4%). Approximately 1000 or more patients were evaluated at each site. The study population consisted of the following race groups: Caucasian (41.2%); Asian (2.3%); Hispanic (9.7%); Native American (1.0%); and other 0.6%. At each site the ThinPrep and conventional Pap were independently reviewed, without knowledge of the corresponding diagnosis. Report forms containing the patient history as well as a checklist of all possible classifications of the Bethesda system were used to record the results of screening. An independent contract research organization (MTRA, Wellsey, MA) was responsible for all data management. An independent pathologist reviewed all discrepant and positive cases in a blinded review. Statistical analysis was performed by the contract research organization, whereby rejecting a null hypothesis of equivalence that indicated a difference between the two methods. When the *P* value was significant ($P < 0.05$), a method was favoured.

## Results

The diagnostic classification for all categories is summarized in Table 32.1, with Table 32.2 summarizing the diagnostic classification for LSIL and more severe diagnoses. The diagnostic data for LSIL and more severe lesions were subjected to statistical analysis at all six of the study sites. These data are presented in Table 32.3. For LSIL and more severe lesions, the diagnostic comparisons statistically favoured the ThinPrep method at four sites and was statistically equivalent at two sites. Overall the diagnostic comparison statistically favoured the ThinPrep method.

An important aspect of this study was the assessment of specimen inadequacy between the ThinPrep and conventional Pap smear. According to the Bethesda system material was classified as satisfactory, satisfactory but limited by . . . (e.g. inflammation, air drying) or unsatisfactory. The specimen adequacy results are shown in Table 32.4. In this study there was a 6.4% difference between the conventional and ThinPrep method in detecting endocervical component. This is similar to previous studies using a split-sample collection methodology. To evaluate the performance of the ThinPrep system in a setting where the sampling device would be directly rinsed into the PreservCyt vial, two studies were performed involving 299 and 484 patients, respectively. In the first study, the 'satisfactory but limited by . . .' absence of endocervical component was 9.36% on ThinPrep slides and 9.4% to conventional Pap smear. In the second study the 'satisfactory but limited by . . .' no endocervical

**Table 32.1** Diagnostic classification table – all categories.

| | | Conventional | | | | | | | |
|---|---|---|---|---|---|---|---|---|---|
| | | Neg | ASCUS | AGUS | LSIL | HSIL | SQ CA | GL CA | Total |
| Thin-layer | Neg | **5224** | 295 | 3 | 60 | 11 | 0 | 0 | 5593 |
| prep | ASCUS | 318 | **125** | 2 | 45 | 7 | 0 | 0 | 497 |
| | AGUS | 13 | 2 | **3** | 0 | 1 | 0 | 1 | 20 |
| | LSIL | 114 | 84 | 0 | **227** | 44 | 0 | 0 | 469 |
| | HSIL | 11 | 15 | 0 | 35 | **104** | 2 | 0 | 167 |
| | SQ CA | 0 | 0 | 0 | 0 | 0 | **1** | 0 | 1 |
| | GL CA | 0 | 0 | 0 | 0 | 0 | 0 | **0** | 0 |
| | Total | 5680 | 521 | 8 | 367 | 167 | 3 | 1 | |

Neg, Normal or negatives; ASCUS, atypical squamous cells of undetermined significance; AGUS, atypical glandular cells of undetermined significance; LSIL, low-grade squamous intraepithelial lesion; HSIL, high-grade squamous intraepithelial lesion; SQ CA, squamous cell carcinoma; GL CA, glandular cell adenocarcinoma.

**Fig. 32.2** Low-grade squamous intraepithelial lesion (LSIL) and more severe diagnoses.

| | | Conventional | | |
| --- | --- | --- | --- | --- |
| | | Neg/ASCUS/AGUS | LSIL + | Total |
| Thin-layer prep | Neg/ASCUS/AGUS | 5985 | 125 | 6110 |
| | LSIL + | 224 | 413 | 637 |
| | Total | 6209 | 538 | |

Neg, Normal or negative; ASCUS, atypical squamous cells of undetermined significance; AGUS, atypical glandular cells of undetermined significance.

**Table 32.3** Statistical analyses – Low-grade squamous intraepithelial lesions (LSIL) and more severe lesions.

| Site | Cases | Thin-layer prep LSIL + | Conventional LSIL + | Increased detection | $P$ value | Method favoured |
| --- | --- | --- | --- | --- | --- | --- |
| S1 | 1336 | 46 | 31 | 48% | 0.027 | ThinPrep |
| S2 | 1563 | 78 | 45 | 73% | < 0.001 | ThinPrep |
| S3 | 1058 | 67 | 40 | 68% | < 0.001 | ThinPrep |
| H1 | 971 | 125 | 96 | 30% | < 0.001 | ThinPrep |
| H2 | 1010 | 111 | 130 | (15%) | 0.135 | Neither |
| H3 | 809 | 210 | 196 | 7% | 0.374 | Neither |
| All sites | | | | | < 0.001 | ThinPrep |

For LSIL and more severe lesions, the diagnostic comparison statistically favoured the ThinPrep method at four sites and was statistically equivalent at two sites. Overall, the diagnostic comparison statistically favoured the ThinPrep method.

**Table 32.4** Specimen adequacy results.

| | | Conventional | | | |
| --- | --- | --- | --- | --- | --- |
| | | Sat | SBLD | Unsat | Total |
| Thin-layer prep | Sat | 4316 | 1302 | 38 | 5656 |
| | SBLB | 722 | 665* | 44 | 1431 |
| | Unsat | 63 | 41 | 32 | |
| | Total | 5101 | 2008 | 114 | |

* 106 slides had scant cellularity that may be associated with the split-sample protocol that used residual sample in the preparation of ThinPrep slides. Sat, satisfactory; SBLB, satisfactory but limited by; unsat, unsatisfactory.

component was 4.96% on ThinPrep slides compared to the historical value of 4.4% in the conventional smear. These studies suggest that with direct-to-vial sampling, the ThinPrep Pap test yields an endocervical component similar to conventional Pap smear.

A variety of benign cellular changes and infections were examined during the trial. In this clinical trial infection was detected in 20.6% of ThinPrep cases, and 20.0% of conventional Pap smears. Reactive cellular changes were noted

**Table 32.5** Statistical analyses of specimen adequacy.

| Site | Cases | $P$ value | Method favoured |
|------|-------|-----------|-----------------|
| S1 | 1386 | < 0.001 | Conventional |
| S2 | 1668 | < 0.001 | ThinPrep |
| S3 | 1093 | < 0.001 | ThinPrep |
| H1 | 1046 | < 0.001 | ThinPrep |
| H2 | 1049 | 0.375 | Neither |
| H3 | 981 | < 0.001 | ThinPrep |
| All sites | | < 0.001 | ThinPrep |

The comparison of specimen adequacy analysis statistically favoured the ThinPrep method at four sites, the conventional at one site, and was statistically equivalent at one site. Overall, the specimen adequacy analysis statistically favoured the ThinPrep method.

in 6.1% with the ThinPrep and 7.0% of conventional Pap smears.

The issue of specimen adequacy was assessed by statistical analysis at each site (Table 32.5). Overall, the specimen adequacy analysis statistically favoured the ThinPrep method.

One pathologist, not involved in the initial diagnosis, served as an independent reviewer for the six clinical sites, receiving both slides from cases where either slide was abnormal or the pair was discrepant. This allows the calculation of a relative sensitivity, providing an alternative to histologic confirmation by biopsy or human papillomavirus testing as a means for determining the relative proportions of abnormals for the two methods. This approach determines the proportion of LSIL or more severe lesions by each method. For the proportion of LSIL or more severe lesions, the ThinPrep method was statistically equivalent at three sites. Overall, the ThinPrep method was statistically favoured. The use of an independent pathologist provides assurance that the increased sensitivity observed with the ThinPrep method does not compromise the specificity of the diagnosis.

## Discussion

Liquid-based collection of the cervical sample, as an alternative to the conventional Pap smear, has been evaluated in a large number of investigator sponsored and independent clinical trials [6–12]. These studies have shown improved performance of the ThinPrep system in the detection of cervical abnormalities. The clinical trial of the ThinPrep system reported in this study is the most rigorously controlled study to date, and uses the ThinPrep 2000, which is the current model of the instrument intended for gynaecological application. Several conclusions can be drawn from this clinical study.

First, and most importantly, for the detection of LSIL or more severe diagnoses the ThinPrep method was statistically favoured over the conventional Pap smear. In screening populations, with relatively low prevalence of disease, the detection was improved by up to 73%, with an average improvement of 63%, as compared to conventional Pap smears. In populations of women with known cervical abnormalities, or at high risk for cervical abnormalities, lesser degrees of improved detection are seen, with an increased detection of up to 30%, and an average of 6%. This difference in improvement reflects the prevalence of disease in the two populations.

The magnitude of improved disease detection by the ThinPrep system in a screening population is attributable to two factors. First, the ThinPrep system improves sampling of the cervix. The entire sample that is collected on the cervical sampling device is rinsed into a preservative solution and available for cytopreparation. This contrasts with the conventional Pap smear, where there is incomplete transference of the cells from the sampling device to the glass slide. Up to 80% of the sample may be discarded [13]. A second, and important factor from the cytologist's perspective, is that the superior morphological presentation of the cells on the ThinPrep slides allows for clear visualization of cell abnormalities and increased ease of detection and classification (Figs 32.1–32.3).

The ThinPrep method also provides for improved specimen adequacy. At the six sites involved in this study, the ThinPrep method showed a reduction in

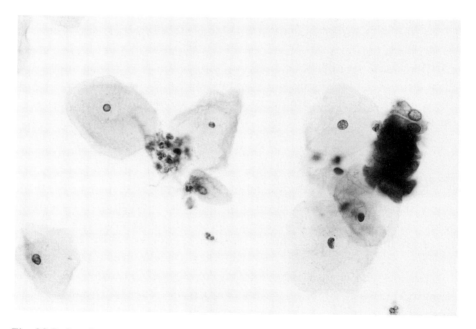

**Fig. 32.1** An advantage of the ThinPrep approach is that cells are deposited on the slide in a thin layer, with minimal overlap. Note the cluster of endocervical cells on the right-hand portion of the photomicrograph. Inflammatory cells, while reduced in number, are still present.

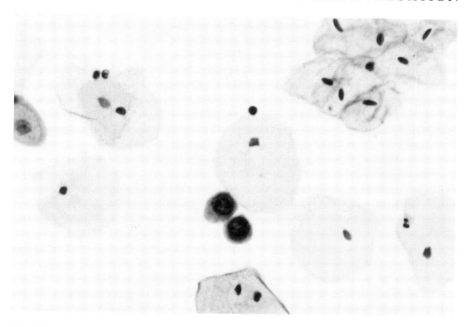

**Fig. 32.2** Small cells from a high-grade squamous intraepithelial lesion are evident on this slide.

the Bethesda system classification 'satisfactory but limited by . . .' by up to 58%, with an average reduction of 29%. This reduction reflects the absence of air-drying, obscuring inflammation, mucus or blood, or thick smears that can accompany conventional smears. In the current clinical study the ThinPrep method was handicapped by the use of residual material on the cervical sampling device. This resulted in 15.8% of the ThinPrep samples lacking endocervical (compared to 9.4% in conventional smears) and 2.1% having scant squamous epithelial component (compared to 0.7% in conventional smears). When a direct-to-vial approach is used in the ThinPrep method, improvement in the ThinPrep specimen adequacy can be anticipated [14]. The identification of inflammation, infection or other benign cellular changes is an important part of the cervical Pap test. When compared to the conventional smear, the ThinPrep method shows equivalent detection of these changes.

Although improved sensitivity of disease detection is an important aspect of any technological change to the Pap smear, it is important that the specificity of the test be maintained. High false-positive results after primary screening or rescreening of putative false-negatives is undesirable, because of both patient anxiety and increased cost due to follow-up examination. Importantly, the independent pathologist review in the current study established that the improved sensitivity of the ThinPrep method did not come at a cost of a loss in specificity.

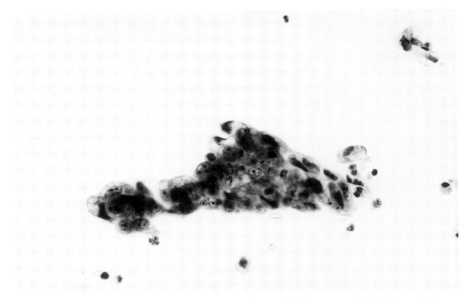

**Fig. 32.3** This cluster of endocervical adenocarcinoma is shown on the ThinPrep slide. Nuclear and cytoplasmic morphology is well preserved.

Other advantages of the ThinPrep method are its adaptability to computer-aided imaging and supplemental testing of the patient cell sample. Additional diagnostic testing of the residual sample can increase the information yielded by the Pap test. For example, identification of *Neisseria gonorrhoeae* or *Chlamydia* infection might be performed by molecular or fluorescent antibody methods. The greatest opportunity, however, is human papillomavirus typing of samples that are morphologically abnormal. Human papillomavirus typing of samples diagnosed as atypical squamous cells of undetermined significance or LGSIL may serve to triage women into conservative follow-up, or colposcopy and biopsy [15]. This determination, based on the types of human papillomavirus DNA that are present, may lead to substantial cost savings and more appropriate patient management.

Finally, ThinPrep slides greatly reduce the difficulty associated with computer-aided imaging of conventional Pap smears. This may facilitate the prescreening or primary screening of cervical samples.

## References

1 Naryshkin S, Davey DD. Terminology of false negative and false positive pap smears: 'they're just worms'. *Diagn Cytopathol* 1996; **14**: 1–3.
2 Gay JD, Donaldson LD, Goellner JR. False-negative results in cervical cytologic studies. *Acta Cytol* 1985; **29**: 1043–1046.

3 Health Care Financing Administration. Medicare, Medicaid and CLIA programs; regulations implementing the clinical laboratory improvement Amendments of 1988: proposed rule. *Fed Registry* 1990; **55**: 20908.

4 Bibbo M, Wied GL. Special issue: new industrial developments in automated cytology. *Acta Cytol* 1996; **40**: 1–132.

5 Zahniser DJ, Sullivan PJ. CYTYC Corporation. *Acta Cytol* 1996; **40**: 37–44.

6 Aponte-Cipriani SL, Teplitz C, Rorat E, Savino A, Jacobs A. Cervical smears prepared by an automated device versus the conventional method. A comparative analysis. *Acta Cytol* 1995; **39**: 623–630.

7 Awen C, Hathway S, Eddy W, Voskuil R, Janes C. Efficacy of ThinPrep preparation of cervical smears: a 1000-case, investigator-sponsored study. *Diagn Cytopathol* 1994; **11**: 33–37.

8 Bur M, Knowles K, Pekow P, Corral O, Donovan J. Comparison of ThinPrep preparations with conventional cervicovaginal smears. Practical considerations. *Acta Cytol* 1995; **39**: 631–642.

9 Hutchinson ML, Agarwal P, Denault T, Berger B, Cibas ES. A new look at cervical cytology. ThinPrep multicenter trial results. *Acta Cytol* 1992; **36**: 499–504.

10 Wilbur DC, Dawson A *et al*. Interpretation of cervical cytology utilizing thin-layer processing: comparison of results with conventional smears. *Lab Invest Mod Pathol* 1992; **66**: 30A.

11 Kish J, Vallera D *et al*. ThinPrep gynecologic study: a review of 488 cases. *Acta Cytol* 1994; **38**: 806.

12 Wilbur DC, Dubeshter B, Angel C, Atkison KM. Use of thin-layer preparations for gynecologic smears with emphasis on the cytomorphology of high-grade intraepithelial lesions and carcinomas. *Diagn Cytopathol* 1996; **14**: 201–211.

13 Hutchinson ML, Isenstein LM, Goodman A *et al*. Homogeneous sampling accounts for the increased diagnostic accuracy using the ThinPrep processor. *Am J Clin Pathol* 1994; **101**: 215–219.

14 Tezuka F, Shuki H, Oikawa H, Higashiiwai H. Numerical counts of epithelial cells collected, smeared and lost in the conventional Papanicolaou smear preparation. *Acta Cytol* 1995; **39**: 837–838.

15 Sherman ME, Schiffman MH, Lorincz AT *et al*. Cytopathologic diagnosis and human papillomavirus testing of cervical specimens collected in PreservCyt: a new paradigm for cervical cancer screening. *J Natl Cancer Inst* 1997; (in press).

# 33: The History of Neural Network Technology in Cytology

## M. E. Boon

## Summary

In this study the history of the first commercialized screening system using neural network technology is described. The story of PAPNET spans 8 years and three continents. The human network involved in the introduction of the concept of neural networks for screening in the medical community is documented in the presented personal careers of five individuals. Out of these personal histories it can be concluded that personal experiences, chance human encounters, personal circumstances and political developments all play a role.

## Introduction

At the time of writing the only commercially available system using neural networks for screening cervical smears is PAPNET, developed and marketed by Neuromedical Systems, Inc. (NSI), a company based in the USA. In our discussion of the history of neural networks in cytology, we will focus on PAPNET and NSI.

For the introduction of a new technology in medical practice, three points are important:

1 There must be an awareness that there is a problem which needs to be solved.

2 A solution to that problem that is technically feasible should be available.

3 There must be a set of people who can interact with each other, each having

*Correspondence*: Dr Mathilde E. Boon, Leiden Cytology and Pathology Laboratory, PO Box 16084, 2301 GB Leiden, The Netherlands.

appreciation of both technology and medical practice. It is important that these people differ in background but have, basically, the same aim.

In this chapter we will present the history of the application of neural network technology in cytology along these lines, providing data of some persons of the early human network involved in the development and clinical testing of PAPNET. The information concerning Mr Rutenberg and Dr Mango was provided by NSI, and that of Drs Koss and Ng predominantly by themselves. The personal history of Dr Boon is derived from the archives of the Leiden Cytology and Pathology Laboratory. Since these were fully accessible, the story of the writer of this article has become disproportionately prominent. Nevertheless, it was decided to keep it intact because it is exemplary for the motivation to make a success of the application of neural networks in medicine.

## Awareness of the problem of the false-negative smear

The problem of the false-negative smear was not very popular amongst the medical profession. At best, the subject is treated with benign negligence. The situation changed dramatically when it was brought into the limelight by Bogdanich in his 1987 article published in the *Wall Street Journal* [1]. The new term 'Pap mill' was coined by him, picturing mass production of erroneous diagnoses by overworked cytotechnologists. The medical bureaucracy woke up and regulatory guidelines were formulated with the aim to improve the performance of US cytology laboratories [2]. Apart from the paperwork thus generated, the laboratory management was plagued by rules concerning the workload of the cytotechnologists. Not only the number of smears to be screened daily by one cytotechnologist was down-regulated to a much lower level than was formerly the custom, but in addition 10% of the smears signed out as negative had to be rescreened.

The rescreening guidelines created their own hurdles. First, it is quite difficult to motivate cytotechs to rescreen with the required unflagging diligence large numbers of smears in which the likelihood of finding abnormal cells is reduced through the initial screening. In this context it is important to mention that a cytotechnologist is completely focused on finding abnormal cells, and if in a working day, or even worse, in a working week, such an event does not take place, there is a slackening of concentration and the danger of habituation lies in wait. The second problem created was a financial one: the income of the cytotechnologist rose steeply after 1988, thus these rescreening requirements became quite costly. Finally, shortage of cytotechnologists in the USA with a high vacancy rate (regionally as high as 42%) [3] made it relevant to search for automated systems which could take over, partly or completely, the burden of rescreening negative smears.

## The availability of neural network technology

Neural network technology had already been available for two decades; however it is, at present, relatively unknown to practising medical doctors. In this context it is interesting to provide the *Lancet* story. In 1994, the reviewer of the *Lancet* criticized a paper on PAPNET in routine practice because the methodology of the neural network was not described to the point where results could be repeated by others. The reviewer wrote that reports on the efficacy of non-disclosed technology should remain in the trade journals which one does not expect to have long-term validity. After a fierce correspondence, the editors of that reputed journal finally decided that the readers of their journal should be informed about this technology. As a consequence, the first review paper on various applications of neural networks in pathology laboratories was published in the *Lancet* in 1995 [4].

Neural networks were first applied for military target recognition. Instead of the serial (single) path of programming utilized by conventional computers, neural computers have thousands of adaptive formed paths linked in parallel, comprising a network conceptually similar to the network of neurons in the human brain. Neural networks can process immense quantities of information while mimicking the neurological ability to learn from experience. Unlike conventional statistical regression models, networks make no assumptions about normal distributions.

The vagaries of the presentation of the cells in cervical smear are almost limitless and the images of normal and abnormal smears are too complex to fit in a precise model system. As a consequence, the construction of formal 'rules' (e.g. a knowledge base) instructing a machine to recognize and correctly interpret the smear is not feasible. This fundamental difficulty is bypassed by neural networks because they can learn complex associations directly from examples without having to know how such an example came to be. Neural networks also display sample tolerance, which is the ability not to err when presented with unusual appearances or smears containing contradictory data. After training on images of a series of normal and abnormal smears, a neural network can recognize images even though they differ considerably from the training set.

In order to apply this to cervical cytology, a person was needed who worked in the defence industry and who was at the same time aware of the false-negative problem. That person was Mr Mark Rutenberg.

## The network of people

In this section we will describe the network of people needed for the introduction of neural network technology in cytology. Part of the information was provided by the persons in question themselves.

## Mr Mark R. Rutenberg

Our story starts in the USA, in the New York area, where Mr Mark Rutenberg lives and works. Mr Rutenberg is the inventor of PAPNET, the first (and only) screening system applying neural network technology, and the founder of the firm NSI, in which his invention was commercialized. Therefore, our story begins with him, in the USA.

First, his educational background, which is as varied as biomedical engineering, neuropsychology, image processing and computer science. He first became involved in investigating the application of computers to cytology while studying biomedical engineering in the early 1970s. At that time, the efforts of his group to automate cytological screening were unsuccessful, but the experience gained by him in that period proved to be very important in his later career.

Prior to founding NSI, Mr Rutenberg was a noted lecturer and consultant in the areas of neural networks and ultrareliable system design. He invented, patented and implemented a highly innovative approach to fault-tolerant system design utilized by the Mark 48 torpedo to prevent accidental detonation. He developed and popularized Integrated Fault Tree Analysis, a technique now mandated by both the Department of Defense and the Food and Drugs Administration (FDA) to protect life-critical systems from the effects of software design error.

During the late 1980s he worked and consulted for several defence contractors in the area of applying adaptive computing to military target recognition. From 1980 to 1988 Mr Rutenberg was responsible for the management and marketing of several advanced defence programmes. His responsibilities included matrix management of the semiautonomous Advanced Program Area composed of engineers, scientists, marketing, finance, legal and manufacturing personnel. The project he worked on concerned large-scale navigation and target recognition computer systems. While working in the defence industry, Mr Rutenberg realized that it might be possible to use neural network technology for the problem he failed to solve in the 1970s, that is, to automate the search for abnormal cells in routinely made smears. Thus the invention of the PAPNET system was the direct result of the fact that somebody who was working at the application of these advanced image recognition techniques for military target identification was also aware of the problems of cervical cytology, that somebody being Mr Rutenberg.

Mark Rutenberg invented the PAPNET testing system in 1987 and founded NSI in 1988. He filed for a patent, which was issued on 23 October 1990. The company has four issued US and nine pending patent applications. Mr Rutenberg has served as the company's chairman, president and chief executive officer since its inception.

Since the problem in the USA was that of rescreening, Mr Rutenberg exclusively thought along these lines and designed the system to be used as a rescreening device. It was found that the system was able to detect even small and rare abnormal cells on conventionally prepared cervical Papanicolaou (Pap) smears, that are likely to be missed in conventional rescreening. This was thought to be such an important asset that it was specifically mentioned in the patent application. Because the idea was that the system should only be used to aid in the rescreening of slides which were diagnosed by manual inspection to be negative and which would otherwise be sent to the laboratory's archive without further examination, Mr Rutenberg could safely claim that there are no risks for the patient involved in PAPNET testing. Theoretically this might be the case if the system would be used for prescreening – a possibility Mr Rutenberg did not yet consider in April 1992, when he met Dr Boon in New York, and even not when NSI applied for FDA approval for the system in 1995.

Mr Rutenberg lived at the time of his invention in the New York area, thus it is not surprising that when he wanted to show his invention to a reputed cytologist, he chose Dr Koss of the Montefiore Hospital in New York. Looking at the data provided by NSI, it seems that at the time he went to Dr Koss, Mr Rutenberg had already filed his first patent on the application of neural networks to cytology.

## Dr Leopold G. Koss

The world-famous US cytologist Dr Koss is not only known for his diagnostic acumen, but also for his long-standing work in automation and quantitation of cytology. He wrote to us that a young Californian pathologist, Dr Thomas Hall, together with Mr Rutenberg, presented the project to him in 1989. The unusual concept was immediately appealing to Dr Koss — the machine searching for cells and the human diagnostician judging the cells. Neural network application to cellular targets, combined with human intellect to clinch the diagnosis, was novel to him. He had spent many years attempting to adapt image analysis to the diagnosis of cancer and he was, at the time he met Mr Rutenberg, convinced that fully automated image analysis would not work on routine smears with the approach used at that moment. Mr Rutenberg told us that he presented a videotape of the system to Dr Koss in his home in Manhattan. Before the video presentation Dr Koss told Mr Rutenberg that if his system failed he could always get a job at 47 Street Photo, a famous discount electric store in New York run by Orthodox Jews. After the show there was no more talk about working at 47 Street Photo.

Dr Koss and his coworkers have been working with the company from its very onset and have performed a great deal of initial research on the performance of the system with a unit in their own laboratory under a grant from the company [5]. The well-documented clinical material of the Montefiore Hospital could be used for clinical testing of the software programs. Dr Koss and his group documented that the machine is very useful in assessing other cytological specimens such as sputum, voided urine and washings and brushings of the oesophagus. Several of the coworkers of NSI have worked with Dr Koss; amongst others the medical director of the company, Laurie Mango. Thus the human network needed for the application of neural networks in cytology was extended to Dr Koss and all his coworkers [6].

## Dr Laurie J. Mango

The young company NSI was in need of a young doctor to add medical know-how, and found this in the person of Laurie J. Mango. Laurie Mango served as a cytology Fellow at the Montefiore Medical Center in New York under Dr Leopold G. Koss. In addition to her medical degree, she holds a BS degree in electrical engineering. This education makes her a medical doctor aware of the possibilities of technology. Prior to joining the company in 1990, Dr Mango was a resident in anatomic pathology at the University of California, San Francisco, where her interest in neuropathology and artificial neural networks brought her into contact with the discipline of neural network technology. In her work in the company she profits from the good contacts with Dr Koss and his staff at the Montefiore Hospital. She contributed to the development of the image-processing algorithms and neural networks used in the PAPNET system, particularly in the evaluation of their performance in a clinical setting. At NSI, she is in charge of all medical affairs of NSI, including the preparation of the PAPNET pre-market approval submission to the FDA. She was involved in the huge rescreening project in several US laboratories in which over 11 000 negative smears were rescreened with the PAPNET method. This large clinical study was needed to acquire FDA approval for using the PAPNET system in the USA as a rescreening test. Note that NSI did not try to get the PAPNET method approved for prescreening. Based on the good results of the rescreening project, the FDA has given clearance in autumn 1995, allowing the PAPNET system to be marketed in the USA for rescreening. Of March 1996, 88 US laboratories are equipped with the PAPNET review stations. All this was achieved thanks to Dr Laurie Mango in her role as medical director [7–15].

## Dr Mathilde E. Boon

Here, our story brings us to the Netherlands where Dr Mathilde E. Boon was raised and educated. She met Dr Koss in 1973 in Miami at the International Congress of Cytology, which she visited when she was a resident in pathology at the university hospital in Leiden. She was introduced to him by a friend of Dr Koss, Dr Naylor. Dr Naylor had taught her cytology in his laboratory in Ann Arbor in 1967–1968, making her a US-trained cytologist when she returned to the Netherlands. Dr Koss was so kind as to write an introduction to her book on urinary cytology in 1977, and advised her on various cytology problems. Dr Boon was the cytologist of the Dr Ploem group in Leiden in the early 1970s [16–18]. This well-known group was aiming at the automation of cervical cytology. In the late 1970s she shared her office with Dr Jan Baak, then a resident in pathology in Delft. In that period, she published several papers on morphometry, in part with Dr Baak [19–24]. With the experiences described, she was aware of the problems of automation and quantitation of cytology, but more is needed to see the necessities of switching to automation of the screening process.

The events of the late 1980s played a key role in further developments. Since it concerns an exemplary case of a false-negative smear and what can happen around it, we will describe it in great detail. In 1988, she was threatened with a claim of US$300 000 due to false-negative diagnosis made in her laboratory. It concerned a smear in which, at rescreening, with foreknowledge of the clinical diagnosis, the staff of the Leiden laboratory could indeed detect groups of small cancer cells. This smear could thus be marked as a truly false-negative smear. However, the staff of the Leiden laboratory was of the opinion that the 'mistake' was understandable since the cancer cells were small and hidden under a thick inflammatory infiltrate. The claimant's lawyer did not agree with this viewpoint and was strengthened in standpoint by a highly damaging report of one of Dr Boon's colleagues in which was stated that the quality of screening in the Leiden laboratory was substandard. This pathologist thought that he was in the position to conclude in his report that the smear had not received the necessary attention of the supervising pathologist of the Leiden laboratory. To make matters worse, he contested that the cancer cells were small and difficult to detect (as Dr Boon claimed). He even went so far as to write that rumours went that the cytotechnologists of the Leiden laboratory screened more smears per day than is allowed in the Netherlands.

The insurance company decided against a law suit and settled the case, being afraid that it was extremely difficult to refute this damaging report. This development was much to the chagrin of Dr Boon, who thought that the opinions voiced by her colleague were totally unjustified. She had no say in the legal proceedings, and consequently the truth was never brought to light in the court room. This frustrating experience triggered her to investigate the problem of false-negative smears in a scientific way. She thought it was all-important to have false negatives screened by unaware cytotechnologists. This was easier said than done, and possibly because of this, no report of such an endeavour could be found in the literature. For this scientific investigation five smears of patients with proven invasive carcinoma, containing cancer cells that were missed by the cytotechnologist and thus erroneously signed out as negative, were used. Dr Boon planted, together with her colleague Dr Madeleine Bosch, over a period of 6 months, one by one, the five false-negative smears in the routine screening load of one of the 12 cytotechnologists. To keep the cytotechnologists completely unaware of what was going on (which was essential for the scientific validity of the test), nobody in the laboratory but Drs Boon and Bosch knew that there were planted smears in the routine screening portions.

Each false-negative smear was planted five times, resulting in 25 test runs. Only once were the cancer cells detected. In all other 24 runs they were missed (again) [25]. The errors made in screening these false-negative smears were due to a combination of a low number of abnormal cells, poor preservation and the small size of the cancer cells. It could be concluded that it was impossible to avoid *all* false-negative diagnoses. Moreover, rescreening of smears signed out as negative, as was done in the USA, is possibly of little or no help in these cases because it is likely that the cancer cells will remain undetected in the second screening round.

With this knowledge Dr Boon was on the look-out for a completely new way of screening. In the summer of 1991, she saw the PAPNET system at an exhibition at the European Congress of Cytology in Turku, Finland. Her husband, the theoretical physicist Dr L.P. Kok, well-versed in the possibilities of neural networks, advised her to try the system on her false-negative smears. This test was very successful [26]; indeed PAPNET was able to detect the small cancer cells overlooked in human screening. However, she was not interested in *rescreening* but in *prescreening*. Therefore she asked Dr Laurie Mango to install a review station in her laboratory to investigate whether the system can be used for this purpose. First, she personally tested in the warm summer of 1992 whether the interactive PAPNET method is successful in cases with positive histology which were detected in human screening. In all unequivocal cases, PAPNET found (pre)cancer cells. The next step was to make a screening protocol, and in autumn 1992, her cytotechnologists were trained one by one on her PAPNET protocol for interactive PAPNET screening.

By August 1994, all smears from the Leiden Cytology and Pathology Laboratory, at that time scanned in the Amsterdam scanning centre of NSI, were screened with this method. By May 1996, the digitized images of 180 000 smears screened by the Leiden group could be linked to the database of the cytological, histological and epidemiological data of the screened women. All analyses performed on this clinical material indicate that, using PAPNET in primary screening, more cases of high-grade lesions and invasive carcinoma are detected than in conventional screening. The PAPNET experience in Leiden is vast and the European scanning centre of NSI is based in Amsterdam, making it simple for Dutch pathologists to have a close look at this application of neural networks in cytology. Nevertheless, as of May 1996, the Dutch Society of Pathology has not voiced its opinion on PAPNET. The excuse is that at this moment Dutch pathologists are fully occupied by the reorganizational problems created by the new governmentally financed screening programmes, leaving no room for contemplations concerning the application of new screening techniques. This (cyto)pathological silence, however, hampers the introduction of this system in other Dutch screening laboratories.

Finally, it should be stressed that Dr Boon has shown that PAPNET can be used for prescreening, for which it was initially not developed and for which no FDA approval was asked for in 1995. This concept of primary PAPNET-assisted screening has been exported to several other European countries, including Germany, Italy and Switzerland [27,28].


## Dr Stephen Ng

Here, our story brings us to the Far East. The epidemiologist Dr Stephen Ng introduced PAPNET in Asia. He is the director of the Hong Kong-based scanning centre of NSI. His wife Marie is a pathologist.

The Ng couple combines knowledge of cytology with epidemiological know-how, and, as will become clear, they have valuable contacts with the high-tech business world of the Far East. A contributing factor of their role in the NSI story was their wish to return from the USA to Hong Kong to witness the transition in 1997. All they needed was a good opportunity, for which they were on the look-out.

The Ngs were both raised and educated in Hong Kong but worked in 1993 in the USA. In April 1993, Dr Ng heard for the first time about NSI, from his wife via her boss, Dr Weiss of the Good Samaritan Hospital. Dr Weiss was an investor in the company, and it seems likely that he shared his positive expectations about NSI with his coworkers. Her interest was further heightened by her conversations with Dr Schreiber, one of the coworkers of Dr Koss, who highly recommended PAPNET to her. All this led to a meeting of the Ngs with Mr Rutenberg, who suggested starting a scanning centre in Hong Kong. This was the chance they were looking for to return to their roots. In the realization of this, Dr Ng's friendship of over 20 years with Hong Kong businessmen, kept intact during the USA years, proved to be a key factor. These college friends had remained in Hong Kong and were active in medical and high-tech business in Hong Kong and China. While quite a few Hong Kong businessmen had left the British crown colony in the past decade, they stayed and had realized an expanding trade, particularly with mainland China.

When they heard about NSI from Stephen Ng, they saw in this novel technology a good business opportunity. Within 2 weeks of the first conversations with the Ngs they went to the USA to meet with Mr Rutenberg. It was agreed upon that they would invest in NSI in return for permission to represent NSI in Hong Kong, China and Singapore. It was also arranged that Dr Ng and his wife would return to Hong Kong to set up a cytology laboratory, making their dream come true.

The years preceding the transition of Hong Kong from crown colony to part of communistic China were years of great uncertainties but, for those who did not refrain from taking risks, this was a period of great opportunities. In 1994, the Ngs could receive Drs Koss, Mango and Boon, who visited the International Pathology Congress in Hong Kong in the autumn of 1994, in the Hong Kong scanning centre of NSI and their well-run cytology laboratories, with leaflets on PAPNET in Chinese. The NSI headquarters had just moved to a brand-new shining high rise, with a wide view over the busy harbour, which was in the process of being remodelled; this mega task performed by Dutch firms. From May 1996, PAPNET is used in several big cities in China, including Beijing, Shanghai, Guangzhoud, Shenzhen, Xian and Nanjing. It is well received but there are not many qualified cytotechnologists or cytopathologists in China. NSI will help to train more cytologists in China to use PAPNET. The Ngs look forward positively to the transition in 1997, with NSI already having a firm foot planted in China.

## Conclusion

Out of these personal histories it can be concluded that personal experiences, chance human encounters, personal circumstances and political developments all play a role in the human network needed for the development and introduction of neural network technology in cervical screening.

## References

1 Bogdanich W. The Pap test misses much cervical cancer through labs' errors. *Wall St J* 1987; Nov 21.
2 Clinical Laboratory Improvement Amendments of 1988. Public Law 100–578. *Fed Reg* 1990; **55**: 9538.
3 Grohs DH. Challenges in cervical cancer screening: what clinicians, patients and the general public need to know. *Acta Cytol* 1996; **40**: 73–80.
4 Dybowski R, Gant V. Artificial neural networks in pathology and medical laboratories. *Lancet* 1995; **346**: 1203–1207.
5 Koss LG, Lin E, Schreiber K, Elgert P, Mango L. Evaluation of the PAPNET cytologic screening system for quality control of cervical smears. *Am J Clin Pathol* 1994; **101**: 220–229.

6  Koss LG. Reducing the error rate in Papanicolaou smears. One laboratory's experience with the PAPNET system. *Female Patient* 1994; **119**: 34–40.

7  Mango LJ, Holund B, Holm K, Schreiber K, Alonzo A, Decker D. Rescreening of 89 'negative' cervical smears preceding invasive carcinoma by the PAPNET cytologic screening system. *Acta Cytol* 1993; **37**: 780.

8  Mango LJ. Computer-assisted cervical cancer screening using neural networks. *Cancer Lett* 1994; **77**: 155–162.

9  Mango LJ, Elgert PA. The PAPNET cytological screening system. *ASCT News* 1994; **15**: 10–13.

10  Mango LJ, Herriman JM. The PAPNET cytological screening system. In: Wied GL, Bartels PH, Rosenthal DL, Schenck U (eds) *Compendium on the Computerized Cytology and Histology Laboratory*. Chicago: Tutorials of Cytology, 1994; pp 320–334.

11  Rosenthal DL, Mango LJ. Applications of neural networks for interactive diagnosis of anatomic pathology specimens. In: Wied GL, Bartels PH, Rosenthal DL, Schenck U (eds) *Compendium on the Computerized Cytology and Histology Laboratory*. Chicago: Tutorials of Cytology, 1994, pp 173–184.

12  Sherman ME, Mango LJ, Kelly D *et al*. PAPNET analysis of reportedly negative smears preceding the diagnosis of a high-grade squamous intraepithelial lesion or carcinoma. *Mod Pathol* 1994; 7: 578–581.

13  Mango LJ, Ivasauskas EY. Computer-assisted cervical cytology using PAPNET testing. In: Wied GL, Keebler CM, Rosenthal DL, Schenck U, Somrak TM, Vooijs GP (eds) *Compendium on Quality Assurance, Proficiency Testing and Workload Limitations in Clinical Cytology*. Chicago: Tutorials of Cytology, 1995, pp 155–166.

14  Mango LJ. Industrial developments in automated cytology; Neuromedical Systems, Inc. *Acta Cytol* 1996; **40**: 53–59.

15  Mango LJ. The FDA review process: obtaining premarket approval for the PAPNET testing system. *Acta Cytol* 1996; **40**: 138–140.

16  Beyer-Boon ME, Hilgevoord-de Ruyter C, Ploem JS, de Voogt HJ. The applicability of acriflavine-SITS stain in urinary cytology. In: Pressman NJ, Wied GL (eds) *The Automation of Cancer Cytology and Cell Image Analysis*. Chicago: Tutorials of Cytology, 1979, pp 207–211.

17  Ploem-Zaaijer JJ, Beyer-Boon ME, Leyte-Veldstra L, Ploem JS. Cytofluorometric and cytophotometric DNA measurements of cervical smears stained using a new bi-color method. In: Pressman NJ, Wied GL (eds) *The Automation of Cancer Cytology and Cell Image Analysis*. Chicago: Tutorials of Cytology, 1979, pp 225–235.

18  de Voogt HJ, Beyer-Boon ME, Ploem JS. The value of DNA-cytophotometry for the refinement of cytologic diagnosis of urothelial carcinoma. *Cancer Cytol* 1979; **19**: 6–7.

19  Baak JPA, Kurver PHJ, de Graaf S, Boon ME. Morphometry for prognosis prediction in breast cancer. *Lancet* 1981; **ii**: 315.

20  Boon ME, Kurver PHJ, Baak JPA, Thompson HT. The application of morphometry in gastric cytological diagnosis. *Virchows Arch [Pathol Anat]* 1981; **393**: 159–164.

21  Boon ME, Kurver PHJ, Baak JPA, Ooms ECM. Morphometric differences between urothelial cells in voided urine of patients with grade I and grade II bladder tumours. *J Clin Pathol* 1981; **34**: 612–615.

22  Baak JPA, Kurver PHJ, de Snoo-Niewlaat AJE, de Graef S, Makkink B, Boon ME. Prognostic indicators in breast cancer – morphometric methods. *Histopathology* 1982; **6**: 327–339.

23  Boon ME, Trott PA, van Kaam H, Kurver PJH, Leach A, Baak JPA. Morphometry and cytodiagnosis of breast lesions. *Virchows Arch [Pathol Anat]* 1982; **396**: 9–18.

24  Van Roon E, Boon ME, Kurver PJH, Baak JPA. The association between precancerous-

columnar and squamous lesions of the cervix: a morphometric study. *Histopathology* 1983; 7: 887–896.

25 Bosch MMC, Rietveld-Scheffers PEM, Boon ME. Characteristics of false-negative smears tested in the normal screening situation. *Acta Cytol* 1992; **36**: 711–716.

26 Boon ME, Kok LP. Neural network processing can provide means to catch errors that slip through human screening of Pap smears. *Diagn Cytopathol* 1993; **9**: 411–416.

27 Boon ME, Kok LP, Beck S. Histologic validation of neural network-assisted cervical screening: comparison with the conventional procedure. *Cell Vision* 1995; **2**: 23–27.

28 Boon ME, Kok MR, Beck S. Consequences of neural network technology for cervical screening: increase of diagnostic consistency and increase of positive scores. *Cancer* 1996; **78**: 112–117.

# 34: A Comparison of Automated and Manual Screening: Theoretical Considerations

## M. E. Sherman

## Summary

Studies demonstrate that computer-assisted systems are effective in identifying cervical smears containing abnormal cells that were missed in conventional screening. The role of these devices in primary screening has not been extensively explored. Theoretical considerations related to the implementation of automated primary screening are explored in this review.

## Introduction

The effectiveness of cytological screening in reducing the incidence of cervical cancer is widely acknowledged. None the less, the Pap smear has an unavoidable false-negative rate related to sampling, screening and interpretation. In particular, the monotony of screening large numbers of normal smears promotes lapses of inattentiveness in which rare cancer cells may be overlooked. The development of computer-assisted instruments capable of identifying abnormal smears has raised hopes that some of the burden of primary screening could be assumed by machines, thus reducing the human effort required to perform this arduous task.

In the USA, two devices, PAPNET [1–8] (Neuromedical Systems Inc., Suffern, NY) and AutoPap® 300QC [9–12] (NeoPath Inc., Redmond, WA) have received Food and Drugs Administration approval for review of smears originally reported as negative. Computer-assisted devices are not currently approved for use in primary screening in the USA. The purpose of this chapter is to provide a theoretical discussion of logistical and economic considerations

*Correspondence*: Dr Mark E. Sherman, The John Hopkins Hospital, Department of Pathology, 600 North Wolfe Street, Baltimore, MD 21287, USA.

relevant to assessing the use of these systems in primary screening. It is recognized that existing computer systems might require modification for use as primary screening devices. For the purposes of the current discussion, however, it is assumed that the operating procedures for using these devices in primary screening would be similar to the ones employed in reviewing previously screened smears.

## PAPNET

In the PAPNET system [1–8], conventionally prepared smears are shipped to a central laboratory for analysis with a device that uses both traditional computer imaging technology and neural network software. For each case, the system identifies 128 images of potentially abnormal cells which are recorded as two screens on a video disk. The disk is returned to the user's facility for review at a workstation equipped with a high-resolution video monitor. Images are reviewed as quadrants of 16 images at low magnification with the option for viewing at a higher power. If abnormal images are identified, the slide is manually screened by a cytotechnologist and forwarded to a pathologist for diagnosis. The cells seen on the screen may be identified on the glass slide using a system of coordinates.

## AutoPap® 300

In the AutoPap® 300 system [9–12] the image analyser is placed in the user's laboratory. Based on a QC score assigned by the user, the AutoPap® selects a predetermined proportion of smears as potentially abnormal. The percentage of slides selected for a given QC score reflects the historical performance of the devices. Slides identified as abnormal with AutoPap® 300 are manually rescreened by a cytotechnologist and the abnormal cases are diagnosed by a pathologist.

## Theoretical considerations related to automated primary screening

Theoretical considerations relevant to evaluating the practicality of using computer systems in primary screening are discussed below.

In the PAPNET system, slides must be shipped to a central facility for processing. Shipping costs are assumed by the manufacturer. The manufacturer also provides shipping boxes with styrofoam liners scored with 100 narrow slits which hold individual slides. In our experience, which includes shipping over 10 000 smears from Costa Rica to the USA, breakage was extremely rare. Loss or breakage of slides would require women to return for a repeat clinical visit to obtain another smear. The AutoPap® is housed in the user's laboratory. Both PAPNET and AutoPap® have been designed to use conventional smears, therefore special slide preparations are not required.

The use of automated computer screeners entails specific costs. In PAPNET testing, costs include a training fee for each potential user, the expense of purchasing or leasing the workstation and a charge for each slide that is examined. In the case of the AutoPap®, there is a fee per slide and costs related to computer disposables and bar coding. Both systems require the cytopathology laboratory to allot a physical space for the equipment.

Hypothetically, some or all of the added costs of using computer systems outlined above could be offset by a reduction in the number of slides requiring manual screening by cytotechnologists. Unofficial estimates provided by Neuromedical Systems, Inc., suggest that cytotechnologists can review approximately 25 000 cases per year with the PAPNET system in a quality assurance application. The AutoPAP® 300 does not present video images for review by the user. The laboratory selects a QC score which corresponds to a historical rate of slide selection. The percentage of slides that would require review for use in primary screening is unknown. Sensitivity data for AutoPap® in quality assurance review of negative smears using different QC scores have been published [9]. A technician is needed to load and unload smears from the instruments, but the screening process itself proceeds automatically. The machine can review about 180 slides per day. Cytotechnologists are required to rescreen the cases selected by the instrument which are then submitted to a pathologist for final diagnosis. The relevant question for cost-effectiveness, therefore, is whether cytotechnologists using these devices plus manual re-screening in indicated cases can increase productivity while maintaining excellent quality.

Evaluating the potential cost-effectiveness of using computer-assisted screening in combination with thin-layer slide preparations is complicated. Thin-layer slides are more expensive to prepare than smears, but require less time for microscopic screening. Would it be cost-effective to use thin-layer slides and computer-assisted devices in combination? Clearly, the computer systems would have to perform with high specificity because the major cost with thin-layer technology is related to slide preparation, not screening. Since thin-layer slides produce excellent cellular fixation with minimal cellular overlapping, the performance of computer-assisted screening devices could be better with these preparations than with smears, but this has not been extensively studied. Most cytologists agree that the appearance of cells in thin-layer slides and smears is somewhat different, suggesting that automated screening devices might require modifications to screen these new preparations optimally.

In summary, the effectiveness of computer systems in primary screening is not known, but preliminary experience with these instruments is promising.

## Unanswered questions about primary screening

The feasibility of using computers for primary screening will ultimately depend on whether these devices permit cost-effective identification of abnormal smears. As with all new technologies, continuous improvement in the performance characteristics of the instruments is ongoing. However, the decision to use these devices in primary screening rather than in quality assurance represents a huge leap in thinking. In quality assurance applications, discovery of any false-negative result represents a benefit. If computers were used in primary screening, any missed abnormality that resulted in a bad clinical outcome would be considered a failure. In addition, the devices described in this report identify potentially abnormal smears, but do not provide a specific diagnosis. Final diagnosis of abnormal cases will ultimately reflect human judgement with all of the attendant uncertainties related to the interpretation of cytological specimens.

## Acknowledgement

The author thanks Neuromedical Systems and NeoPath for helpful input in the preparation of this chapter. Dr Sherman has been affiliated with institutions that have had contractual agreements with Cytyc Corp., Boxborough, MA (George Washington University) and Neuromedical Systems, Inc., Suffern, NY (Johns Hopkins Medical Institutions).

## References

1 Boon ME, Kok LP. Neural network processing can provide means to catch errors that slip through human screening of Pap smears. *Diagn Cytopathol* 1993; **9**: 411–416.

2 Boon ME, Kok LP, Nygaard-Nielsen M, Holm K, Holund B. Neural network processing of cervical smears can lead to a decrease in diagnostic variability and an increase in screening efficacy: a study of 63 false negative smears. *Mod Pathol* 1994; **7**: 957–961.

3 Koss LG, Lin E, Schreiber K, Elgert P, Mango L. Evaluation of PAPNET cytologic screening system for quality control of cervical smears. *Am J Clin Pathol* 1994; **101**: 220–229.

4 Ouwerkerk-Noordam E, Boon ME, Beck S. Computerized-assisted primary screening of cervical smears using the PAPNET method: comparison with conventional screening and evaluation of the role of the cytologist. *Cytopathology* 1994; **5**: 211–218.

5 Sherman ME, Mango LJ, Kelly D *et al*. PAPNET analysis of reportedly negative smears preceding the diagnosis of a high-grade squamous intraepithelial lesion or carcinoma. *Mod Pathol* 1994; **7**: 578–581.

6 Mango LJ. Neuromedical Systems, Inc., *Acta Cytol* 1996; **40**: 53–59.

7 Mango LJ. The FDA review process: obtaining premarket approval for the PAPNET testing system. *Acta Cytol* 1996; **40**: 138–140.

8 Rosenthal DL, Acosta D, Peters RK. Computer-assisted rescreening of clinically important false negative cervical smears using the PAPNET testing system. *Acta Cytol* 1996; **40**: 120–126.

9  Colgan TJ, Patten SF, Lee JSJ. A clinical trial of the AutoPap® 300 QC system for quality control (QC) of cervico-vaginal cytology in the clinical laboratory. *Acta Cytol* 1995; **39**: 1191–1198.

10  Patten Jr SF, James JSJ, Nelson AC. NeoPath, Inc. NeoPath Autopap® 300 automatic screener system. *Acta Cytol* 1996; **40**: 45–52.

11  Patten Jr SF. The FDA process form the perspective of a cytologist in industry. *Acta Cytol* 1996; **40**: 141–142.

12  Wilbur DC, Bonfiglio TA, Rutkowski MA, *et al.* Sensitivity of the AutoPap® 300 QC system for cervical cytologic abnormalities. Biopsy data confirmation. *Acta Cytol* 1996; **40**: 127–132.

# 35: Cooperation of the Image Analyser and the Cytologist

## M. E. Boon

## Summary

In interactive semiautomatic screening procedures, the cytologist has to co-operate with the image analyser. We have gained experience with the PAPNET system (over 150 000 smears), using it for primary screening. We found that not only did the detection of carcinoma-*in-situ* and invasive carcinoma increase significantly, but also diagnostic consistency improved. When PAPNET is used, the cytologist has to decide which of the 128 images should be chosen for the summary screen of 16 images. Our hypothesis was that human factors are important in this decision-making process, and in the synthesis of the summary screen of the system with the light microscopic cell images. If a cytotechnologist (CT) performs suboptimally, the positive scores will be influenced negatively.

In this study we present PAPNET's screening data for human papilloma-virus (HPV) and cervical intraepithelial neoplasia (CIN) III for the years 1992, 1993 and 1994 of two of our CTs (CT1 and CT2) who were the same age and had the same screening experience. We show that a dramatic life event that happened in 1992 to CT1 can be traced in the height of her positive scores. These findings confirm our hypothesis and illustrate that novel techniques should not be introduced to distraught CTs.

## Introduction

In the last decade of this century, the computer has become an indispensable piece of equipment in diagnostic laboratories. Recently, neural network computing has become available. Like the vertebrate brain, artificial neural

*Correspondence*: Dr Mathilde E. Boon, Leiden Cytology and Pathology Laboratory, PO Box 16084, 2301 GB Leiden, The Netherlands.

networks are good at recognition, adaptation and (rough) optimization. Their architecture is highly parallel, robust and fault-tolerant. By contrast, the traditional computer is good at addition, multiplication, If (. . .) then (. . .)else (. . .) instructions. Its architecture is more serial (although parts are parallel) and rather fragile.

The PAPNET system, using neural networks, aids in detecting abnormal cells in the smear. Out of the 300 000 or more cells, 128 images are displayed, which are ranked by the system to have the highest level of potential abnormality. Out of these 128 images, 16 'most suspicious images' can be selected by the CT on a summary screen, further condensing the diagnostic information. Apart from the 'new' information provided by the system through collecting the diagnostic information on one video screen, the CT can find the abnormal cells in the smears using $x/y$ coordinates. In other words, one can simultaneously profit from the light microscopic and the video images. The final diagnosis is reached through a synthesis of the summary screen and the light microscopic images.

Neural network-assisted screening reduces the amount of redundant visual information, but intensive attention must be given to the 128 video images. First, video images are not identical to microscopical images. Additionally, the CT has to appreciate the selection of PAPNET, which might differ from the selection that the CT would have made. If a CT is too rigid, and disappointed that the video screen did not display the cells she favours most, the CT is not able to take full advantage of the information presented on the screen. It is clear that personality structures are important here. In addition, personal life events may play a role in how a CT performs with PAPNET.

From the above descriptions it can be deduced that PAPNET-assisted screening is a semiautomatic screening procedure. The artificial neural network and the human physiological neural network have to work together in an optimal way in order to get optimal positive scores. In the Leiden Cytology and Pathology Laboratory, we have gained extensive experience on this semiautomatic system. Our Dutch view on PAPNET is summarized in Table 35.1. Using PAPNET, more cases of carcinoma-*in-situ* and invasive carcinoma are detected (Table 35.2). In the most recent study, we showed that primary PAPNET screening leads to increase in diagnostic consistency [1], in other words, the outcome of the screening is less dependent on the person who does the screening (Table 35.3).

All screeners involved can profit from the fact that with PAPNET visualization of the cancer cells is improved and the diagnostic hard signs (e.g. the cancer cells) and soft signs (background features related to a cancerous process) can be brought together on the summary screen. By highlighting the soft signs, PAPNET elevates the level of expectation of cancer cells. Nevertheless, humans are still involved, and therefore, in an extreme situation, in which

**Table 35.1** A Dutch view on PAPNET.

PAPNET detects cancer cells in false-negative smears [2]

PAPNET can be used for interactive primary screening [3]

PAPNET rescreening leads to a decrease in diagnostic variability and an increase in screening efficacy [4]

PAPNET detects adenocarcinoma of the endocervix overlooked in human screening [5]

PAPNET interactive primary screening leads to higher histological scores for carcinoma-*in-situ* and invasive carcinoma [6]

PAPNET interactive primary screening leads to an increase in diagnostic consistency [1]

**Table 35.2** Histological validation: PAPNET vs. conventional.

|  | PAPNET (n = 35 876) | Conventional (n = 42 134) |
|---|---|---|
| Severe dysplasia | 68 (0.19%) | 72 (0.17%) |
| Carcinoma-*in-situ** | 43 (0.12%) | 29 (0.07%) |
| Invasive carcinoma* | 24 (0.07%) | 13 (0.03%) |

*Difference between PAPNET and conventional is significant [6].

**Table 35.3** Mean and coefficient of variability for cervical intraepithelial neoplasia (CIN) I–II and $\geq$ CIN III (in %) of seven CTs in 1992, 1993 and 1994.

| Group | PAPNET (n = 65 527) | | Conventional (n = 25 767) | |
|---|---|---|---|---|
|  | Mean | CV | Mean | CV |
| CIN I–II | 1.59 | 0.21 | 1.43 | 0.23 |
| $\geq$ CIN III* | 0.52 | 0.03 | 0.35 | 0.09 |

CV, Coefficient of variability = inversely correlated with diagnostic consistency.
* Difference between PAPNET and conventional screening is significant [1].

a CT is completely distraught, learning to work with this novel approach to cytology might be suboptimal.

In the current study, we will present the screening data for HPV and CIN III of two of the seven cytotechnologists involved in the screening in 1992, 1993 and 1994 to test the hypothesis that human factors are important in the screening results of PAPNET. Our data are unique, because only in our laboratory has the new PAPNET technology been used over a long period of time, allowing observation of time-related changes in screening patterns. Moreover, one of our CTs was completely distraught when she started working with PAPNET; thus the effect of such an extreme state of mind can be evaluated in our data.

## Materials and methods

The Leiden Cytology and Pathology Laboratory receives cervical smears from general practitioners. In September 1992, PAPNET-assisted screening commenced. In 1992, 1993 and 1994, 78 691 cases were screened via PAPNET by 12 CTs, of which seven (female) CTs are involved in this analysis because each of them had screened a substantial number of smears in this period of time. Their total PAPNET screening load in 1992 was 7388 smears, in 1993 23 620, and in 1994 34 568. These data were used in our latest study concerning consistency of screening [1]. Out of the seven CTs, two (CT1 and CT2) were selected for the current analysis. CT1 and CT2 were the same age, were supervisors, and had the same screening experience (Table 35.4). The life of CT2 was without upheavals in the period 1992–1994. In 1992, dramatic events took place in the personal life of CT1, almost shattering her completely. We could observe that around 1994 she more or less found her balance. CT2 was chosen as a control for CT1. The other five CTs were younger and/or had less screening experience and accordingly were less suited as a control for CT1.

**Table 35.4** Background information on cytotechnologist (CT)1 and CT2.

|  | CT1 | CT2 |
|---|---|---|
| Age | 50 | 57 |
| Sex | F | F |
| Supervisor (Y/N) | Y | Y |
| Number of years being a CT | 25 | 22 |
| Total screened smears | 125 000 | 110 000 |
| Total number of PAPNET smears in 1992–1994 | 6303 | 7412 |

In 1992 four of the seven CTs participated in PAPNET screening (including CT1 and CT2); in 1993 six of the seven were involved; and finally in 1994 all seven participated.

Each day, the incoming smears are randomly divided between the CTs, so that each CT has her own portion to screen. There is no bias as to which CT receives which portion to screen.

For both HPV and CIN III, the PAPNET-positive scores were calculated per 100 PAPNET-screened smears for 1992, 1993 and 1994, respectively. These scores are referred to in the text as total scores when calculated for the screening efforts of all seven CTs.

In addition, for CT1 and CT2, the positive scores for HPV and for CIN III were calculated for 1992, 1993 and 1994, over the portion of smears screened by CT1 or CT2, respectively. We refer to these scores as CT1 and CT2 scores.

## Results and discussion

In Table 35.5, the positive scores for HPV are presented. Of the 7388 smears screened in 1992, the total score for HPV was 1.42; that of CT1 and CT2 was much lower, 0.55 and 0.58, respectively. In 1993, with 23 620 smears being screened, and in 1994, with 34 568 smears, the scores for CT1 and CT2 were also more lower than the total score. It is clear that these two very experienced cytotechnologists, CT1 and CT2, both scored consistently lower for HPV than their younger coworkers. The HPV scores for CT1 showed some fluctuations in time, which were very similar to the variations found in the scores of CT2. In short, in the data on HPV, the performance of CT1 and CT2 was similar.

**Table 35.5** Positive scores for human papillomavirus (HPV) and cervical intraepithelial neoplasia (CIN) III per 100 screened women.

| | Total | | CT1 | | CT2 | |
|---|---|---|---|---|---|---|
| | *n* | Score (%) | *n* | Score (%) | *n* | Score (%) |
| *HPV* | | | | | | |
| 1992 | 7388 | 1.42 | 1100 | 0.55 | 863 | 0.58 |
| 1993 | 23 620 | 0.77 | 2146 | 0.33 | 2146 | 0.44 |
| 1994 | 34 568 | 0.88 | 3057 | 0.33 | 3057 | 0.30 |
| *CIN III* | | | | | | |
| 1992 | 7388 | 0.55 | 1100 | 0.18 | 863 | 0.46 |
| 1933 | 23 620 | 0.56 | 2146 | 0.14 | 2146 | 0.58 |
| 1994 | 34 568 | 0.55 | 3057 | 0.59 | 3057 | 0.59 |

CT, Cytotechnologist.

The picture for CIN III is completely different. Here, the CT1 and CT2 data are dissimilar in 1992 and 1993. In addition, we see that in 1992, 1993 and 1994, the scores of CT2 resemble the total scores, all being around 0.50. Thus, in contrast to HPV, CT2 scored for CIN III the same as her younger colleagues. Let us have a closer look at the CT1 scores. In 1992, the year when she had totally lost her mental equilibrium, her CIN III score was only a third of that of CT2, that is 0.18 versus 0.46. One year after, it still was even lower, 0.14, with a CIN III score for CT2 of 0.58. In other words, in these two years CT1 performed suboptimally in her PAPNET screening for CIN III. In 1994, when she regained her balance, as was noted by her coworkers, her CIN III score rose to the optimal level of 0.59, and was exactly the same as the CT2 score.

## Conclusion

This investigation has shown that dramatic life events can influence positive scores of PAPNET-assisted screening for CIN III but not for HPV.

## References

1 Kok MR, Boon ME. Consequences of neural network technology for cervical screening: increase in diagnostic consistency and positive scores. *Cancer* 1996; **78**: 112–117.
2 Boon ME, Kok LP. Neural network processing can provide means to catch errors that slip through human screening of Pap smears. *Diagn Cytopathol* 1993; **9**: 411–416.
3 Ouwerkerk-Noordam E, Boon ME, Beck S. Computer-assisted primary screening of cervical smears using the PAPNET method: comparison with conventional screening and evaluation of the role of the cytologist. *Cytopathology* 1994; **5**: 211–218.
4 Boon ME, Kok LP, Nygaard-Nielsen M, Holm K, Holund B. Neural network processing of cervical smears can lead to a decrease in diagnostic variability and an increase in screening efficacy: a study of 63 false-negative smears. *Mod Pathol* 1994; 7: 957–961.
5 Boon ME. A Dutch view on American cytology in the headlines. *Diagn Cytopathol* 1995; **12**: 87–89.
6 Boon ME, Kok LP, Beck S. Histologic validation of neural network-assisted cervical screening: comparison with the conventional procedure. *Cell Vision* 1995; **2**: 23–27.

# 36: Advantages and Limitations of Automated Screening Systems in Developing and Developed Countries

## E. McGoogan

## Summary

Automated screening systems must be evaluated in the context of local cervical screening programmes to assess their impact on the sensitivity, specificity and cost-effectiveness of each programme before they are introduced. The deficiencies which limit sensitivity and specificity should be identified for each programme and consideration given as to whether the introduction of automated systems would address these deficiencies. Since conventional Papanicolaou (Pap) smear screening programmes are expensive and automated devices are usually cost-increasing, it is unlikely that they would be cost-effective in developing countries where basic health care measures and empowerment of women would have a much greater effect on the mortality from cervical cancer.

## Introduction

The aim of a cervical screening programme is to eradicate invasive squamous carcinoma by identifying and treating all women with preinvasive neoplasia. Cancer of the uterine cervix is the most common cancer in developing countries and the second most common cancer among women worldwide. Eighty per cent of new cases occur in women in the developing countries and more than 80% present at the late stages (stage 3 or stage 4), with only a 20% 5-year survival worldwide. Detection at a preinvasive or early invasive stage results in easier treatment and a greatly improved prognosis. Most cervical cancers present in women over 40 years of age.

*Correspondence*: Dr Euphemia McGoogan, Department of Pathology, University of Edinburgh Medical School, Teviot Place, Edinburgh EH8 9AG, UK.

Opportunistic screening (i.e. without an organized, population-based, call-and-recall invitation of women in the screening age group) has failed to achieve a marked reduction in mortality from invasive cancer in developed countries [1]. Failure to screen regularly all women in the at-risk age group and deficiencies in the quality of the sample sent to the laboratory have been identified as the major limitations of the sensitivity of a cervical screening programme [2]. In addition, the success of the programme is limited by a reluctance among women to present themselves for regular tests, the ability of laboratory staff to identify correctly smears containing abnormal cells, deficiencies in following up and managing women with identified abnormalities in their smears and in the failure to cure all women treated for preinvasive disease.

The quality of the screening test is limited by inadequate sampling of appropriate cells from the cervix, poor transfer and non-random transfer of the cellular material on to the glass slide [2,3]. Microscopic assessment is limited by poor preparation and fixation of the smear as well as by the repetitive nature of the task and the training and continuing competence of the cytotechnologist. The laboratory assessment is further limited by the skill of the cytopathologist in interpreting any unusual or doubtful cells identified [4].

## New automated technologies

Can automation help? There are three main areas of development which may be considered:

1   New thin-layer technologies which may permit adjuvant testing of cervical scrape samples.

2   Automated scanning devices for use as primary screeners or for quality control of conventional microscopic primary screening.

3   Computer-assisted conventional microscopy to assist the human observers in their assessment of the slide.

### Thin-layer preparation

The new thin-layer technology can address some of the sampling, transfer, preparation and fixation problems encountered in conventional screening [3,5–10]. This should improve the quality of the specimen presented to the cytotechnologist and result in increased accuracy of assessment. Thin-layer preparations offer the advantage that the sample removed from the cervix is rinsed from the sampler into a transport fluid so that the cells are preserved in an optimal state and is prepared by skilled technical staff in the laboratory. In addition, all the cellular material removed from the cervix is sent to the laboratory. Excess blood, inflammatory exudate and debris can be removed before representative randomized sampling of cells as a thin layer on a small area of the slide. The belief is that thin-layer preparations could reduce the number of inadequate tests and can be screened more easily, quickly and efficiently than conventional smears. The new thin-layer technology, since it is in a liquid specimen, also facilitates adjuvant tests such as human papillomavirus (HPV) testing and typing, hybrid capture, *Chlamydia* and other pathogen detection, etc. [3,11].

One disadvantage of using thin-layer technology in developing countries is that it requires containers of transport medium to be distributed to the clinics where smears are being taken. There they require to be stored under appropriate conditions before being transported back to laboratory centres once the samples have been collected. The transport and storage of liquids can prove difficult in developed countries and may be a major problem in developing countries. This fluid is methanol-based and can evaporate and, in some pilot studies, the supplies have 'disappeared' or been stolen for their alcohol content.

The thin-layer technologies impose an additional preparation resource on laboratories. Some new robotic devices have been developed to prepare these thin layers but none are yet ideal and all require expert maintenance and skilled staff to run them [10,12]. In addition, thin-layer technology requires plastic rather than wooden samplers to be used; these are much more expensive than the wooden Ayre's spatula [3]. In summary, the disadvantages of thin-layer technology are that it necessitates a change in smear-taking practice and equipment; there are problems associated with the transport of liquid specimens; they require an additional laboratory resource for preparation and, if thin layers are to be assessed by conventional microscopy, cytotechnologists require thorough retraining since the interpretation of these thin-layer slides differs from that of conventional smears.

## Automated scanning devices

Computerized scanning devices may be designed for use in primary screening or for quality control of conventional microscopic primary screening [12–15]. In primary screening mode they should require less human resource than conventional microscopy and be cost-effective. This can only be achieved if the false-negative and false-positive rates are decreased or, at least, not increased. Manufacturers claim automated scanners will influence the false-negative rate but there is concern that this will be at the expense of the false-positive rate. Unless they can identify a reasonable percentage of samples which do not require human assessment, automated primary screening devices are cost-increasing. In quality control mode, these devices are expensive and increase the cost of each test significantly and also the skilled cytotechnologist resource so they are unlikely to be of value to developing countries. There is also great debate as to whether this is a cost-effective method of laboratory quality control even in developed countries.

Scanning devices may be located on site in local laboratories or in centralized national or international facilities. If they are located on site they must be kept in a special environment with a reasonably well-controlled temperature and humidity and a stable electrical supply. They also require technical expertise to maintain the systems at optimum performance. If the scanning devices are not on site then the samples or slides require to be despatched in batches to the centralized facility, resulting in longer delays in returning the result to women. After a time delay, the women may no longer be identifiable or traceable when the result is available. For interactive scanning devices there is a second phase where the selected digitized images must be assessed on computer monitor by a skilled cytotechnologist. These are in very short supply, particularly in developing countries.

### Computer-assisted conventional microscopy

Computer-assisted conventional microscopy using systems such as Pathfinder or AcCell 2000 assists the primary screener in ensuring that the whole of the slide has been scanned and allows the human to attach electronic labels to individual cells [16,17]. These labels can be used for quality control, training and continuing education purposes. Such devices add an extra cost to the equipment used by each cytotechnologist which may place them beyond the reach of many developing countries. Their value in developed countries is still to be fully assessed.

### Cervical screening in developing countries — is there a role for the new technologies?

In developed countries with non-organized cervical screening policies and in the early days of population-based cervical screening programmes, most invasive cancers of the uterine cervix appear in the unscreened population. As organized programmes become effective in covering all of the population at risk, the percentage of invasive cancers in the screened population increases until these are in the vast majority. Cervical cancers in the screened population may result from deficiencies in smear-taking, laboratory assessment, follow-up and treatment and are often a result of failures having occurred at multiple levels. Targeting the laboratory aspects of the programme alone will not significantly change the sensitivity of the overall cervical screening programme.

The health priorities and economics in developing countries are targeted at control of communicable diseases and the population explosion and cancer has a low priority. In many developing countries there are major problems with identifying the population at risk. Population registers do not exist and major confusions arise in the names used by women in different countries and cultures. Addresses do not follow those systems recognized in developed countries and it may be impossible to communicate directly or indirectly with women except at the time of initial contact. In some areas there are social and religious limitations on the acceptability of vaginal examinations. It may therefore not be feasible to attempt regularly to screen all the population. For this reason the World Health Organization suggested a 'once in a lifetime' screen for women at the age interval 35–40 years to achieve the most cost-effective outcome in developing countries [18]. However, the health care services in developing countries rarely have adequate facilities for colposcopy and investigation of women with preinvasive disease and facilities for follow-up and even treatment are extremely limited. The social costs of identifying cervical intraepithelial neoplasia (CIN) in women must also be considered if this will result in marital or family problems. It is patently unethical to identify women with early or preinvasive disease if the resource is not available to provide effective treatment.

One must not lose sight of the fact that the sensitivity of a cervical screening programme is influenced by the failure of the programme to reach all the population at risk, failure of the Pap test to detect all abnormal women, failure to set the interval or frequency of screening to catch rapidly growing cancers, failure to follow up women with abnormalities identified in a Pap test, failure to cure all women treated for preinvasive disease and failure continuously to audit and monitor the programme. Health education is also important so that women have a realistic expectation of what screening can offer and what a negative smear result means for them as an individual.

Until each of these components can be addressed to a satisfactory level, it would not be cost-effective to introduce conventional cervical screening programmes into developing countries. Established programmes should put their energies into improving population coverage and quality of smear-taking since improvements in the overall quality of the programme are most likely to be achieved in these areas. Automation in the laboratory should be considered, but only if this can be done without increasing the cost of the overall programme. There is an urgent need for large independent trials of the sensitivity, specificity and economic aspects of the use of automated devices by authors working in routine laboratory settings and who do not owe allegiance to the commercial company concerned in manufacturing or marketing the device. These should be submitted to high-ranked journals which have stringent referee procedures before publication.

## References

1 Day NE. Screening for cancer of the cervix. *J Epidemiol Community Health* 1989; **43**: 103–106.

2 Hutchinson ML, Isenstein LM, Goodman A *et al*. Homogeneous sampling accounts for the increased diagnostic accuracy using the ThinPrep processor. *Am J Clin Pathol* 1994; **101**: 215–219.

3 McGoogan E, Reith A. Would monolayers provide more representative samples and improved preparations for cervical screening? Overview and evaluation of systems available. *Acta Cytol* 1996; **40**: 107–119.

4 Koss LG. The Papanicolaou test for cervical cancer detection: a triumph and tragedy. *JAMA* 1989; **261**: 737–743.

5 Grohs HK, Zahniser DJ, Geyer JW. Standardization of specimen preparation through mono/thin-layer technology. In: Grohs HK, Husain OAN (eds) *Automated Cervical Cancer Screening*, vol. II. New York, Igaku-Shoin, 1994, pp 176–185.

6 Hutchinson ML, Agarwal P, Denault T, Berger B, Cibas ES. A new look at cervical cytology: ThinPrep multicenter trial results. *Acta Cytol* 1992; **36**: 499–504.

7 Laverty CR, Farnsworth A, Thurloe JK, Bowditch RC. The importance of the cell sample in cervical cytology: a controlled trial of a new sampling device. *Med J Aust* 1989; **150**: 432–436.

8 Linder J. The coming era of cytologic automation. *Am J Clin Pathol* 1991; **96**: 293–294.

9 Vassilakos P, Cossali D, Albe X, Alonso L, Hohener R, Puget E. Efficacy of monolayer preparation for cervical cytology. Emphasis on suboptimal specimen. *Acta Cytol* 1995; **39**: 368.

10 Wilbur DC, Cibas ES, Merritt S, James P, Berger BM, Bonfiglio TA. ThinPrep processor clinical trials demonstrate an increased detection rate of abnormal cervical cytologic specimens. *Am J Clin Pathol* 1994; **101**: 209–214.

11 Hall S, Wu T-C, Field AL, Sherman M, Erozan Y. Suitability of ThinPrep specimens for immunocytochemistry and gene amplification by polymerase chain reaction. *Acta Cytol* 1992; **36**: 585.

12 Knesel EA, Geyer JW, Gahm T, Nguyen T, Fischer J, Dörrer R. The Roche cytology systems: Cyto-Rich and Autocyte. In: Grohs HK, Husain OAN (eds) *Automated Cervical Cancer Screening*, vol. II. New York: Igaku-Shoin, 1994, pp 294–303.

13 Anderson TL. Automated screening of conventional Papanicolaou smears. The Autopap® 300QC systems. In: Wied GL, Bartels PH, Rosenthal DL, Schenck U (eds) *Compendium on the Computerized Cytology and Histology Laboratory*. Chicago: Tutorials of Cytology, 1994, pp 306–311.

14 Mango LJ, Herriman JM. The PAPNET cytological screening system. In: Wied GL, Bartels DL, Rosenthal PH, Schenck U (eds) *Compendium on the Computerized Cytology and Histology Laboratory*. Chicago: Tutorials of Cytology, 1994, pp 320–334.

15 Schumann JL. Standardization of specimen acquisition for automated Pap smear screening. In: Grohs HK, Husain OAN (eds) *Automated Cervical Cancer Screening*, vol. II. New York: Igaku-Shoin, Tokyo, 1994, pp 165–175.

16 Berver BM. Statistical quality assurance in cytology. The use of the Pathfinder to continuously assess screener process control in real time. *Acta Cytol* 1996; **40**: 97–106.

17 Grohs DH, Gombrich PP, Domanik RA. Meeting the challenges in cervical screening: the AcCell series 2000 automated slide handling and data management system. *Acta Cytol* 1996; **40**: 26–36.

18 WHO. *Cytological Screening in the Control of Cervical Cancer: Technical Guidelines*. Geneva: World Health Organization, 1988.

# Section 6
# Human Papillomavirus Testing

# 37: Methods of DNA Hybridization and their Clinical Applicability to Human Papillomavirus Detection

A. T. Lörincz

## Summary

Given the subjective and variably inaccurate nature of the Papanicolaou (Pap) smear, it is time to consider widespread use of human papillomavirus (HPV) DNA testing to supplement our cervical cancer prevention efforts. HPV DNA testing by probe technology has evolved over the past 15 years from relatively crude, labour-intensive and insensitive methods to sophisticated, highly sensitive tests with good clinical utility. Two main tests dominate the landscape today: polymerase chain reaction (PCR) and Hybrid Capture. With these tests, it is possible to detect any of over 70 different HPV types, but from a clinical perspective only tests for carcinogenic HPV types are likely to be used frequently. Older tests, such as Southern blot and dot blot, have been all but abandoned, except for esoteric use.

Both Hybrid Capture and PCR appear suitable for routine clinical use. In the case of Hybrid Capture, the test is quantitative and is available in standardized kit format, while PCR is usually qualitative and kits for HPV are still under development. Substantial data now indicate that HPV DNA testing has clinical utility in the management of women with mildly abnormal Pap smears. A second, more important use is in population screening. Several studies are underway (such as the Costa Rica study) to validate the use of HPV testing as a primary screen for cervical cancer precursors, either in conjunction with the Pap smear or as a stand-alone test.

Test procedures and equipment continue to evolve at a rapid pace. The ultimate goal is superior sensitivity and specificity in a simple, fully automated format with turnkey software for test runs, data analysis and report generation.

*Correspondence*: Dr Attila T. Lörincz, Digene Corporation, 2301-B Broadbirch Drive, Silver Spring, MD 20904, USA.

The overall picture is one of great promise; it seems we are on the verge of a major paradigm shift in disease detection and prognosis in the not too distant future. Automated, molecular-based tests are likely to take the forefront in detecting or confirming many human diseases and will become indispensable in most areas of medicine.

## Introduction

Nucleic acid-based probe tests are the most advanced form of biochemical diagnostic testing methodology available today. It is possible to detect minute amounts of target molecules by means of ultrasensitive amplification procedures that are impossible to match by any other physical or chemical means. Probe technology permits simple, highly accurate quantitation of target molecules over wide dynamic ranges spanning 5–6 logs or more. This is becoming very important for monitoring viral infections such as human immunodeficiency virus (HIV) burden measurements and disease prognosis in acquired immunodeficiency syndrome (AIDS) patients [1] and for detecting clinically relevant levels of HPV infection. Target-amplified tests like PCR are best suited to the ultrasensitive detection of very low levels of DNA or RNA molecules. Signal-amplified tests such as Hybrid Capture are best suited to quantitative or semiquantitative applications and for diseases with higher levels of pathogen.

A substantial body of work by several research groups had, by the early 1990s, demonstrated that certain HPVs – mainly types 16, 18, 31, 33, 35, 39, 45, 51, 52 and 56 – were responsible for the majority of cervical cancers in Europe and North America [2–5]. These early findings were later confirmed and extended by more formal epidemiological studies [6] and generalized to most remaining geographical regions of the world [7]. Recent studies show the merit of HPV DNA testing for routine clinical use [8–12].

The Pap smear is a good screening tool for cervical cancer and has served us well. However, it is not without substantial problems; it misses 20–30% or more of cervical intraepithelial neoplasia (CIN) II–III and cancers. HPV DNA testing can help here as it has good sensitivity for detecting neoplastic disease missed by the Pap [8,9,12–14]. Another interesting application is for identifying latent HPV infection where lesions are not discernible by traditional means. A majority of these cases develop or are discovered to have squamous intraepithelial lesions (SIL) within 3–4 years (Schiffman *et al.*, unpublished data) [10,11]. Such information can permit efficient grouping of women according to disease risk.

Another problem area in Pap classification is the meaning of HPV effect. This diagnosis is based on the presence of koilocytes on a smear and is presumed to reflect the presence of HPV. However, even experts may be misled by artefacts that closely mimic HPV-containing cells. Overcalls in Pap smears are common [8,13,15–17] and usually precipitate a search by the clinician for the culprit lesion with the potential for overcall of the subsequent biopsies. In addition to being wasteful of medical resources, a further adverse result of such actions is emotional fall-out for women [18] who may mistakenly assume that they are infected by a sexually transmitted cancer virus and may look for an explanation from their partners or feel themselves demeaned by the experience.

## Basics of probe technology

The ways in which molecules of DNA and RNA behave in aqueous solutions, as they pertain to the essentials of probe tests, have been described in detail in earlier reviews [19,20]. Key to all probe tests is an exquisitely specific recognition of target nucleic acid sequences by complementary nucleic acid sequences called probes. Under normal physiological conditions, nucleic acid polymers exhibit a strong attraction for their partners and preferentially exist as stable double-stranded forms. These double-stranded molecules can be separated into single-stranded forms by well-known physical or chemical means. Then, as desired, the strands can be induced to resort into new probe–target pairs, which are detectable.

## Kinds of probe tests

Probe tests may be divided into three broad groups: non-amplified tests, target-amplified tests and signal-amplified tests. Within these groups different test formats are possible. The non-amplified tests, such as the dot blot, Southern blot or filter *in situ* hybridization (FISH), are seldom used today. Among target-amplified tests, the best known is PCR which is the progenitor target amplification test. Signal-amplified tests like the Hybrid Capture system (HCS) have proven themselves to be sensitive, accurately quantitative, robust and suitable for routine clinical use. Table 37.1 lists some nucleic acid tests.

## Hybrid Capture system

HCS is an *in vitro*, solution hybridization, signal-amplified test for detecting DNA or RNA targets (Fig. 37.1) [21,22]. For HPV detection, it is formatted as a solution hybridization of RNA probes with DNA targets that is followed by an immunologically based 'back-end' similar to an enzyme-linked immunosorbent assay (ELISA). The test derives its high sensitivity from several independent sources. First, in HCS the entire genome of the virus is the usual target of

**Table 37.1** Test methods for DNA or RNA targets.

| Test category | Test name |
|---|---|
| Target amplification* | Polymerase chain reaction (PCR) |
| | Ligase chain reaction (LCR) |
| | Nucleic acid sequence-based amplification (NASBA) |
| | Strand displacement amplification (SDA) |
| Signal amplification† | Hybrid Capture system (HCS) |
| | Branched DNA (bDNA) |
| No amplification | Southern blot (SB)‡ |
| | Dot blot (DB)§ |
| | Filter *in situ* hybridization (FISH) |
| | Reverse Southern blot (RSB)‖ |
| | Northern blot (NB)¶ |
| | *In situ* hybridization (ISH)** |

* Can be adapted for detecting either DNA or RNA targets. Some, such as NASBA, are better suited for RNA.
† Solution hybridization tests that can be adapted for detecting either DNA or RNA targets; especially suitable for accurate quantitation.
‡ Filter-based hybridization test for detecting DNA after electrophoresis.
§ Filter-based hybridization test for detecting crude DNA or RNA.
‖ A filter-based test in which the probe is immobilized to the filter and the target in solution drives the reactions; the reverse format leads to a large loss of sensitivity.
¶ Similar to Southern blot, but directed to RNA targets.
** This test is for detecting DNA or RNA in tissue sections or cells. All other tests in this table are *in vitro* tests that do not retain morphology.
From Lörincz [34] with permission.

choice. Long single-stranded RNA probes are used to hybridize efficiently with all 8000 nucleotides of the HPV DNA genome. RNA–DNA hybrids are more stable than DNA–DNA hybrids, and the use of single-stranded RNA probes avoids unwanted side reactions. Second, a source of added sensitivity for HCS is the use of RNA–DNA antibodies that are conjugated to multiple molecules of alkaline phosphatase. These antibody conjugates recognize short stretches of RNA–DNA hybrid in a specific but non-sequence-dependent manner such that thousands of antibodies can coat a single genomic hybrid of HPV DNA. Third, each immobilized alkaline phosphatase enzyme reacts with numerous molecules of the chemiluminescent dioxetane substrate per minute to produce a steady stream of photons that are counted by the photomultiplier tube of a luminometer. Fourth, the HCS test readily accepts large amounts (10–20% or more) of clinical material into the reaction without inhibition of the assay. Thus, HCS to some extent benefits from natural amplification of virus in the host organism that tends to produce a large amount of HPV in a large volume of the clinical material, that will nevertheless translate to a small quantity of virus if only a minuscule fraction of the specimen can be placed into the reaction.

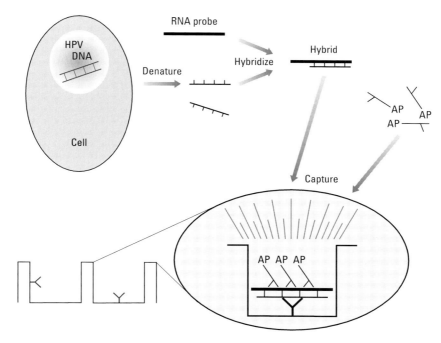

**Fig. 37.1** HCS employs unlabelled full genomic human papillomavirus (HPV) RNA probes that are hybridized in solution with denatured target DNA from specimens. Resulting RNA–DNA hybrids are captured on the surface of microplate wells by an immobilized antibody that specifically recognizes RNA–DNA hybrids. Captured RNA–DNA hybrids are reacted with a second antibody conjugated to alkaline phosphatase (AP). Detection is accomplished by addition of a chemiluminescent dioxetane-based substrate [33]. As the substrate is cleaved by the bound alkaline phosphatase conjugate, light is emitted in a long-lived glow reaction and measured in relative light units (RLUs) using a microplate luminometer. Emitted light intensity is proportional to the amount of target DNA in the specimen and is usually expressed as a ratio of the signal to the positive control (abbreviated as RLU/PC). A linear range of quantitation is achievable over approximately 4 logs. Although there is some curvature of the dose–response line at low and at very high target concentrations, the use of carefully selected standards permits quantitation of HPV DNA in the range of $5 \times 10^3$ to $5 \times 10^7$ genomes with a single assay, and repeat testing with additional dilutions can extend the high end to virtually any desired level. From Lörincz [21] with permission.

Formally to evaluate the performance of a prototype HCS assay, aliquots of cervical specimens from 199 women were tested by a prototype HCS assay in three independent laboratories. These clinical specimens were derived from a study described earlier [17]. The results of the study showed HCS to be a simple, reliable test suitable for routine use [22]. Pairwise interlaboratory agreement ranged from 87% to 94% and $\kappa$ values from 0.61 to 0.83, with no clearly superior results from any laboratory.

An improved version of HCS that provides increased sensitivity, reproducibility and ease of use has been developed recently. In this new test, called hybrid capture microplate (HCM), some notable changes are the replacement of the capture tubes with a removable strip microtitre plate and the addition of several new probes for high-risk HPVs. With these added probes, HCM can now detect 13 different carcinogenic HPV types (16, 18, 31, 33, 35, 39, 45, 51, 52, 56, 58, 59 and 68) which represent virtually all important cancer-causing HPV types worldwide [7]. Other formulation changes have increased the analytical sensitivity of HCM by about 50-fold over HCS, such that HCM is capable of detecting as few as 1000 HPV genomes per assay. A valuable attribute of HCM is its dynamic range of quantitation of over 4 logs.

## Polymerase chain reaction

The approach taken by target-amplified tests is to create extra copies of the desired target sequence prior to detection of these amplicons by more traditional methods (Fig. 37.2) [23,24]. In PCR, the target DNA is selectively amplified through repeated cycles of denaturation, primer hybridization and primer extension. Target DNA concentration rises exponentially and, after 30 cycles, over 1 000 000 copies of the target DNA will be produced. Hence, as few as 10–100 HPV DNA molecules can be amplified and detected within a biopsy or smear containing $5 \times 10^4$ cells. Thus, PCR has been used to detect HPV DNA in Pap smears and in single sections of paraffin-embedded tissue biopsies from CIN and cervical cancer [25]. The amplified DNA products (amplicons) are detected, either by conventional methods (dot blot or Southern blot), by ethidium bromide staining and visualization by the naked eye of the specific amplified DNA fragment following gel electrophoresis, or by oligonucleotide probes in an ELISA format.

There are many alternative sets of primers for detecting HPV by PCR. Two commonly used sets are consensus primer pair MY09 MY11 [26] and the general primers GP5 GP6 [27]; both primer sets amplify regions in the conserved L1 open reading frame. Several other sets of primers have been reported in the literature, such as consensus E1 primers [28] and type-specific E6 primers [29], but their use is not widespread enough to permit a clear evaluation of their performance or utility for clinical use. The MY primer pair produces a PCR amplicon of about 450 nucleotides, whereas the GP primer pair produces an amplicon of about 140 nucleotides from a region of L1 that overlaps with MY. There is still some debate as to which HPV PCR method is better. It seems that both methods are fairly equivalent for *in vitro* use, but the GP primers are better for amplification of targets from paraffin-embedded sections, as the longer MY amplicons are not synthesized as efficiently because of formalin cross-linking in the tissue. The use of PCR for clinical applica-

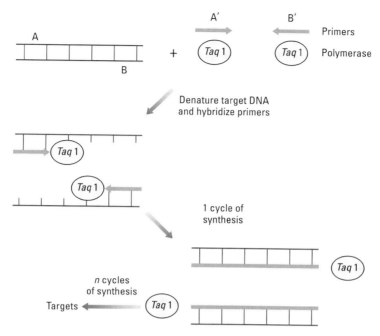

**Fig. 37.2** Polymerase chain reaction (PCR) synthesis is performed as follows: double-stranded target DNA is denatured to allow the two primers (A' and B') to hybridize specifically to their complementary DNA target sequences (A and B), usually a few hundred nucleotides apart. The primers direct synthesis towards each other by means of a polymerase enzyme such as *Taq* 1, converting the initial two DNA target strands into four target strands, upon which another PCR cycle can be performed. After $n$ cycles, one target will become $(1 + E)^n$ amplicons, where $E$ is the efficiency of the amplification and is a number between 0 and 1. In an ideal PCR with 100% efficiency, $E = 1$. Usually the value of $E$ is 0.7–0.8. From Lörincz [34] with permission.

tions is reviewed by Meijer *et al.* (Chapter 38), Cuzick *et al.* (Chapters 42 and 43) and Villa *et al.* (Chapter 44), hence, I will focus only on results with HCS and HCM.

## Clinical applications of Hybrid Capture

Five clinical studies of patient management using HPV DNA testing by HCS have been completed [8,12,13,15,30]. The studies examined the utility of HPV DNA detection as an adjunct to the Pap smear for managing women with previous atypical squamous cells of undetermined significance (ASCUS) or low-grade squamous intraepithelial lesion (LSIL) Pap smears. The general study design was to obtain specimens of exfoliated cervical cells for HPV DNA testing, and perform a repeat Pap smear just prior to colposcopy. Histopathology was used as the reference standard definition of prevalent cervical disease.

Three studies employed the recommended specimen collection devices (swabs or cone brush) for HPV DNA testing. The fourth study [30] compared the use of a cervicovaginal lavage to the use of a cytobrush. The fifth study [13] examined the use of a liquid cytology transport medium (PreservCyt, Cytyc Corp., Boxborough, MA, USA) that is compatible with both HPV DNA testing and a Pap slide from the same specimen. This latter method is particularly interesting, as it permits HPV DNA testing to be performed from routine Pap screening specimens, thus eliminating an additional office visit.

Selected results of the studies are shown in Table 37.2. I chose to focus on two interesting measures of test utility, namely test sensitivity for cervical disease of grades CIN II, CIN III or cancer ($\geqslant$ CIN II) and number of colposcopies required per case detected. The Pap smear and HCS appear equivalent in sensitivity, with some studies showing a slight advantage for HCS and others showing a slight advantage for the Pap smear. Interestingly, in four of the five studies, HCS was better at predicting women with $\geqslant$ CIN II than the Pap smear, which is somewhat surprising given the HPV literature of the last 5 years [23]. In all studies, the combination of HCS and the Pap smear was better than either alone, generally reaching a sensitivity of over 95% for important cervical disease. Although colposcopy was the most sensitive method by definition (it was assumed, perhaps incorrectly, the colposcopy detected all relevant cervical disease), it required, on average, about 30% more colposcopies per case of $\geqslant$ CIN II detected than the other options.

HCS has been employed as the main HPV test in a recent National Cancer Institute study in Costa Rica (Schiffman *et al.*, unpublished data). The study is a population-based screening study of 10 000 women residing in Guanacaste province, a high-incidence area for cervical cancer. Each cohort member has been screened with conventional cytology, thin-layer cytology (ThinPrep, Cytyc Corp.), Cervicography, and the first-generation HCS test. Women with any abnormal morphological test were referred to colposcopy and biopsies were taken of any cervical tissues suspected to contain CIN or cancer. The histopathology and cytopathology went through multiple levels of review by a panel of expert pathologists to determine the most correct final diagnosis. HCS testing was done blinded to the other results in my laboratory. An initial analysis of the first 8000 women showed HCS to be quite sensitive for detecting CIN III. Of 22 cases of CIN III, 82% (18/22) were positive for high-risk HPVs. In this initial evaluation, the Pap smear was less sensitive, detecting on average about 65% of the 22 cases of CIN III. However, the overall referral rate to colposcopy based on the Pap smear was 3.3% and for HCS it was 5.5%, as would be expected due to the presence of latent HPV infection. Additional analyses of the data for all 10 000 women, which now include CIN

**Table 37.2** (HCS) appears to be a useful tool for managing women with atypical squamous cells of undetermined significance (ASCUS) Papanicolaou (Pap) smears: results of five recent studies.

| Study (≥ CIN II/total) | Protocol | % Sensitivity | Colposcopies per ≥ CIN II | Referral Pap* |
|---|---|---|---|---|
| Cox *et al.* (1995) [8] (15/217) | Colposcopy | 100 | 14.5 | |
| | Pap smear | 73 | 6.1 | |
| | HCS | 93† | 5.3 | ASCUS |
| | Pap + HCS | 100 | 7.1 | |
| Wright *et al.* (1995) [12] (50/398) | Colposcopy | 100 | 8.0 | |
| | Pap smear | 80 | 5.1 | |
| | HCS | 78 | 5.3 | ASCUS or SIL |
| | Pap + HCS | 96 | 5.9 | |
| Hatch *et al.* (1995) [15]‡ (126/311) | Colposcopy | 100 | 2.5 | |
| | Pap smear | 75 | 2.3 | |
| | HCS | 74 | 1.8 | SIL |
| | Pap + HCS | 91 | 2.2 | |
| Hall *et al.* (1996) [30]§ (15/75) | Colposcopy | 100 | 5.0 | |
| | Pap smear | 87 | 4.2 | |
| | HCS | 93 | 4.0 | ASCUS or SIL |
| | Pap + HCS | 100 | 4.1 | |
| Ferenczy *et al.* (1996) [13] (47/364) | Colposcopy | 100 | 8.3 | |
| | Pap smear | 87 | 5.1 | |
| | HCS | 77 | 4.8 | ASCUS or SIL |
| | Pap + HCS | 95 | 5.4 | |

CIN, Cervical intraepithelial neoplasia; SIL, squamous intraepithelial lesion.
* This Pap smear was the basis of the original referral of the women for colposcopy.
† The sensitivity of HCS was 100% when human papillomavirus (HPV) 39 and 58 were added to the probe mix, indicating the importance of an expanded probe set for HPV. The other studies in the table did not have HPVs 39 or 58 as part of the probe test.
‡ End-point was based on CIN II–III.
§ Data are for high-risk HPV types only.
Adapted from Lörincz [21] with permission.

II as well as difficult cases of CIN III, show the HCS performance to be somewhat reduced. The overall sensitivity for 44 cases of CIN II–III was 75%. It is possible that the negative cases of CIN II–III either had lower levels of HPV DNA as a biological phenomenon or were sampled poorly and thus the HCS results suffered. Further studies with the more sensitive HCM test and with PCR will hopefully reveal the true nature of these currently HPV-negative cases of CIN II–III.

## Recent results with the HCM test

Two preliminary clinical studies have been performed with the more sensitive HCM. The first study (Chesebro *et al.*, personal communication) was similar in design to the Hatch and Hall studies of Table 37.2, except that concurrent Pap smears were not taken. Sensitivity of HCM for CIN II–III was 92% (36/39) and required 3.5 colposcopies per high-grade CIN confirmed on histology, while 4.1 colposcopies were required to reach 100% sensitivity for CIN II–III. In a second ongoing study (Cox *et al.*, personal communication), only sensitivity data are currently available for HCM: of CIN I, 91% (88/97) were detected; of CIN II, 96% (24/25) were detected; and of CIN III, 100% (8/8) were detected. Vaginal and vulvar high-grade lesions were also detected at 95% or better sensitivity in this study.

It appears that HCM has consistently high sensitivity for ⩾ CIN II in a fairly large group of specimens from two different study sites in the USA, with an average of 95% sensitivity among a combined set of 72 histologically confirmed lesions.

## General considerations

A review of the literature shows variation in the reported performance of HPV probe tests relative to each other and to histology. In many studies the HCS and PCR tests show excellent sensitivity and specificity for detecting disease [7,8]. In other studies, the correlations are not as good [12,15,23,31]. There are many possible reasons for these variations. PCR in particular is prone to inhibitory substances that can interfere with amplification; however, the problem with PCR is usually excessive false positives [23,31]. In the case of HCS, inhibition and false positives are not problems, but specimen adequacy is critical to avoid false negatives. In my experience, sampling is an important area that requires careful attention. The optimal method of cervical sampling has still not been determined. Some essential elements to consider are proper access to CIN II–III lesions deep in the endocervical canal, especially in older women. Brush devices appear better at cutting through mucus or other material to access HPV-infected cells. Thus, careful and standardized sampling should be learned by every clinician wishing to use HPV tests in screening and patient management. Dacron swabs are not optimal; cotton swabs and lavages should be avoided.

Another reason for poor agreement between accurate HPV DNA tests and histology may lie more with the subjectivity of the histopathology than with a lack of adequate sensitivity or specificity of the molecular HPV tests [32], particularly when the molecular tests are known to be capable of detecting a wide spectrum of HPV types with high sensitivity and specificity. CIN II is usually lumped with CIN III, and it is possible that overcall on histology may place some CIN I/LSIL into the CIN II–III group. Since CIN I/LSIL is often associated with low-risk or novel HPV types, the result will appear as a false negative for a probe test that detects only carcinogenic HPV types. In some instances, variants of immature squamous metaplasia or other artefacts could be misread as CIN II–III.

## Future directions

Incorporation of HPV testing into routine clinical practice should be considered a boon for both developed and developing nations. Ultimately, full automation will make routine HPV testing for triage and mass screening substantially less expensive and more accurate than repeat Pap smears, as it will virtually eliminate human error and subjectivity of interpretation. A very attractive way to incorporate HPV testing into routine patient management is to perform a ThinPrep Pap smear and to follow with HPV DNA testing on cells remaining in the PreservCyt liquid, if the result from the cytologist is ASCUS. Two recent studies (Sherman *et al.*, unpublished; [13]) show that this strategy works efficiently.

## Acknowledgements

The author is Scientific Director of Digene Corporation, the company that manufactures the Hybrid Capture test. He wishes to thank all his scientific and medical colleagues – and in particular J. Thomas Cox MD, Mark E. Sherman MD, and Mark H. Schiffman MD – for providing results from unpublished studies. The author also wishes to thank his staff for excellent work in developing the Hybrid Capture test and for help in numerous epidemiological and clinical investigations, in particular Allison Cullen MS, Alice Corrigan PhD and Iwona Mielzynska PhD. Special thanks go to Katherine Mack for her tireless dedication to the preparation of papers and reviews.

## References

1 Cao Y, Qin L, Zhang L *et al*. Virologic and immunologic characterization of long-term survivors of human immunodeficiency virus type 1 infection. *N Engl J Med* 1995; **332**: 201.

2 Durst M, Gissmann L, Ikenberg H *et al*. A papillomavirus DNA from a cervical carcinoma and its prevalence in cancer biopsy samples from different geographic regions. *Proc Natl Acad Sci USA* 1983; **80**: 3812.

3 Fuchs PG, Girardi F, Pfister H. Human papillomavirus DNA in normal metaplastic, preneoplastic and neoplastic epithelia of the cervix uteri. *Int J Cancer* 1988; **41**: 41.

4 Lörincz AT, Temple GF, Kurman RJ *et al*. Oncogenic association of specific human papillomavirus types with cervical neoplasia *J Natl Canc Inst* 1987; **79**: 671.

5 Lörincz AT, Reid R, Jenson AB *et al*. Human papillomavirus infection of the cervix: relative risk associations of 15 common anogenital types. *Obstet Gynecol* 1992: **79**: 328.

6 Munoz N, Bosch FX, de Sanjose S *et al*. The causal link between human papillomavirus and invasive cervical cancer: a population-based case-control study in Colombia and Spain. *Int J Cancer* 1992; **52**: 743.

7 Bosch FX, Manos MM, Munoz N *et al*. Prevalence of human papillomavirus in cervical cancer: a worldwide perspective. *J Natl Canc Inst* 1995; **87**: 796.

8 Cox JT, Lörincz AT, Schiffman MH *et al*. Human papillomavirus testing by hybrid capture appears to be useful in triaging women with a cytologic diagnosis of atypical squamous cells of undetermined significance. *Am J Obstet Gynecol* 1995; **172**: 946.

9 Cuzick J, Szarewski A, Terry G *et al*. Human papillomavirus testing in primary cervical screening. *Lancet* 1995; **345**: 1533.

10 Koutsky LA, Holmes KK, Critchlow CW *et al*. A cohort study of the risk of cervical intraepithelial neoplasia grade 2 or 3 in relation to papillomavirus infection. *N Engl J Med* 1992; **327**: 1272.

11 Lörincz AT, Schiffman MH, Jaffurs WJ *et al*. Temporal associations of human papillomavirus infection with cervical cytologic abnormalities. *Am J Obstet Gynecol* 1990; **162**: 645.

12 Wright TC, Sun XW, Koulos J. Comparison of management algorithms for the evaluation of women with low-grade cytologic abnormalities. *Obstet Gynecol* 1995; **85**: 202.

13 Ferenczy A, Franco E, Arseneau J *et al*. Diagnostic performance of Hybrid Capture human papillomavirus deoxyribonucleic acid assay combined with liquid-based cytologic study. *Am J Obstet Gynecol* 1996; **175**: 651.

14 Reid R, Greenberg MD, Lörincz A *et al*. Should cervical cytologic testing be augmented by cervicography or human papillomavirus deoxyribonucleic acid detection? *Am J Obstet Gynecol* 1991; **164**: 1461.

15 Hatch KD, Schneider A, Abdel-Nour MW. An evaluation of human papillomavirus testing for intermediate- and high-risk types as triage before colposcopy. *Am J Obstet Gynecol* 1995; **172**: 1150.

16 Klinkhamer PJJ, Vooijs GP, de Haan AFJ. Intraobserver and interobserver variability in the diagnosis of epithelial abnormalities in cervical smears. *Acta Cytol* 1988; **32**: 794.

17 Sherman ME, Schiffman MH, Lörincz AT *et al*. Toward objective quality assurance in cervical cytopathology: correlation of cytopathologic diagnoses with detection of high-risk human papillomavirus types. *Am J Clin Pathol* 1994; **102**: 182.

18 Campion MJ, Brown JR, McCance DJ *et al*. Psychosexual trauma of an abnormal cervical smear. *Br J Obstet Gynaecol* 1988; **95**: 175.

19 Hames BD, Higgins SJ. (eds) *Nucleic Acid Hybridisation: A Practical Approach*. Oxford: IRL Press, 1985.

20 Meinkoth J, Wahl G. Hybridization of nucleic acids immobilized on solid supports. *Anal Biochem* 1984; **138**: 267.

21 Lörincz A. Hybrid Capture method for detection of human papillomavirus DNA in clinical specimens. *Papillomavirus Rep* 1996; 7: 1–5.

22 Schiffman MH, Kiviat NB, Burk RD *et al*. Accuracy and interlaboratory reliability of human papillomavirus DNA testing by Hybrid Capture. *J Clin Microbiol* 1995; **33**: 545.

23 Bauer HM, Ting Y, Greer CE *et al*. Genital human papillomavirus infection in female university students as determined by a PCR-based method. *JAMA* 1991; **265**: 472.

24 Mullis KB, Faloona FA. Specific synthesis of DNA *in vitro* via a polymerase-catalyzed chain reaction. *Meth Enzymol* 1987; **155**: 335.

25 Griffin NR, Dockey D, Lewis FA *et al*. Demonstration of low frequency of human papillomavirus DNA in cervical adenocarcinoma and adenocarcinoma *in situ* by the polymerase chain reaction and *in situ* hybridization. *Int J Gynecol Pathol* 1991; **10**: 36.

26 Ting Y, Manos MM. Detection and typing of genital human papillomaviruses. In: Innis MA, Gelfand DH, Sninsky JJ *et al.* (eds) *PCR Protocols: A Guide to Methods and Applications.* San Diego: Academic Press, 1990, p 356.

27 Van den Brule AJC, Meijer CJLM, Bakels V *et al.* Rapid detection of human papillomavirus in cervical scrapes by combined general primer-mediated and type-specific polymerase chain reaction. *J Clin Microbiol* 1990; **28**: 2739.

28 Gregoire L, Arella M, Campione-Piccardo J *et al.* Amplification of human papillomavirus DNA sequences by using conserved primers. *J Clin Microbiol* 1989; **27**: 2660.

29 Shibata DK, Arnheim N, Martin WJ. Detection of human papillomavirus in paraffin-embedded tissue using the polymerase chain reaction. *J Exp Med* 1988; **167**: 225.

30 Hall S, Lörincz A, Shah F *et al.* Human papillomavirus DNA detection in cervical specimens by Hybrid Capture: correlation with cytologic and histologic diagnoses of squamous intraepithelial lesions of the cervix. *Gynecol Oncol* 1996; **62**: 353.

31 Hinchliffe SA, van Velzen D, Korporaal H *et al.* Transience of cervical HPV infection in sexually active young women with normal cervicovaginal cytology. *Br J Cancer* 1995; **72**: 943.

32 Robertson AJ, Anderson JM, Beck JS *et al.* Observer variability in histopathological reporting of cervical biopsy specimens. *J Clin Pathol* 1989; **42**: 231.

33 Pollard-Knight D, Simmonds AC, Schaap AP *et al.* Nonradioactive DNA detection on Southern blots by enzymatically triggered chemiluminescence. *Ann Biochem* 1990; **185**: 353.

34 Lörincz AT. Molecular methods for the detection of human papillomavirus infection. In: Lörincz AT, Reid R (eds) *Human Papillomavirus.* Philadelphia: W.B. Saunders, 1996, p 707.

# 38: Human Papillomavirus Testing for Primary Cervical Cancer Screening

C. J. L. M. Meijer,[1] L. Rozendaal,[1] J. C. van der Linden,[1] Th. J. M. Helmerhorst,[2] F. J. Voorhorst[3] & J. M. M. Walboomers[1]

## Summary

Epidemiological and *in vitro* studies clearly establish that some specific human papillomaviruses (HPVs) play an aetiopathogenetic role in cervical carcinogenesis. This has consequences for cervical cancer screening. Strategies can be developed based on the following working hypothesis:

1 The transient presence of HPV in a large number of women with normal cytology indicates that these women can clear a cervical HPV infection without obtaining cervical lesions.

2 A substantial number of cervical HPV infections result in an HPV-associated cervical intraepithelial neoplasia (CIN) lesion.

3 In young women under the age of 30 years more than 90% of these HPV-associated CIN lesions regress spontaneously, whereas in middle-aged women, substantially fewer lesions regress, due to viral persistence.

4 Only women with persistent high-risk HPV infections are at risk of obtaining cervical cancer.

We advocate a combined screening with HPV testing in conjunction with classical Papanicolaou (Pap) smears after the age of 30 years. Under this age, due to the relatively high prevalence of high-risk HPV, we suggest primary screening by Pap smear cytology only. In this group HPV testing is advocated only for women with abnormal cells.

This proposed screening strategy for women > 30 years with cervical cytology in conjunction with HPV testing will result in a more effective

*Correspondence*: Professor C. J. L. M. Meijer, Department of Pathology, Free University Hospital, De Boelelaan 1117, 1081 HV Amsterdam, the Netherlands.
[1]Department of Pathology and [2]Department of Gynaecology and Obstetrics, [3]Department of Epidemiology and Biostatistics; Free University Hospital Amsterdam, De Boelelaan 1117, 1081 HV Amsterdam, The Netherlands.

screening programme with fewer screening rounds and fewer referrals to gynaecologists for colposcopy.

## Introduction

In the Netherlands nationwide cervical cancer screening programmes began in 1976, and they still continue. Every year 800 000 cervical smears are taken in the context of these nationwide screening programmes. Cytomorphological examination of Pap smears has resulted in a significant decrease in the incidence of cervical carcinoma [1].

Despite the triumph of the Pap smears in cervical cancer prevention, it is error-prone. Due to its subjective nature, it is difficult to maintain reproducibility and continuously requires highly trained cytotechnicians and cytopathologists. The number of false-negative smears for cervical cancer and high-grade squamous intraepithelial lesions (SILs) is at least 15%. Moreover, the specificity of the test is relatively low (70%), resulting in a worrying number of false-positive smears [2–5]. Epidemiological and *in vitro* studies have clearly established that some specific HPV play an aetiopathogenetic role in cervical carcinoma [6,7].

Therefore, the question to be asked is whether screening for cervical cancer can be done more efficiently when HPV testing is included. In answering this question we have to present data which emphasize that HPV testing can be used for screening for cervical cancer and its specific precursor lesions.

## HPV and (pre)malignant cervical lesions

**1** Worldwide analyses showed that in cervical cancer (92.3%) high-risk HPV types can be found [8]. HPV 16 and 18 are the most prevalent. In our hands, due to the selection of well-presented tissue, the percentage of cervical cancer which appeared to be positive for HPV is higher than 98% [9–11].
**2** In all cases of carcinoma-*in-situ* of the cervix high-risk HPV types have been found [12].
**3** In smears from patients with cervical dysplasia (dyskaryosis), an increasing prevalence of HPV was detected, ranging from 70% in mild to moderate dyskaryosis to 85% in severe dyskaryosis [10,12,13].

## HPV in women with cytomorphologically normal smears

After HPV prevalence data in premalignant cervical lesions and cervical cancer became available the first important question was: What is the prevalence of HPV in women with cytomorphologically normal smears? Our group showed that in women with normal smears the prevalence of all HPV types is age-related, decreasing from 20% in women aged between 20 and 25 years to 6% in women ⩾ 30 years. High-risk HPV types decrease from 10% in women between 20 and 35 years to 4% in women ⩾ 30 years old [14,15]. Similar age-dependent prevalence trends were also found in studies performed by others [16,17], indicating that HPV infections are very common among young women and that these infections frequently resolve spontaneously. Next we compared the HPV age-related prevalence data to the cytology screening results of the British Columbia cohort study [18] as analysed by Oortmarssen and Habbema [19]. These authors could only explain the British Columbia data by assuming that regression of cervical premalignant lesions is age-dependent. Using their computer model they estimated that 84% of the premalignant lesions regress in women under the age of 34 years whereas in women older than 34 years only 40% regress.

## Working hypothesis

Combining these cytology data with the HPV age prevalence results, our own contribution in case-control studies [11,20] and our own experience we have developed the following working hypothesis:

1  The transient presence of HPV in a large number of women with normal cytology indicates that these women can clear a cervical HPV infection without obtaining cervical lesions.

2  A substantial number of cervical HPV infections result in an HPV-associated CIN lesion.

3  In young women under the age of 30 years, more than 90% of these HPV-associated CIN lesions regress spontaneously, whereas in middle-aged women substantially fewer lesions regress, due to viral persistence.

4  Only women with persistent high-risk HPV infections are at risk of obtaining cervical cancer.

## Progression dependent on persistent HPV infection

To support this working hypothesis, a retrospective study [21] was performed and a prospective study was initiated [22] to see whether the presence of certain HPV types was associated with progression of cervical lesions. Both studies clearly showed that only women with persistent high-risk HPV types show progression to CIN III and are at risk of developing cervical cancer. Women with abnormal cytology with low-risk HPV types or HPV-negative smears do not show progression during the follow-up time (up to 36 months). Instead, these women mainly showed regression and a small number showed stable disease. A recent update of this study (up to 5 years) yields identical results.

The results of the study of Ho *et al.* [23] are in agreement with our findings concerning progression and they show that regression of a considerable number of the CIN lesions is associated with resolution of the HPV infection. Our working hypothesis is further corroborated by follow-up studies of women with normal cytology in relation to HPV status, which show that HPV infection is the most dominant risk factor for predicting CIN [24,25]. Moreover, studies using archival cervical smears previously taken from women who developed cervical cancer show that the same oncogenic HPV types as detected by polymerase chain reaction (PCR) on cervical cancer biopsy can be found in these preceding smears up to 7 years before the diagnosis of cervical cancer [26]. Since in these studies no smears with a longer follow-up time than 7 years were tested, we have now initiated a study in which smears are used from women with cervical cancer more than 10 years before the diagnosis of cervical cancer.

In conclusion, with all these data in mind we believe that enough data have now been collected to argue that HPV testing should be added to Pap smear reading to improve the specificity and sensitivity of cervical cancer screening.

## Choice of HPV test for screening on cervical cancer

Several HPV tests are currently available [9]. Of these, Virapap, Hybrid Capture, and PCR-based HPV tests are commonly used. In our opinion the test must be reproducible, robust, easy to handle and suitable for mass screening. Moreover, the test should be very sensitive because a substantial number of carcinomas and severe dysplasia contain low viral copy number. Only a PCR-based HPV test can meet the last criterion and therefore our choice is a PCR-based HPV method [27–29]. In the near future a PCR-based non-radioactive HPV detection method suitable for mass screening of cervical smears will be available [30,31] which meets the criteria mentioned before.

## Screening: HPV testing versus Pap smear reading

With the data presented above in mind, the first question which arises is whether HPV testing can replace Pap smear reading in primary screening for cervical cancer [32]. Although prospective follow-up studies of Remmink *et al.* [22] and Ho *et al.* [23] clearly show that no progression of cervical lesions is found in the absence of high-risk HPV types and presumably HPV-negative cervical cancers are very rare, gynaecologists are at the moment not willing to replace Pap smear reading with HPV testing as a primary screening tool.

The main reasons are:

1  Gynaecologists do not feel confident with the wait-and-see policy of HPV-negative CIN lesions they formerly used to treat.

2    The legal problems gynaecologists and pathologists have met in the past with inappropriate Pap smear reading and successive treatment.

Therefore, HPV testing must be used in conjunction with Pap smear reading in primary screening for cervical cancer.

## Screening by HPV testing in conjunction with cytology

This will lead to a more efficient way of screening since both techniques, which detect different items (i.e. abnormal cells and high-risk HPV types), strengthen each other in the detection of abnormal cells. This will lead to a better selection of high-risk cases.

In this context it is important that we found that *rescreening* of high-risk HPV-positive and cytomorphologically normal cervical smears of women > 30 years (4% of the total number of smears) yields an abnormal Pap classification in 7% of smears (Van der Linden *et al.*, unpublished results). Interestingly, rescreening of the HPV high-risk negative smears yields very low percentages (< 1%). As well as greater efficiency, HPV testing can also serve as a tool for *quality control* of Pap smear reading.

## HPV infection in normal Pap smears identifies patients at risk for development of severe dysplasia

This is further substantiated by the findings of Rozendaal *et al.* [24]. In this study a group of 1622 women with *normal* cytology for a period of 40 months (range 3–73) was analysed.

They found that, from the 86 patients who were HPV high-risk positive at the start of the study, 6 developed CIN III. In contrast, in the HPV-negative group ($n = 1536$), only 1 developed CIN III. This means that women with HPV high-risk positive normal smears have 115 times (95% confidence interval 14–970) greater chance of developing severe dysplasia than women with HPV high-risk negative normal smears. From this cohort 6-year follow-up data are also available of 800 women with an initial HPV high-risk negative cytomorphologically normal Pap smear. It appeared that in this group no CIN III could be detected, indicating that the time between initial HPV infection and the development of CIN III is at least 6 years. These findings strongly underline our working hypothesis about the relation of HPV infection and CIN lesion and stress the importance of testing on HPV high-risk types in primary screening as an adjunct to cytology. Moreover, they show that HPV infection precedes the development of CIN lesions. Interestingly, 2 patients of the 6 who developed strong dysplasia had, after rescreening, mild to moderate dysplastic cells in their smear, again showing that HPV rescreening of high-risk HPV positive smear can serve as quality control for Pap smear reading.

## Which patients?

The question is, which patients should participate in the screening programme and how many times during their life-time? In the Netherlands until 1995 all women aged between 35 and 55 years participated in a 3-yearly cervical cancer screening programme. In 1996 the age has been changed to women between 30 years and 60 years, while the interval has been increased to 5 years. This is based on a cost-effectiveness analysis by the Institute of Public Health Rotterdam [33]. When HPV is added to Pap smear reading, one must keep in mind that the prevalence of high-risk HPV types in patients younger than 30 years of age is relatively high and the specificity for detection of progressive CIN lesions is very low. Therefore we advocate HPV testing in conjunction with cytology screening for women > 30 years.

## Interval

From the results of the nationwide screening programmes in the Netherlands it was calculated that it takes 13.1 years to develop cervical cancer from normal cytology [34]. As already discussed, in the preceding paragraph, our results of the 6-year follow-up of HPV high-risk positive cytomorphological normal women indicate that it takes at least 6 years to develop CIN III lesions and that patients who have been negative for both high-risk HPV and abnormal cells on Pap smear have a decreased risk for developing CIN lesions as compared to women who had normal smears, as tested by a Pap smear alone. At the moment we do not have evidence for significant time differences in the development of CIN lesions for certain high-risk HPV types. Taken together, the available data indicate that the interval between two successive rounds of cervical cancer screening can be at least 6 years or even maybe increased to 8–10 years by combining cytology and HPV testing.

Studies leading to a more exact time interval are currently underway. They concern HPV testing of archival Pap smears from women who developed cervical cancer and analysis of clinical follow-up data of women with cytomorphologically normal smears tested for HPV and cytology for three successive triannual screenings.

## Cost benefits

Economically, HPV testing is also beneficial. The higher price of primary screening caused by adding HPV testing will be easily compensated for by the longer interval between successive screening rounds. Due to more efficient screening, the HPV-negative, cytologically negative group can be screened less frequently. Instead of 5 years, a time interval of probably 8–10 years can be advised because nearly all patients who will develop severe dysplasia are detected by HPV testing at a very early stage. The advice given to women with HPV high-risk positive, cytologically negative smears is rescreening for HPV and cytology after 1 year. Also the costs for rescreening this group of women are compensated for by the increased interval of screening of the women with HPV-negative, cytomorphologically normal smears.

Another important factor in economics is the referral to gynaecologists. In the proposed screening programme all severe dysplasias (> Pap IIIb) are referred to the gynaecologists for colposcopy. Furthermore, only women with smears classified as mild to moderate dysplasias (Pap IIIa and atypical squamous cells of undetermined significance (ASCUS) Pap II), who are high-risk HPV positive are sent to the gynaecologist. Now the procedure is that women who show mild to moderate dysplasia twice in 6 months are referred to the gynaecologists, together with all women with strong dysplasia or more. In the Dutch setting of cervical screening this saves about 150 referrals to gynaecologists in 10 000 women (manuscript in preparation). Compared with the results of the follow-up studies, this finding is further substantiated by the fact that among high-risk HPV positive women with ASCUS and normal cytology, a high proportion of histological CIN III lesions can be found [35].

## Individual compliance of women

The design outlined here is very woman-friendly. Both the increased time interval for successive screening rounds, resulting in fewer repetitive smears, and the lower referral rate of women to gynaecologists are better tolerated by women participating in the new screening programme. Perhaps this may result in greater participation of women in screening programmes.

## What about women under 30 years of age?

Although the prevalence of cervical cancer in this group is relatively low, and this group does not participate in the screening programme, they constitute a problem for the clinician. Since the prevalence of high-risk HPV in this group of women is about 10%, it can be expected that the specificity to predict progressive CIN lesions is too low. Therefore in this group we advise clinical Pap smear reading. Severe dysplasia or higher means referral to gynaecologists whereas mild to moderate dysplasia means rescreening, including HPV testing within 6 months. Women with cytomorphologically abnormal cells and high-risk HPV types are sent to the gynaecologist. Those who are not high-risk HPV positive and have slight to moderate dysplasias are rescreened after a year. Women with cytomorphologically normal high-risk HPV-type positive smears are rescreened after a year with HPV testing and cytology.

## Women in developing countries

The considerations outlined above are clearly defined for developed countries. However, in underdeveloped countries the prevalence of cervical cancer and its precursor lesions is much higher and follow-up is often difficult. Therefore different options have to be worked out. Before making definite strategies we tentatively suggest performing just one non-radioactive PCR HPV test using general primers on smears of women at the age of 30–40 years. Those women who are high-risk HPV positive are sent for colposcopy and, if necessary, treatment can follow immediately. In this way a considerable reduction in the prevalence of cervical cancer can be expected of about 70%. Moreover, this procedure can be performed with a limited number of well-trained cytotechnicians.

## Acknowledgement

The authors would like to thank Hanna van Soest for typing the manuscript. We are also grateful to Professor P. Kenemans for continuous interest in our work. Part of the work presented in this chapter was supported by grants of the Praeventiefonds (28-1502,2), the Dutch Cancer Society (IKA-VU-96-1151) and the Ziekenfondsraad.

## References

1 Van de Graaf Y. *Screenings for cervical cancer. The Nijmegen project*. Doctoral thesis, 1987.
2 Koss LG. The Papanicolaou test for cervical cancer detection: a triumph and a tragedy. *JAMA* 1989; **261**: 737–743.
3 Devessa SS, Young JL, Brinton LA, Fraumen JF. Recent trends in cervix uteri cancer. *Cancer* 1989; **64**: 2184–2190.
4 Coppleson LW, Brown B. Estimation of the screening error rate from the observed detection rates in repeated cervical cytology. *Am J Obstet Gynecol* 1974; **119**: 953–958.
5 Wied GL, Bartels PH, Bibbo M, Bolbler CM. Frequency and reliability of diagnostic cytology of the female genital tract. *Acta Cytol* 1980; **25**: 543–549.
6 IARC Working group. IARC monographs on the evaluation of carcinogenic risks. Human papillomavirus. *IARC Sci Publ* 1995; 64, Lyon.
7 Zur Hausen H. Molecular pathogenesis of cancer of the cervix and its causation by specific human papillomavirus types. In: Zur Hausen H (ed) *Human Pathogenic Papillomaviruses*. Berlin: Springer Verlag, 1994, pp 131–156.
8 Bosch FX, Manos MM Muñoz N. *et al*. Prevalence of human papillomavirus in cervical smears: a worldwide perspective. *J Natl Cancer Inst* 1995; **87**: 796–802.
9 Walboomers JMM, De Roda Husman AM, Snijders PJF *et al*. Detection of genital human papillomavirus infections. Critical review of methods and prevalence studies in relation to cervical cancer. In: Stern PL, Stanley MA (eds) *Human Papillomaviruses and Cervical Cancer. Biology and Immunology*. Oxford: Oxford University Press, 1994, pp 41–71.

10  Van den Brule AJC, Walboomers JMM, Du Maine M, Kenemans P, Meijer CJLM. Difference in prevalence of human papillomavirus genotypes in cytomorphologically normal cervical smears is associated with a history of cervical intra-epithelial neoplasia. *Int J Cancer* 1991; **48**: 404–408.

11  Eluf-Neto J, Booth M, Muñoz N, Bosch FX, Meijer CJLM, Walboomers JMM. Human papillomavirus and invasive cervical cancer in Brazil. *Br J Cancer* 1994; **69**: 114–119.

12  Roda Husman AM de, Walboomers JMM, Meijer CJLM *et al*. Analysis of cytomorphologically abnormal cervical scrapes for the presence of 27 mucosotropic human papillomavirus genotypes, using polymerase chain reaction. *Int J Cancer* 1994; **56**: 802–806.

13  Meijer CJLM, Snijders PFJ, Van den Brule AJC, Helmerhorst ThJM, Remmink AJ, Walboomers JMM. Can cytological detection be improved by HPV screening? In: Monsonego J (ed) *Challenges of Modern Medicine*, vol 9. *Papillomavirus in Human Pathology*. Rome: Ares-Serono Symposia Publications, 1995, pp 493–497.

14  Melkert PJW, Hopman E, Brule AJC van den *et al*. Prevalence of HPV in cytomorphologically normal cervical smears as determined by the polymerase chain reaction is age-dependent. *Int J Cancer* 1993; **53**: 919–923.

15  Roda Husman AM de, Walboomers JMM, Hopman E *et al*. Prevalence in cytomorphologically normal cervical scrapes of pregnant women as determined by PCR: the age-related pattern. *J Med Virol* 1995; **46**: 97–102.

16  Bauer HM, Ting Y, Green CE *et al*. Genital human papillomavirus infection in female university students as determined by a PCR based method. *JAMA* 1991; **265**: 472–477.

17  Evander M, Edlund K, Gustafsson A *et al*. Human papillomavirus infection is transient in young women: a population based cohort study. *J Infect Dis* 1995; **171**: 1026–1030.

18  Boyes DA, Morrison B, Know EG, Draper GJ, Miller AB. A cohort study of cervical cancer screening in British Columbia. *Clin Invest Med* 1982; **5**: 1–29.

19  van Oortmarssen GJ, Habbema JDF. Epidemiological evidence for age-dependent regression of pre-invasive cervical cancer. *Br J Cancer* 1991; **64**: 559–564.

20  Krüger-Kjaer SK, Van den Brule AJC, Bock JE *et al*. Human papillomavirus – the most significant risk determinant of cervical intraepithelial neoplasia. *Int J Cancer* 1996; **65**: 601–606.

21  Gaarenstroom KN, Melkert P, Hopman E *et al*. Human papillomavirus DNA and genotypes: prognostic factors for progression of cervical intraepithelial neoplasia. *Int J Gynecol Cancer* 1994; **4**: 73–78.

22  Remmink A, Walboomers JMM, Helmerhorst ThJM *et al*. The presence of persistent high risk HPV genotypes in dysplastic cervical lesions is associated with progressive disease: natural history up to 36 months. *Int J Cancer* 1995; **61**: 306–311.

23  Ho GY, Buck RD, Klein *et al*. Persistent genital human papillomavirus infection as a risk factor for persistent cervical dysplasia. *J Natl Cancer Inst* 1995; **87**: 1365–1371.

24  Rozendaal L, Walboomers JMM, Van der Linden JC *et al*. High risk human papillomavirus in cytomorphological normal cervical smears has a high predictive value for development of severe dysplasia. *Int J Cancer* 1996; **68**: 766–769.

25  Schiffman MH, Bauer HM, Hooieren RN *et al*. Epidemiologic evidence showing that human papillomavirus infection causes most cervical intraepithelial neoplasia. *J Natl Cancer Inst* 1993; **85**: 958–964.

26  Walboomers JMM, Roda Husman AM de, Snijders PJF *et al*. Human papillomavirus in false negative archival cervical smears: implications for screening for cervical cancer. *J Clin Pathol* 1995; **48**: 728–732.

27  Van den Brule AJC, Snijders PJF, Meijer CJLM, Walboomers JMM. PCR based detection of genital HPV genotypes: an update and future perspectives. *Papillomavirus Rep* 1993; **4**: 95–99.

28  Roda Husman AM de, Walboomers JMM, Brule AJC van den, Meijer CJLM, Snijders

PJF. The use of general primers GP5 and GP6 elongated at their 3' ends with adjacent highly conserved sequences improves human papillomavirus detection by polymerase chain reaction. *J Gen Virol* 1995; **76**: 1057–1062.

29 Jacobs MV, Brule AJC van den, Snijders PJF, Meijer CJLM, Walboomers JMM. Group-specific differentiation between high- and low-risk HPV genotypes by GP-PCR and two cocktails of oligonucleotide probes. *J Clin Microbiol* 1995; **33**: 901–905.

30 Jacobs MV, Brule AJC van den, Snijders PJF, Meijer CJLM, Walboomers JMM. A non-radioactive PCR enzyme-immunoassay enables a rapid identification of HPV 16 and 18 in cervical smears after GP5 + /6 + PCR. *J Med Virol* 1996; **49**: 223–229.

31 Jacobs MV, Van den Brule AJC, Kjaer SK *et al*. A general primer GP5 + /6 + mediated PCR-EIA for rapid detection of oncogenic human papillomavirus DNA in normal and abnormal cervical scrapes. *J Clin Microbiol* (in press).

32 Meijer CJLM, Van den Brule AJC, Snijders PJF, Helmerhorst ThJM, Kenemans P, Walboomers JMM. Detection of human papillomavirus in cervical scrapes by the polymerase chain reaction in relation to cytology: possible implications for cervical cancer screening. In: Muñoz N, Bosch XF, Shah KV, Meheus A (eds) *The Epidemiology of Cervical Cancer and Human Papillomavirus*. Lyon: IARC Science Publications 1992, pp 271–281.

33 Van Ballegooijen M, Koopmanschap MA, Habbema JDF. The management of cervical intraepithelial neoplasia (CIN): extensiveness and costs in the Netherlands. *Eur J Cancer* 1995; **31A**: 1672–1676.

34 Van Oortmarssen GH, Habbema JDF, Van Ballegooijen M. Predicting mortality from cervical cancer after negative test smears results. *BMJ* 1995; **305**: 449–453.

35 Cuzick J, Szarewski A, Terry G *et al*. Human papillomavirus testing in primary cervical screening. *Lancet* 1995; **345**: 1533–1536.

# 39: Human Papillomavirus DNA Testing Using Liquid-based Cytology

A. Ferenczy[1] & E. L. Franco[2]

## Summary

Liquid-based cytology samples are suitable for human papillomavirus (HPV) DNA testing.

We used the Thin-Prep method and Hybrid Capture HPV DNA assay in 364 women who were referred to colposcopy for an abnormal Papanicolaou (Pap) smear, e.g. atypical squamous cells of undetermined significance (ASCUS) or worse.

The combination of Thin-Prep cytology and HPV DNA testing detected accurately 95% of patients with histologically proven squamous intraepithelial lesions (SIL). Conversely, the negative predictive value of double-testing was in the order of 97%. We have shown, furthermore, that the specificity of Thin-Prep cytology–HPV DNA testing combination was significantly better than that of the cytology and a hypothetical, random adjunct test combination for detecting either invasive cancer or its precursors.

In conclusion, the combination of Thin-Prep cytology and HPV DNA testing is a sensitive method for screening and diagnosing clinically significant cervical lesions.

## Introduction

The central role of HPV infection in the pathogenesis of cervical carcinoma and its precursors, named low- and high-grade squamous intraepithelial lesions

*Correspondence*: Dr Alex Ferenczy, [1]Department of Pathology, Sir Mortimer B. Davis Jewish General Hospital, 3755 Côte Ste Catherine Road, Montreal, Quebec, Canada H3T 1E2. [2]Department of Oncology, McGill University, 546 Pine Avenue West, Montreal, QC, Canada H2W 1S6.

(LGSIL, HGSIL) has been abundantly documented in the past 10 years [1,2]. Persistent or progressive SILs are associated with persistent, high levels of high oncogenic risk HPV DNA, particularly in women aged 25 years and older [3]. Women aged 30–35 years old are most likely to have incident HGSIL/CIN III [4].

Cervical cytology is currently the most widely used screening test for the detection of cervical carcinoma and its precursors; its widespread use has contributed to a 63% decrease in mortality from cervical cancer in the past 50 years [5]. Unfortunately, cervical cytology as a screening test is not perfect as it fails to detect on average 20% of individuals with disease [6]. About one-third of the false-negative smears are due to laboratory reading errors and two-thirds to sampling errors by the physicians taking a cell sample from the cervix uteri [5].

Another problematic area in cervical pathology relates to the management of women with an ASCUS or LGSIL smear [7]. New epidemiology confirms the traditional view held by many that the majority of women with minor-grade cytological abnormalities revert to normal; only about 15% of them remain with LGSIL with the potential to progression to HGSIL [4,8]. Another 15% of women with an initial low-grade lesion may in fact have an HGSIL on colposcopy and biopsy [9].

It is clear today that only a small proportion of women with HPV infection have clinically significant disease and it is also clear that cytology is a relatively insensitive test to detect cervical cancer precursors and invasive lesions. Furthermore, it is generally agreed that two imperfect screening tests in combination provide for better diagnostic performance than each test taken alone [10]. Since HPV DNA is found in over 90% of cervical cancer and its precursor lesions, it seems logical to combine cytology with HPV DNA testing to improve the sensitivity and negative predictive value of screening for cervical neoplasia [7].

Using quantitative HPV testing and limiting the combination screening approach to women between the ages of 25 and 35, in whom persistent lesions are prevalent, may have high specificity and positive predictive value as well [4]. Furthermore, an HPV DNA-based diagnostic triage may better identify the small group of women with progressive-type LGSIL amongst women with an initial ASCUS/LGSIL smear [9–13].

A potential problem with double-testing, however, is related to the expense which is associated with the return visit for HPV testing. The development of liquid-based cytology methods seems to be a highly attractive means of circumventing this problem. Indeed, recent studies have shown that the traditional manual method for taking a cellular sample results in the loss of up to 80% of the collected cells by discarding them with the collection device. Using this new technology, all of the cells are retained by suspending them in a collection tube which contains a cell preserver solution (PreservCyt/Cytyc Corporation, USA). The collection vial is then transported to the laboratory and the residual cellular material (after processing Thin-Prep slides for routine cytology) can then be used for HPV DNA testing. Double-testing could be used in women between the ages of 25 and 35 and in those with minor-grade cytological atypia.

A feasibility study using liquid-based cytology for HPV DNA testing has been performed in our laboratory [10]. We found that PreservCyt cytology samples were suitable for HPV DNA testing with the Hybrid Capture HPV DNA assay (Digene Diagnostics, Inc., Silver Spring, MD, USA).

In a series of 364 women referred to colposcopy because of an abnormal smear diagnosis, we found a good correlation between HPV DNA quantitation and histological grade of SIL; increasing levels (20/pg of HPV DNA/ml sample) were associated with a statistically significant increased likelihood of detecting HGSIL than lower levels. Similar results were obtained by others using conventional cytology and HPV DNA sampling kits [9,11–13].

Tables 39.1 and 39.2 contain the diagnostic performance indices for cytology and HPV DNA alone and a combination, respectively. For Thin-Prep cytology combined with HPV DNA testing, the combination method improved detection rates of cervical disease in all histological categories over either Thin-Prep slide or HPV DNA testing alone. It was of particular interest to find that the combination approach detected 95% of patients with HGSIL.

**Table 39.1** Diagnostic performance indices (%) for repeat cytology and human papillomavirus (HPV) testing as independent screening tools in women referred for an atypical squamous cells of undetermined significance (ASCUS) or worse Papanicolaou (PAP) smears.

| Lesions detected* | Method | Sensitivity | Specificity | Predictive value | |
|---|---|---|---|---|---|
| | | | | Positive | Negative |
| HGSIL and invasive cancer | Cytology | 87.5† | 57.0† | 36.5 | 94.2 |
| | HPV | 75.3 | 63.7 | 37.2 | 90.0 |
| HGSIL | Cytology | 86.8† | 57.0† | 35.1 | 94.2 |
| | HPV | 76.6 | 63.7 | 36.4 | 91.0 |
| LGSIL, HGSIL and invasive cancer | Cytology | 78.0† | 73.6 | 75.5 | 76.2† |
| | HPV | 66.3 | 77.5 | 75.6 | 68.7 |
| LGSIL and HGSIL | Cytology | 77.5† | 73.6 | 75.0 | 76.2 |
| | HPV | 66.7 | 77.5 | 75.3 | 69.3 |

* Based on histological ascertainment.
† Significant difference (P < 0.05) between cytology and HPV testing. HGSIL, low-grade squamous intraepithelial lesion; LGSIL, low-grade squamous intraepithelial lesion. From Ferenczy et al. [10] with permission.

**Table 39.2** Screening performance of a combination of repeat cytology and human papillomavirus (HPV) testing among women referred for colposcopy because of an abnormal Papanicolaou (PAP) smear.

| Lesions detected* | | Sensitivity | Specificity | Predictive value | |
|---|---|---|---|---|---|
| | | | | Positive | Negative |
| HGSIL and invasive cancer | Observed | 95.1 (88.0–98.1)† | 47.2 (41.5–53.0) | 33.9 (28.1–40.3) | 97.1 (92.8–98.9) |
| | Expected‡ | 93.1 | 31.4 | 27.7 | 94.2 |
| HGSIL | Observed | 94.8 (87.4–98.0) | 47.2 (41.5–53.0) | 32.7 (26.9–39.1) | 97.1 (92.8–98.9) |
| | Expected | 92.8 | 31.4 | 26.6 | 94.2 |
| LGSIL, HGSIL and invasive cancer | Observed | 87.7 (82.2–91.7) | 64.6 (57.3–71.3) | 72.2 (66.1–77.7) | 83.3 (76.2–88.6) |
| | Expected | 87.8 | 40.6 | 60.7 | 76.2 |
| LGSIL and HGSIL | Observed | 87.4 (81.8–91.5) | 64.6 (57.3–71.3) | 71.7 (65.5–77.3) | 83.3 (76.2–88.6) |
| | Expected | 87.6 | 40.6 | 60.1 | 76.2 |

* Based on histological ascertainment.
† Range in parentheses represents the 95% confidence interval.
‡ Assuming a combination of cytology and a hypothetical random adjunct test yielding the same prevalence of positive results as HPV testing. HGSIL, High-grade squamous intraepithelial lesion; LGSIL, low-grade squamous intraepithelial lesion. From Ferenczy et al. [10] with permission.

**Table 39.3** Diagnostic performance of Thin-Prep smear with and without human papillomavirus (HPV) DNA testing for detecting high-grade squamous intraepithelial lesions HGSIL (47/364).

| Referral Pap | Diagnostic tests | % Sensitivity | Number of colposcopies required per HGSIL patient |
|---|---|---|---|
| ≥ASCUS | Colposcopy | 100 | 8.3 |
| | Thin-Prep | 87 | 5.1 |
| | HPV | 77 | 4.8 |
| | Thin-Prep + HPV | 95 | 5.4 |

Pap, Papanicolaou; ASCUS, atypical squamous cells of undetermined significance.

The high negative predictive value of the combination approach was noticeable, as double-negative results indicated a very low risk of missing HGSIL and/or cancer — in the order of 3% (Table 39.2). The study showed, furthermore, that due to the high sensitivity of the combination method for detecting HGSIL, the number of colposcopies needed to evaluate HGSIL cases can be reduced by nearly 50% (Table 39.3).

Another interesting finding was comparison of cytology/HPV DNA testing combination with cytology and a hypothetical random adjunctive test. Indeed, in theory the combination of an adjunctive test to cytology may simply be a function of increased sensitivity by chance alone rather than the genuine in-built superior diagnostic performance of the adjunctive test. It can be seen from Table 39.2 that, although the sensitivity was similar by both methods, the specificity of the Thin-Prep cytology/HPV DNA testing was significantly better than that of the cytology/random test combination in all of the diagnostic combinations.

In view of the feasibility study results obtained, it may be useful to undertake further studies on a large number of patients to compare cost-effectiveness of the liquid-based Thin-Prep cytology/HPV DNA combination in a screening capacity, focusing on older women, in whom persistent and/or progressive SILs are prevalent. Thanks to the high negative predictive value of the combination method — 97% absence of significant lesions — substantial savings in health care funds may be realized and, by virtue, it will be possible to increase safely screening cytological intervals. The same may be the case for diagnostic triage protocols; using the combination alternative (rather than cytology follow-up or colposcopy for all) for women with minor-grade cytology atypia, it is possible to eliminate a return office visit for HPV DNA testing and decreasing unnecessary colposcopy by at least 30%. Large-scale studies are underway to substantiate and hopefully validate the preliminary results of our study and hypotheses generated thereof.

## References

1 IARC working group on the evaluation of carcinogenic risks to humans. *Human Papilloma Viruses*. Lyon, France: IARC Science Publications, 1995.

2 Lorincz AT, Reid R, Jenson AB *et al*. Human papillomavirus infection of the cervix: relative risk associations of 15 common anogenital types. *Obstet Gynecol* 1992; **79**: 328.

3 Ho GY, Burk RD, Klein S *et al*. Persistent genital human papillomavirus infection as a risk factor for persistent cervical dysplasia. *J Natl Cancer Inst* 1995; **87**: 1365.

4 Schiffman MH. Recent progress in defining the epidemiology of human papillomavirus infection and cervical neoplasia. *J Natl Cancer Inst* 1992; **84**: 394.

5 Miller AB, Anderson G, Brisson J *et al*. Report of a national workshop on screening for cancer of the cervix. *Can Med Assoc J* 1991; **145**: 1301–1325.

6 Koss LG. Cervical (Pap) smear. New directions. *Cancer* 1993; **71**: 1406.

7 Ferenczy A. Viral testing for genital human papillomavirus infections: recent progress and clinical potentials. *Int J Gynecol Cancer* 1995; **5**: 321.

8 Nasiell K, Roger V, Nasiell M. Behavior of mild cervical dysplasia during long term follow-up. *Obstet Gynecol* 1986; **67**: 665.

9 Wright TC, Sun XW, Koulos J. Comparison of management algorithms for the evaluation of women with low-grade cytology abnormalities. *Obstet Gynecol* 1995; **85**: 202.

10 Ferenczy A, Franco E, Arseneau J *et al*. Diagnostic performance of Hybrid Capture HPV DNA assay combined with liquid-based cytology. *Am J Obstet Gynecol* 1996; **175**: 651.

11 Cox JT, Lorincz AT, Schiffman MH *et al*. Human papillomavirus testing by hybrid capture is useful in triaging women with a cytologic diagnosis of ASCUS. *Am J Obstet Gynecol* 1995; **172**: 946.

12 Cox JT, Schiffman MH, Winzelberg AJ *et al*. An evaluation of human papillomavirus testing as part of referral to colposcopy clinics. *Obstet Gynecol* 1992; **80**: 389.

13 Hatch KD, Schneider A, Abdel-Nour MW. An evaluation of human papillomavirus testing for intermediate- and high-risk types as triage before colposcopy. *Am J Obstet Gynecol* 1995; **172**: 1150.

# 40: Human Papillomavirus Testing for Diagnostic Triage of Minor-grade Cytological Abnormalities: The European Perspective

T. A. J. Mould & A. Singer

## Summary

A total of 250 000 Papanicolaou (Pap) smears are reported as minor cytological abnormalities annually in the UK. At present these women are kept under cytological surveillance until a second smear is abnormal. Arguments to recommend immediate colposcopy for these women have not caused any change in policy as yet. An intermediate strategy using a second test to triage women into those who can safely stay under cytological surveillance and those who require immediate colposcopy has received much discussion. The involvement of human papillomavirus (HPV) in the development of cervical cancer, and the ability of high levels of HPV DNA accurately to predict cervical lesions, make HPV DNA testing an obvious choice for this test. Commercial kits such as SHARP and Hybrid Capture using quantitative PCR or modern solution hybridization techniques respectively are the assays of choice. Hybrid Capture has been shown in reports from the USA and in work from the UK to have a good sensitivity in detecting from this population those women with high-grade lesions.

Widespread clinical uptake of HPV DNA probing as a triage test has yet to occur, principally due to perceived extra cost to the screening programme and the belief that these tests are exclusively the domain of specified research laboratories. Results from large prospective trials to be undertaken in both the USA and the UK are awaited to resolve these problems.

*Correspondence*: Professor A. Singer, Department of Women's Health, F Block, Whittington Hospital, Highgate Hill, London N19 5NF, UK.

## Introduction

In the UK, 5.5 million Pap smear tests are performed annually, of which 2.4% show mild dyskaryosis and 2.2% show borderline dyskaryosis. These figures increase in younger women, and a total of over 250 000 smears are reported as minor cytological abnormalities annually. Present guidelines from the Royal College of Obstetricians and Gynaecologists recommend referral to colposcopy after two mildly abnormal smears, but there is a substantial body of opinion that immediate referral after one abnormal smear is more appropriate. A compromise strategy is to use a triage test to select which women should be referred for immediate colposcopy and which can be left to cytological surveillance. HPV DNA testing has been proposed as this triage test in view of the role of HPV in cervical carcinogenesis and the ability of high levels of HPV to predict cervical disease. However, worries about potentially increased costs and suspicion of HPV testing due to earlier results using inappropriate methodology such as filter *in situ* hybridization (FISH) mean that HPV testing is still confined to research institutes.

## The argument for a triage test

There remains a dilemma as to the best management strategy for women with minor cytological abnormalities on their Pap smear. Many of these minor Pap smear abnormalities will represent the early and usually transient effects of HPV infection. Up to 50% of them will return to normal and 19% will have no visible lesion, making immediate colposcopy in these women an unnecessary procedure [1,2]. Also the cost of performing immediate colposcopy on all women with minor abnormalities may be excessive for the potential number of cancers prevented and the local facilities may not be able to keep up with the demand for colposcopy [3]. Finally, referral to colposcopy may result in over-treatment, as up to 52% of women with a mildly abnormal Pap smear treated by loop diathermy in a 'see-and-treat' clinic may have no CIN in the loop specimen [4].

The dilemma is that cross-sectional and retrospective studies show that up to 50% of women with minor abnormalities of their Pap smear have cervical intraepithelial neoplasia (CIN) II or III and this rate has been confirmed in prospective trials [5–8]. One retrospective trial showed that the rate of the abnormality did not depend on the number of mildly dyskaryotic smear tests before referral [8].

The ultimate answer to determine the validity of each management strategy is by randomized studies. One such study has recently reported that cytological surveillance is safe and cancers will not develop undetected in women in this system [6]. Cross-sectional and retrospective studies also suggest that cytological surveillance is safe both individually and on a population basis [1,9]. Furthermore, the risk of invasive disease seems to be the same in women who have had colposcopy and those who have had cytological surveillance [1]. This may be because early invasive changes can be missed at colposcopy [10].

However, Flannelly *et al.* [6] reported that only a quarter of the women with an initial mildly abnormal Pap smear avoided colposcopy after 2 years of cytological surveillance, and thus this management policy was not cost-effective. Furthermore, retrospective studies consistently show that women with mildly abnormal Pap smears are at high risk of developing invasive cancer of the cervix, with a higher rate of invasive cancer than women who have never had abnormal cervical cytology [11].

## Reason for using HPV DNA testing as the triage test

HPV DNA testing provides an objective, automatable test to predict the presence of cervical disease. Furthermore, HPV may provide a marker to predict whether a lesion is likely to progress or regress. No clinician using colposcopy, histology, cytology or any other technique is able to predict the outcome of a cervical lesion and thus many women with non-progressive lesions are being overtreated.

## HPV DNA testing methodology

In expert hands, Southern blots are sensitive and specific HPV tests. However, they are arduous procedures and have no applicability to the testing of routine clinical samples. Dot blots are a rapid and easier method of analysing samples and have become available in commercially available kits (Virapap and Vira-type, Digene Diagnostics), but are expensive due to the use of $^{32}$P isotope in the detection system. *In situ* hybridization (ISH) targets intracellular nucleic acids within histological material on specially treated glass slides. ISH is less sensitive than Southern blot or dot blot and will only identify the presence of HPV DNA rather than the type.

PCR is an excellent tool for epidemiological studies as the amplification means that extreme sensitivity can be achieved, but this sensitivity produces two problems. First, the epidemiological specificity of the test will become low and traces of HPV DNA can be detected in 40–50% of normal women. These traces may represent previously resolved HPV infections and have little clinical significance. Recent studies have shown that the likelihood of a positive HPV DNA result reflecting the presence of CIN is directly proportional to the virus load [12,13]. Thus, PCR is most useful when restricted to the analytical sensitivity of Southern blot at $5 \times 10^4$ HPV DNA molecules per specimen. Second, amplification of minuscule amounts of contaminating HPV DNA can produce very high false-positive rates and many studies performed before stringent sterility rules were introduced were quite unreliable and not reproducible. Some of these studies have been retracted [14]. Thus, PCR is an invaluable research tool but may be too sensitive and liable to contamination to be used in the everyday clinical setting, despite advances in contamination control.

Nevertheless, a PCR-based HPV detection kit, known as the SHARP signal system, is available (Digene Diagnostics, USA). The use of a commercial kit of this kind means that standardized and reproducible results may be possible in a clinical setting. Furthermore, this technology is readily automated [15] but so far it has only been tested by expert research virologists in a designated laboratory [13].

Modern forms of solution hybridization are simple-to-perform procedures with good sensitivity. A commercially available form of solution hybridization using a non-radioactive detection system, Hybrid Capture (Digene Diagnostics, USA), is comparable to the best Southern blot methodology, with an accuracy of 92% or greater [16,17]. This particular product includes RNA probes to detect HPV DNA types 16, 18, 31, 33, 35, 45, 51, 52, 56 and thus it would be hoped that its clinical sensitivity is high. Although false positives can still occur with this method, it is much less prone to contamination than amplification techniques and should be suitable for clinical use.

## Efficacy of HPV DNA testing as a triage test

In women presenting to colposcopy with mild cytological abnormalities, semiquantitative HPV testing detected 57% of those with CIN II–III using HPV 16 alone [18] and 67% using types 16, 18, 31 and 33 [19]. Combining HPV 16, 18, 31, 33 testing with a repeat Pap smear increased the sensitivity to 94% but decreased the specificity from 88% to 55% [19].

Hybrid Capture has been used in the USA on women presenting with ASCUS or low-grade SIL [20–22]. Its sensitivity to detect CIN II or above was reported to be between 74 and 93%. Combining a repeat smear and Hybrid Capture increased the sensitivity to between 91 and 100%.

In the UK, Hybrid Capture has been trialed at our unit using colposcopy and histology as the gold standard assessment of the cervix. A total of 180 women referred with either borderline or mildly dyskaryotic smears had a swab taken for quantitative detection of oncogenic HPV DNA types. Sensitivity to detect CIN II or above was 91% with a negative predictive value for high-grade lesions in this population of women of 93%. The specificity was 56% with a positive predictive value of 66%. The low specificity is of less concern when using the test in a high-risk population such as this where high-grade lesions may be present in as many as 30% of women.

Concerns reported in the American journals that Hybrid Capture missed a proportion of frankly invasive or necrotic tumours were not confirmed by a trial on 38 histologically confirmed cervical cancers in women recruited in Recife, Northern Brazil. Of the 38 women, 37 had a positive Hybrid Capture test. The laboratory analysis was performed by a gynaecologist (TM) for both of these trials, showing the robustness of the test, and that the test can be used effectively by personnel without specific virological research training.

## Present usage of HPV DNA testing

HPV DNA testing has not been started in mainstream clinical use in the UK. This results from a scepticism about the oncogenic role of HPV in cervical carcinogenesis, the perceived extra cost of a triage test and the view that the test remains the realm of the research laboratory. Previous misleading studies using FISH and early PCR damaged the reputation of HPV DNA testing and it is taking time for this to change. Furthermore, the similarities between the now discredited herpes simplex cervical cancer oncogenesis theory and the present-day HPV evidence remain too close for some observers. The expense of the present HPV DNA tests still represents a considerable increase in initial expenditure and until trials show that its use will decrease the incidence of cervical cancer, or be cost-effective by improving the efficiency of the screening programme, uptake of the test will be slow. Large-scale trials involving HPV testing in women with minor Pap smear abnormalities are being planned both in the USA and the UK.

In conclusion, triaging of minor Pap smear abnormalities is an appropriate way of dealing with the increasing numbers of these smears. HPV DNA testing is a objective test which has been shown to be extremely sensitive in this population of women. Perceived problems with additional cost and repeatability and validity of HPV DNA testing are preventing widespread use.

## Acknowledgements

The authors would like to thank Linda Ho and George Terry of the Middlesex Hospital Academic Virology Department, London, UK for their help and advice in the HPV DNA testing.

## References

1 Robertson JH, Woodend BE, Crozier EH, Hutchinson J. Risk of cervical cancer associated with mild dyskaryosis. *BMJ* 1988; **297**: 18–21.
2 Shafi MI. Cytological surveillance avoids treatment. *BMJ* 1994; **309**: 590–591.
3 Roberts CJ, Farrow SC, Charney MC. Cost of saving a life by cervical screening. *Lancet* 1985; **ii**: 950.

4 Murdoch JB, Grimshaw RN, Monaghan JM. Loop diathermy excision of the abnormal cervical transformation zone. *Int J Gynecol Cancer* 1991; **1**: 105–111.

5 Bolger BS, Lewis BV. A prospective study of colposcopy in women with mild dyskaryosis or koilocytosis. *Br J Obstet Gynaecol* 1988; **95** 1117–1119.

6 Flannelly G, Anderson D, Kitchener HC *et al.* Management of women with mild and moderate cervical dyskaryosis. *BMJ* 1994; **308**: 1399–1403.

7 Stewart CJR, Livingstone D, Mutch A. Borderline nuclear changes in cervical smears; a cytological review of 200 cases with histological correlation. *Cytopathology* 1993; **4**: 339–346.

8 Soutter WP, Wisdom S, Brough AK, Monaghan JM. Should patients with mild atypia in a cervical smear be referred for colposcopy? *Br J Obstet Gynaecol* 1986; **93**: 70–74.

9 Cooper P, Kirby AJ, Spigelhaiter DJ, Whitehead AL, Patterson A. Management of women with a cervical smear showing a mild degree of dyskaryosis: a review of policy. *Cytopathology* 1992; **3**: 331–339.

10 Benedet JL, Anderson GH, Boyes DA. Colposcopic accuracy in the diagnosis of microinvasive and occult invasive carcinoma of the cervix. *Obstet Gynecol* 1985; **65**: 557–562.

11 Soutter WP. Immediate referral to colposcopy is safer. *BMJ* 1994; **309**: 591–592.

12 Cuzick J, Terry G, Hoe L, Hollingsworth T, Anderson M. Human papillomavirus DNA in cervical smears as predictor of high-grade cervical cancer. *Lancet* 1992; **339**: 959–960.

13 Terry G, Ho L, Jenkins D *et al.* Definition of human papillomavirus type 16 DNA levels in low and high grade cervical lesions by a simple polymerase chain reaction technique. *Arch Virol* 1993; **12**: 123–133.

14 Tidy JA, Farrell PF. Retraction: human papillomavirus subtype 16b. *Lancet* 1989; **ii**: 1535.

15 Terry G, Ho L, Szarewski A, Cuzick J. Semi-automated detection of human papillomavirus DNA of high and low oncogenic potential in cervical smears. *Clin Chem* 1994; **40**: 1890–1892.

16 Sun X-Y, Ferenczy A, Johnson D *et al.* Evaluation of the Hybrid Capture human papillomavirus deoxyribonucleic acid detection test. *Am J Obstet Gynecol* 1995; **173**: 1432–1437.

17 Lorincz AT. Diagnosis of human papillomavirus infection by a new generation of molecular DNA assays. *Clin Immunol Newslett* 1992; **12**: 123–127

18 Bavin PJ, Giles JA, Deery A *et al.* Use of semi-quantitative PCR for human papillomavirus DNA type 16 to identify women with high grade cervical disease in a population presenting with a mildly dyskaryotic smear. *Br J Cancer* 1993; **67**: 602–605.

19 Mansell ME, Ho L, Terry G, Singer A, Cuzick J. Semi-quantitative human papillomavirus DNA detection in the management of women with minor cytological abnormality. *Br J Obstet Gynaecol* 1994; **101**: 807–809.

20 Cox JT, Lorincz AT, Schiffman MH, Sherman ME, Cullen A, Kurmen R. Human papillomavirus testing by hybrid capture appears to be useful in triaging women with a cytological diagnosis of atypical squamous cells of undetermined significance. *Am J Obstet Gynecol* 1995; **172**: 946–954.

21 Hatch KD, Schneider A, Abdel-Nour MW. An evaluation of human papillomavirus testing for intermediate- and high-risk types as triage before colposcopy. *Am J Obstet Gynecol* 1995; **172**: 1150–1157.

22 Wright TC, Sun XW, Koulos J. Comparison of management algorithms for the evaluation of women with low-grade cytological abnormalities. *Obstet Gynecol* 1995; **85**: 202–210.

*New Developments in Cervical Cancer Screening and Prevention* (ed. Franco & Monsonego), pp. 360–363

# 41 : Use of Human Papillomavirus Typing for Quality Assurance of Cytological Diagnosis

M. E. Sherman, [1,2] M. H. Schiffman[2] & A. T. Lorincz[3]

## Introduction

The term atypical squamous cells of undetermined significance (ASCUS) was introduced in the Bethesda system (TBS) to provide pathologists with a term to designate smears that fall in the grey zone between reactive changes and a definite cervical cancer precursor (squamous intraepithelial lesion or SIL) [1]. Because patients with ASCUS are difficult to manage clinically, quality assurance measures have focused on ensuring that pathologists use the ASCUS diagnosis sparingly, while maintaining accuracy in classifying cases as reactive or SIL.

Various measures have been proposed to evaluate the performance of cytology laboratories. Review of reportedly negative smears preceding the diagnosis of high-grade SIL and correlation of discrepant smears and biopsies are mandated by federal regulations and represent useful measures [2]. Interim guidelines suggest that rates of ASCUS should be less than 5% in most populations, with a ratio of ASCUS to SIL of about two or three to one [3]. Recently, we have observed consistent associations between the diagnosis of smears using TBS and human papillomavirus (HPV) typing [4]. These data suggest that HPV testing may be useful for quality control of the ASCUS smear.

## Correlation of cytological diagnoses with HPV typing

To explore the relationship between TBS diagnoses and HPV typing, we selected 200 smears originally diagnosed as atypical that were included in a

*Correspondence*: Dr Mark Sherman, [1]Department of Pathology, The John Hopkins Hospital, 600 North Wolfe Street, Baltimore, MD 21289, USA. [2]Division Cancer Epidemiology and Genetics, National Cancer Institute, Bethesda, MD, USA; [3]Digene Corporation, Silver Spring, MD, USA.

National Cancer Institute-sponsored cervical cancer screening study [4]. Samples were obtained with an Ayre spatula and an endocervical brush and prepared as single smears fixed in ethanol and stained with a modified Papanicolaou technique. At the time of the clinical examination, a 10 ml lavage was obtained for future HPV DNA testing using multiple methods, including Southern analysis, a polymerase chain reaction-based method and the Hybrid Capture tube test (Digene Corp., Silver Spring, MD). All HPV testing methods yielded similar results [5]. Five cytopathologists independently classified the smears according to TBS. Correlation of these diagnoses with HPV DNA detection is described below.

The reviewers classified 38–62% of the smears as negative, 16–39% as ASCUS and 21–28% as SIL. Thus, all of the reviewers classified a significant percentage of the originally atypical smears as normal. The ASCUS rate varied more than two to one between reviewers. Interobserver agreement between reviewers was poor, with only 29% five-way agreement. There was not a single smear unanimously classified as ASCUS by the panel.

The pattern of HPV DNA detection across TBS diagnostic categories was similar for each reviewer. In every pathologist's review, the overall detection of HPV DNA was lowest in women with negative smears, highest in women with SIL and intermediate in frequency in cases of ASCUS. Detection of cancer-associated types of HPV DNA was about 10% in negative smears, 25–35% in ASCUS smears and about 60% in SIL using Southern analysis. The detection of low-risk HPV DNA was about 20% in each diagnostic category for every reviewer. Therefore, the detection of low-risk HPV DNA was unrelated to cytopathological diagnosis. However, cytopathological diagnosis was strongly related to the detection of cancer-associated HPV types. HPV DNA was detected in 100% of cases unanimously diagnosed as SIL by the five panelists. The detection of cancer-associated HPV types was extremely rare in cases in which the five pathologists agreed that the smear was negative.

Studies demonstrate that approximately 90% of SIL and cancer are related to HPV infection [6,7]. The observation that detection rates of cancer-associated HPV DNA are highest in women with SIL, lowest in women who are normal and intermediate in frequency in patients with ASCUS indicates that TBS categories stratify patients according to cancer risk. From a public health point of view, these data support the effectiveness of TBS for classifying cervical smears.

## HPV testing for quality assurance

The extraordinarily consistent relationship between diagnoses of negative, ASCUS and SIL in TBS and the detection of cancer-associated HPV types suggests that pathologists could evaluate their diagnostic performance through a correlation experiment as described above [4]. This could be achieved by obtaining cervical swabs from 500 patients participating in a general screening programme. The swabs would be stored at $-20°C$ until the smears had been screened and diagnosed. Then, all of the abnormal smears and 50–100 normal smears would be selected and the corresponding frozen specimen thawed and tested for cancer-associated types of HPV DNA. Failure to detect the highest rate of cancer-associated HPV types in SIL, the lowest frequency in normals and an intermediate frequency in ASCUS would suggest that TBS criteria had been misapplied. In particular, liberal, non-specific use of the ASCUS category would result in a low rate of HPV DNA detection in these specimens, similar to that found in normals. Once established, the study set could be reused multiple times by different cytotechnologists and pathologists.

## Biological implications of HPV testing

This study and related work have other implications for TBS classification. Most importantly, these data indicate that nearly all SIL is related to HPV infection. Previous studies failing to detect a high rate of HPV infection in patients with a cytological diagnosis of SIL most likely reflect cytological misclassification or insensitive HPV testing. A second important conclusion of this work is that infection with cancer-associated HPV types accounts for the majority of *bona fide* SIL. Therefore, it is unlikely that testing for low-risk HPV types will contribute significantly to patient management. However, testing women with ASCUS cytology for the presence of cancer-associated HPV DNA may help identify women with equivocal smears who have an underlying SIL and require immediate colposcopy [8].

## Summary

Various measures have been suggested for quality assurance of cervical smears. Data suggest that correlating cytopathological diagnoses with the detection of cancer-associated HPV types yields useful information about diagnostic performance.

## Acknowledgements

George Washington University has had contractual arrangements with Cytyc Corp. and Digene Corp. Dr Lorincz is a paid employee with Digene.

## References

1  National Cancer Institute Workshop. The revised Bethesda system for reporting cervical/

vaginal cytologic diagnoses: report of the 1991 Bethesda workshop. *JAMA* 1991; **267**: 1892.

2 Clinical Laboratory Improvement Amendments of 1988: final rule. *Fed Reg* 1992; **57**: 7001–7186.

3 Kurman RJ, Henson DE, Herbst AL *et al*. Toward optimal laboratory use. Interim guidelines for management of abnormal cervical cytology. *JAMA* 1994; **271**: 1866–1869.

4 Sherman ME, Schiffman MH, Lorincz A *et al*. Toward objective quality assurance in cervical cytopathology. Correlation of cytopathologic diagnoses with detection of high-risk human papillomavirus types. *Am J Clin Pathol* 1994; **102**: 182–187.

5 Schiffman MH, Kiviat NB, Burk RD *et al*. Accuracy and reliability of human papillomavirus DNA testing by Hybrid Capture. *J Clin Microbiol* 1995; **33**: 545–550.

6 Schiffman MH, Bauer HM, Hoover RN *et al*. Epidemiologic evidence that human papillomavirus causes most cervical intraepithelial neoplasia. *J Natl Cancer Inst* 1993; **85**: 958–963.

7 Bosch FX. Manos MM, Munoz N *et al*. Prevalence of human papillomavirus in cervical cancer: a worldwide perspective. *J Natl Cancer Inst* 1995; **87**: 796–802.

8 Cox JT, Lorincz AT, Schiffman MH *et al*. Human papillomavirus testing by Hybrid Capture appears to be useful in triaging women with a cytologic diagnosis of atypical squamous cells of undetermined significance. *Am J Obstet Gynecol* 1995; **172**: 946–954.

# 42: Estimates of the Cost Impact of Introducing Human Papillomavirus Testing into a Cervical Screening Programme

J. Cuzick & P. Sasieni[1]

## Summary

Based on available data from the British cervical screening programme and studies on human papillomavirus (HPV) testing, cost estimates for introducing HPV testing into routine screening have been made. It is assumed that screening with cytology only requires a 3-year interval, but that if HPV testing were also added to cytology for women over the age of 30 the interval could be safely extended to 5 years. HPV testing is also assumed substantially to reduce the number of inadequate smears, from 7.9% to 1%. The increased detection rate associated with a stringent HPV test (with an assumed 4% positive rate in women with negative cytology) is balanced by the fewer number of women screened each year, leading to a similar number of colposcopies and only slightly more biopsies and treatments. However, the routine screening rate is reduced by 40%, leading to an estimated saving of £30 million/year from the current costs of the programme, which are estimated at around £130 million/year.

In this study we have made estimates of the cost impact on the British cervical screening programme of introducing HPV testing as part of routine screening in women over the age of 30 and simultaneously increasing the screening interval from 3 to 5 years. Some districts already operate a 5-year screening interval, but in many of these districts the majority of women are screened more frequently. For the purposes of this analysis, we therefore assume that these figures are appropriate to a 3-year interval and make comparisons of a pure 3-year interval with cytology only with a 5-year interval

*Correspondence*: Dr Jack Cuzick, Imperial Cancer Research Fund, PO Box 123, Lincoln's Inn Fields, London WC2A 3PX, UK.
[1]Imperial Cancer Research Fund, Lincoln's Inn Fields, London WC2A 3PX, UK.

using both cytology and HPV testing. Data are not available to make precise calculations, but the analysis presented below is based on the best available information and assumes HPV testing is performed in the most efficient possible manner.

## Cytology only

Table 42.1 shows the cytological diagnosis of screening smears taken in England from 1 April 1994 to 31 March 1995 [1], along with the estimated referral and treatment outcomes. The target population of eligible women aged 25–64 was 12 million and just over 4.5 million smears were taken, although some of these were for women outside this age band. Of these, 7.9% were inadequate and required repeating (corresponding to 8.6% of adequate smears). Just over 3.7 million women had an adequate smear and for the last adequate smear recorded in this period 94.4% were negative, 4.4% showed borderline on mild changes, 0.7% showed moderate dyskaryosis and 0.6% showed severe dyskaryosis or worse (Table 7; Department of Health [1]). Another report based on laboratory returns (Table 11; Department of Health [1]) indicated that 36.9% of all smears classified as mild or borderline were actually mild dyskaryosis. Thus, overall we estimate that 2.8% of all adequate screening smears are borderline and 1.6% are classified as mild dyskaryosis.

In order to estimate the follow-up resources associated with a mild or borderline smear, the subsequent history of 100 women with an initial

**Table 42.1** Current outcomes of screening with 3-yearly cytology only.

| | Routine smears (%) | Extra smears before colposcopy (factor) | Colposcopy (proportion of first column) | Biopsy (proportion of first column) | Treatment (proportion of first column) |
|---|---|---|---|---|---|
| Negative | 3 544 575 (94.4) | | | | |
| Borderline | 104 569 (2.8) | 198 681 (1.9) | 31 371 (0.3) | 20 914 (0.2) | 12 548 (0.12) |
| Mild | 61,137 (1.6) | 97 812 (1.6) | 30 568 (0.5) | 24 454 (0.4) | 18 341 (0.3) |
| Moderate | 25 005 (0.7) | | 25 005 (1.0) | 22 504 (0.9) | 12 502 (0.5) |
| Severe (positive) | 20 842 (0.6) | | 20 842 (1.0) | 20 842 (1.0) | 16 674 (0.8) |
| | | | | | |
| *Total* | | | | | |
| Adequate | 3 756 128 (100) | | | | |
| Inadequate | (8.6) | 322 187 | | | |
| | | | | | |
| Total | 3 756 128* (100) | 618 680 | 107 786 | 88 714 | 60 065 |

* A total of 4.5 million smears were taken in 1994–1995, corresponding well to this number of routine smears: about 600 000 pre-colposcopy smears and 200 000 post-colposcopy smears.

borderline result and 100 women with an initial mild result was examined at Southend District Hospital by Dr E.F. Fowler. For borderline changes 30% of these women had colposcopy within the next 5 years preceded by an average of 1.6 smears. If we assume that the women not receiving colposcopy would have received an average of two smears before being discharged, this group would on average have required 1.9 extra smears per woman. On colposcopy, 12 women were found to have cervical intraepithelial neoplasia (CIN) II–III, yielding a 12% overall treatment rate. We assume that women with borderline smears (two-thirds of those attending for colposcopy) received a biopsy at some stage; the remaining 10% had no visible lesion at colposcopy.

Similarly, 51% of women with mild dyskaryosis proceeded to colposcopy and 30% were found to have CIN II–III. Sixty-four extra smears were taken before referral to colposcopy, and if we again assume two additional smears before return to routine screening in the 49 women not progressing to colposcopy, this gives 1.6 extra smears per woman with mild dyskaryosis. Again, we assume 10% of women with mild dyskaryosis had no visible lesion on colposcopy and the rest (40%) were biopsied at colposcopy.

In accordance with national guidelines [2], we assume that all women with moderate or severe dyskaryosis received immediate colposcopy. We also assume the biopsy rates were 90% and 100% respectively and that treatment for CIN II–III or worse is required in 50% and 80% respectively. These figures are consistent with those found in the literature [3–5].

In summary, just over 3.7 million women received an adequate smear in 1994–1995. Although some health authorities were operating a 5-year recall service, most used a 3-year interval and for the sake of definiteness, we assume these figures relate to a 3-yearly screening policy. Several studies have shown that the protection afforded by cytological screening begins to wane after 3 years [6,7]. The data do not provide enough details to separate routine screening smears from repeats, but probably about 5% of these women received repeat smears from abnormalities found in previous years. Nevertheless, all the smears may give rise to further investigations and we estimate that an additional 618 680 smears would be needed to repeat inadequate smears and follow-up patients with borderline/mild changes. We also estimate that a total of 107 786 colposcopies would result from the abnormalities found, leading to 88 714 biopsies and 60 065 treated cases of CIN II–III.

## Cytology plus HPV testing

Table 42.2 shows a projected outcome of a policy of 5-yearly screening using both cytology and HPV testing for women aged 30 or more. Women aged less than 30 would receive two screens by cytology alone, nominally at ages 23 and 26, followed by a screen using HPV and cytology at age 30 and 5-yearly

**Table 42.2** Project outcomes of screening with 5-yearly cytology and human papillomavirus (HPV) testing in women over age 30.

| | Routine smears (%) | Extra smears (factor) | Colposcopy (proportion of first column) | Biopsy (proportion of first column) | Treatment (proportion of first column) |
|---|---|---|---|---|---|
| Negative | 2 055 150 (91.2) | | | | |
| HPV only (age > 30) | 66 600 (3.1) | 66 600 (1) | 44 356 (0.67) | 40 000 (0.6) | 26 640 (0.4) |
| Borderline HPV-negative | 50 400 (2.2) | 49 500 (1) | 5040 (0.1) | 4000 (0.08) | 2016 (0.04) |
| Borderline HPV-positive | 12 600 (0.6) | | 12 600 (1) | 10 000 (0.79) | 5670 (0.45) |
| Mild HPV-negative | 19 800 (0.9) | 19 800 (1) | 3960 (0.2) | 3500 (0.18) | 2772 (0.14) |
| Mild HPV-positive | 16 200 (0.7) | | 16 200 (1) | 12 000 (0.74) | 8100 (0.5) |
| Moderate | 15 750 (0.7) | | 15 750 (1) | 14 175 (0.9) | 7875 (0.5) |
| Severe | 13 500 (0.6) | | 13 500 (1) | 13 500 (1) | 10 800 (0.8) |
| *Total* | | | | | |
| Adequate | 2 250 000* (100) | | | | |
| Inadequate | | 22 500 (0.01) | | | |
| Total | 2 250 000 (100) | 158 400 | 111 406 | 97 175 | 63 873 |

* Based on 60% of the 3 756 128 routine smears in the current programme.

thereafter until age 65. The use of HPV testing may also allow screening to be stopped early or conducted even less frequently in older women (e.g. one test at 50 and one at 60 if no previous abnormalities), but this is not considered here. It is difficult to make steady-state predictions about the abnormality rates for many reasons, so these estimates are somewhat hypothetical. High initial detection rates have been well-documented [5,8], but it is difficult to quantify the extent to which this will lead to lower detection rates on subsequent screening rounds. Follow-up studies employing HPV testing as part of the referral policy will be needed to examine this.

The biggest savings arise from increasing the screening interval from 3 to 5 years, resulting in 40% fewer screening smears. Samples are rarely inadequate for HPV testing (we assume 1%) and if smears inadequate for cytology (about 8%) but adequate for HPV are assumed to be adequate for screening, further savings can be made.

Positivity rates are assay-dependent and several different management strategies are possible. The expected outcome is outlined in Fig. 42.1 for women with negative smears and in Fig. 42.2 for those with mild or borderline smears. We have only considered additional follow-up for cytology-negative

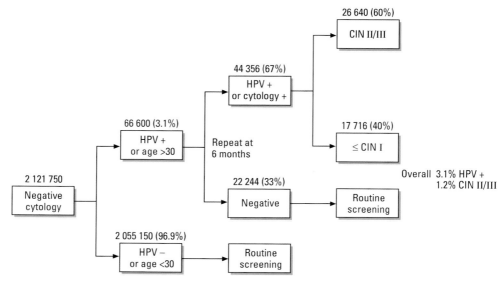

**Fig. 42.1** Anticipated disease states (negative cytology). HPV, human papillomavirus; CIN, cervical intraepithelial neoplasia.

but HPV-positive women if they are aged over 30 years. We have also assumed a stringent criterion for positivity, as in Cuzick *et al*. [5], in which only types 16, 18, 31, 33 are screened for and a high level of virus in the smear is required. Based on the result of that study, approximately 4% of women aged > 30 will be positive for HPV and negative on cytology. This corresponds to 3.1% of all screened women. We propose to manage them, by a repeat test at 6 months and referral of all women who are still positive or who develop any cytological abnormality (assumed to be 67%). The remaining one-third who are negative on cytology and HPV testing are returned to routine 5-yearly screening.

We assume that the *rate* of borderline, mild, moderate and severe smears will be as before. This is a compromise to allow for high rates due to a longer interval and lower rates due to disease previously screened out by HPV-positive, cytology-negative cases. Based on our previous work [5], it is estimated that 20% of borderline smears will be HPV-positive. These women will all be referred for colposcopy and 45% will be found to have CIN II–III. The remaining HPV-negative women (80%) will have a follow-up smear and HPV test at 1 year. It is assumed that 10% will be positive for one of these tests. They will be referred to colposcopy and 4% (40% of 10%) will be CIN II–III. The remaining negative women will be returned to routine screening (Fig. 42.2).

For women with mild smears, it is assumed that 40% will be HPV-positive, and they will be referred immediately for colposcopy, at which time 50% will be found to have CIN II–III. The remaining HPV-negative women will have a

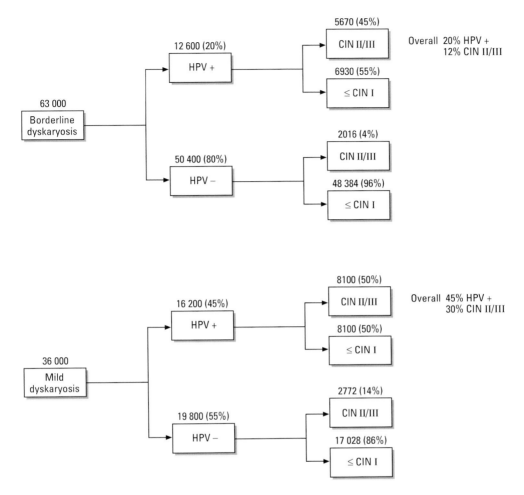

**Fig. 42.2** Anticipated disease states (mild/borderline cytology). HPV, human papillomavirus; CIN, cervical intraepithelial neoplasia.

repeat smear for cytology and HPV at 6 months. It is assumed that 20% will be positive and will be referred for colposcopy and 14% will be found to have CIN II–III. All women with moderate or severe dyskaryosis or worse will be referred for colposcopy regardless of HPV status and their yield of disease will be as before (Fig. 42.2).

## Costs

Based on estimates computed by Havelock [9] we assume that the cost of taking a smear is £15, and the cost of staining and reading it is £10; a colposcopy costs £50 and the histology for a biopsy is £30 and that for a loop excision is £50. We assume that referral for colposcopy on average will result in two colposcopies and two extra follow-up smears for a total cost of £150 plus histology costs. Based on current experience, the cost of an HPV assay is taken as £10, although this may decrease with a larger volume of use. Based on these estimates and the calculations summarized in Tables 42.1 and 42.2, the annual costs of the two strategies are estimated in Table 42.3 for the English programme. Based on these estimates the English programme is estimated to cost £131 million. Substantial savings are potentially available by introducing HPV testing, and extending the screening interval to 5 years. The main savings are due to the lengthening of the screening interval, which more than compensates for the extra cost of the test but savings are also made from a reduced number of follow-up and inadequate smears. Only small increases in the cost of colposcopy and histology are incurred, but these figures depend on the steady-state abnormality rate for routine smears and this is difficult to estimate accurately at the moment.

These estimates suggest an overall potential saving of £30 million if HPV testing were introduced and a 5-year screening interval was adhered to. This does not include the savings in cost and inconvenience to the women associated with less frequent screening.

**Table 42.3** Estimated costs of different aspects of two screening strategies based on the current performance of the English programme and recent human papillomavirus (HPV) testing studies.

| Activity | Cost (£ thousands) based on the English programme | | |
| --- | --- | --- | --- |
| | 3-yearly cytology | 5-yearly cytology and HPV testing | Difference |
| Routine screening @ £25/ smear or £35/smear with HPV testing | 93 903 | 72 750* | −21 153 |
| Extra smears due to inadequate smear or follow-up @ £25/ smear or £35 with HPV testing | 15 467 | 5419 | −10 048 |
| Colposcopy and all follow-up costs @ £150/referral | 16 168 | 16 711 | 543 |
| Biopsy @ £30 | 2661 | 2915 | 254 |
| Treatment @ £50 plus CIN | 3003 | 3194 | 191 |
| Total | 131 202 | 100 989 | −30,213 |

* HPV testing only for age 30 or over (1 650 000 smears).
CIN, Cervical intraepithelial neoplasia.

## Cancer incidence rates

The most recent available figures for the UK suggest that there are about 3500 cases of cervix cancer in women under the age of 70 and 1100 cases in older women. Sasieni *et al.* [7] estimated that without any screening the rate in women under 70 would be about 75% higher, so that there would have been 6100 cases in this age group if screening was not implemented. It was also estimated that 1250 further cases could be prevented if full coverage and adherence to follow-up protocols were achieved. Thus, about 2300 cases would still occur in women aged less than 70. Based on the increased detection rates associated with HPV screening, it is reasonable to estimate that 40% or 900 of these cases of cancer might be avoided if HPV testing were introduced.

## Conclusion

It can be seen from the analysis that the introduction of HPV testing into screening offers the prospect of greatly reduced costs, due to the use of a longer screening interval, yet many still pick up more disease and reduce invasive cancer rates by detecting lesions which are silent on cytology, usually because of the difficulty of complete sampling of the transformation zone in screening smears. This is consistent with the fact that HPV is part of the causative sequence in almost all cervix cancers, but the latency is long, indicating that sensitive but infrequent screening would be efficient. However, to maintain specificity and cost-effectiveness, HPV testing must be carefully quality-controlled and referral in cytology-negative patients should be limited to persistent high-level lesions associated with the most predictive high-risk types (currently HPV 16, 18, 31 and 33).

## References

1 Department of Health. Cervical Screening Programme, England: 1994–1995. *Statistical Bulletin* 1996; **3**.
2 Duncan ID (ed) *Guidelines for Clinical Practice and Programme Management*. Oxford: National Coordinating Network, NHS Cervical Screening Programme, 1992.
3 Flannelly G, Anderson D, Kitchener HC *et al.* Management of women with mild and moderate cervical dyskaryosis. *BMJ* 1994; **308**: 1399–1403.
4 Cuzick J, Terry G, Ho L, Hollingworth T, Anderson M. Type-specific human papillomavirus DNA in abnormal smears as a predictor of high-grade cervical intraepithelial neoplasia. *Br J Cancer* 1994; **69**: 167–171.
5 Cuzick J, Szarewski A, Terry G *et al.* Human papillomavirus testing in primary cervical screening. *Lancet* 1995; **345**: 1533–1537.
6 IARC working group on the evaluation of cervical cancer screening programmes. Screening for squamous cervical cancer: duration of low risk after negative results of cervical cytology and its implication for screening policies. *BMJ* 1986; **293**: 659–664.

7 Sasieni PD, Cuzick J, Lynch-Farmery E and the NCN working group. Estimating the efficacy of screening by auditing smear histories of women with and without cervical cancer. *Br J Cancer* 1996; **73**: 1001–1005.

8 Reid R, Greenberg MD, Lorincz A *et al*. Should cervical cytologic testing be augmented by cervicography or human papillomavirus deoxyribonucleic acid detection? *Am J Obstet Gynecol* 1991; **164**: 1461–1471.

9 Havelock C. *The Cost of the Cervical Screening Programme – An Activity-based Approach. NCN Report on Costings*. Oxford: National Coordinating Network, NHS Cervical Screening Programme, 1994.

# 43: Viral Load as a Surrogate for Persistence in Cervical Human Papillomavirus Infection

## J. Cuzick

## Summary

Most cervix cancer is thought to arise from human papillomavirus (HPV) infection. However, most infections are transient and the development of a persistent HPV infection is a key step in cervical carcinogenesis. Persistence can only be measured by repeated screening and the extent to which high levels of high-risk types of HPV can predict persistence is examined. Viral load was a particularly good predictor of persistence and disease for HPV 16. Good correlations were also found for types 18, 31 and 33 but they were not as strong as for type 16. The correlation may be much weaker for other types.

## Introduction

Transient HPV infections are very unlikely to lead to integration of viral DNA into the human genome or to other DNA damage. Thus, persistence of the virus is crucial if it is to have a carcinogenic effect and several studies have documented the importance of persistence in the progression of cervical lesions [1–4]. This is also a key step in hepatitis B-induced liver cancer and in that case antibodies to the viral surface antigen provide a reliable marker for persistence. No such marker exists for HPV and the only way to be certain about persistence is to test for the virus on several occasions. This is clearly undesirable from a screening point of view and similar requirements related to low-grade cytological changes have caused great anxiety and expense in their management. As yet poorly understood cellular changes seem to be associated with persistence [5] and one of these is permissive replication of the virus

*Correspondence*: Dr Jack Cuzick, Imperial Cancer Research Fund, PO Box 123, Lincoln's Inn Fields, London WC2A 3PX, UK.

leading to relatively high levels of virus in infected cells. Typically this corresponds to about $10^5$ copies in a smear, which is about 0.1 copies per cell in the smear and probably about 1–10 copies per infected cell.

Most of the evidence linking 'high-level' infection to persistence is indirect and is based on the progression sequence shown in Fig. 43.1. Most HPV infections are transient, but occasionally the virus escapes immune surveillance and a persistent infection ensues. The factors related to persistence are not well understood but have been linked to human leukocyte antigen (HLA) type [6], smoking [7], other venereal infections [8] and sequence variants of HPV [4]. Once the virus becomes persistent, there is a much greater chance that it can disrupt the non-cellular regulation functions, either by integration into a suitable location or by direct actions of the E6 and E7 proteins. Once cellular control mechanisms have been damaged, uncontrolled proliferation can take place, leading to high-grade cervical intraepithelial neoplasia (CIN) and invasive cancer. Other cocarcinogens are probably required, but to date none have been clearly identified, although smoking has been suggested by a multitude of studies.

Thus the demonstration that 'high-level' infection is associated with high-grade CIN implies that it is also associated with persistence. Several studies offer evidence for this.

Based on a technique developed by Terry *et al.* [9], Cuzick *et al.* [10,11] showed that in women with cytological abnormalities, HPV positivity at a high level (especially type 16) was strongly related to high-grade CIN (Table 43.1). In contrast, low-level positivity had very little predictive value for CIN II–III (Table 43.1), occurring in similar percentages of women with high-grade lesions as was found in this group overall. The results for HPV 16 were particularly striking: 93% (39/42) of women with high-level infection had CIN II–III compared to 46% (7/16) of women with low-level infection and 36% (27/75) who were negative for HPV 16. Bavin *et al.* [12] also reported high predictive values for HPV 16 in women with mild dyskaryosis on cytology.

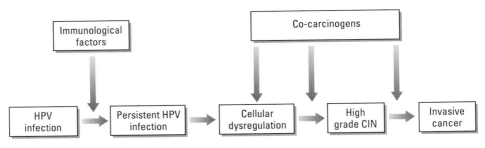

Fig. 43.1 Schematic diagram of the steps in HPV-induced cervix cancer.

**Table 43.1** Number of patients with high and low levels of specific human papillomavirus (HPV) types by histological diagnosis.

| Histology | No. of patients | HPV positivity and level | | | | | | | | | |
| | | HPV 16 | | HPV 18 | | HPV 31 | | HPV 33 | | HPV 35 | |
| | | Low | High | Low | High | Low | High | Low | High | Low | High |
|---|---|---|---|---|---|---|---|---|---|---|---|
| CIN III | 61 | 5 (1) | 36 (10) | 8 (6) | 4 (2) | 5 (3) | 14 (5) | 1 (0) | 7 (5) | 0 | 2 (0) |
| CIN II | 12 | 2 (1) | 3 (2) | 1 (0) | 2 (1) | 0 | 0 | 0 | 4 (1) | 0 | 0 |
| CIN I | 13 | 3 (1) | 0 | 3 (2) | 0 | 1 (0) | 3 (0) | 2 (0) | 1 (0) | 1 (0) | 0 |
| HPV infection or HPV 1 | 11 | 2 (0) | 1 (1) | 0 | 0 | 0 | 2 (1) | 0 | 2 (2) | 0 | 0 |
| Normal | 36 | 4 (1) | 2* (1) | 3 (1) | 3 (1) | 0 | 1 (0) | 1 (0) | 2 (0) | 0 | 2 (2) |
| Total | 133 | 16 (4) | 42 (14) | 15 (9) | 9 (4) | 6 (3) | 20 (6) | 4 (0) | 16 (8) | 1 (0) | 4 (2) |

Numbers in parentheses indicate number with multiple infections, where the other type(s) were 'high-level'. Multiple infections are included for each positive type and thus are represented at least twice in the table.

*One case was pregnant.

CIN, Cervical intraepithelial neoplasia.

From Cuzick et al. [11] with permission.

**Table 43.2** Positive predictive value for CIN II–III of human papillomavirus (HPV) testing for high-risk types using different cut-off levels using Hybrid Capture in a population of women with atypical squamous cells of undetermined significance (ASCUS) smears.

| Level (relative light units; RLU) | Negative | 1–5 | 5–20 | > 20 |
|---|---|---|---|---|
| Positivity for CIN II–III (%) | 1/136 (1) | 0/22 (0) | 2/22 (9) | 12/37 (32) |

From Cox *et al.* [13].

**Table 43.3** Positive predictive value for cervical intraepithelial neoplasia (CIN) II–III of semiquantitative human papillomavirus (HPV) testing and cytology among 1985 evaluable women undergoing routine screening: a total of 81 women were found to have CIN II–III.

| | HPV testing | | Cytology | |
|---|---|---|---|---|
| Type | True positive/test high-level positive (%) | Grade | | True positive/test positive (%) |
| HPV 16 | 36/66 (55%) | Severe | | 17/18 (94%) |
| HPV 18 | 8/24 (33%) | Moderate | | 10/23 (43%) |
| HPV 31 | 20/46 (43%) | Mild | | 10/29 (34%) |
| HPV 33 | 7/22 (32%) | Borderline | | 8/58 (14%) |
| HPV 16 or 31 | 55/111 (50%) | Moderate or severe | | 27/41 (66%) |
| HPV 16, 18, 31 or 33 | 61/146 (42%) | Any dyskaryosis | | 45/128 (35%) |

From Cuzick *et al.* [14] with permission.

**Table 43.4** Relationship of persistence to type of human papillomavirus (HPV) and underlying disease state.

| | HPV 16 | | | HPV 18 | | | HPV 31 | | |
|---|---|---|---|---|---|---|---|---|---|
| Diagnosis | Transient | Persistent | Weakly persistent | Transient | Persistent | Weakly persistent | Transient | Persistent | Weakly persist |
| <CIN I | 5 | 8 | | 2 | 5 | 1 | 6 | 3 | 1 |
| CIN I | | 7 | | 1 | 2 | 2 | 3 | 2 | 0 |
| CIN II | 1 | 14 (1,3) | | | 1 | 0 | 2 | 11 (10,1) | 0 |
| CIN III + | | 20 (1,0) | 1 | | 2 (1,0) | 1 | 2 | 5 | 1 |
| Total | 6 | 49 (2,3) | 1 | 3 | 10 (1,0) | 4 | 13 | 21 | 2 |

Numbers in parentheses denote number of cases with multiple types, and number of cases where disease was found only at subsequent follow-up.
CIN, cervical intraepithelial neoplasia.

Cox *et al.* [13] using the Hybrid Capture system in a group of women with borderline (atypical squamous cells of undetermined significance or ASCUS) smears also found level to be an important predictor of high-grade CIN (Table 43.2). They found that levels above 20 relative light units (RLU) gave a positive predictive value (PPV) for CIN II–III of 30%, levels between 5–20 RLU gave a PPV of 9%, whereas lower values had no predictive value. However even the 1 RLU cut-off is higher than we have used for PCR.

In the first screening study of women attending for routine screening smears, Cuzick *et al.* [14] also found high-level infections from four high-risk types to be predictive of high-grade CIN (Table 43.3). Over 40% of the cases of CIN II–III were negative on cytology and another 10% only had borderline changes. Thus high levels of selected high-risk types are predictive of high-grade CIN even in the absence of cytological abnormalities. Further analysis indicates that most of these infections were persistent, at least over the short term.

To examine the relationship of level to persistence further, the findings of a repeat HPV test taken at colposcopy, usually 2–4 months after the referral test, are shown in Table 43.4. Infections were classified as transient if the next test was negative, weakly persistent if low levels were found or persistent if high levels were again found. A few cases were subsequently found to have a high level of a different type but not the original type. These were classified as persistent-mixed types. Two individuals with two persistent types were included twice.

It can be seen that most high-level infections were persistent. This was most clearly true for HPV 16 where 49 of 56 (88%) high-level infections were persistent and another case was weakly persistent. Persistence was more

**ble 43.3** (*Contd.*)

| | HPV 33 | | Negative or low level followed by | | | | | | Persistent-mixed type |
| nsient | Persistent | Weakly persistent | Negative or no follow-up | 16 | 18 | 31 | 33 | Multi | |
|---|---|---|---|---|---|---|---|---|---|
| | 5 | | 37 | 1 | | 1 | | | 1 |
| | 4 | | 18 | 1 | 2 | 1 | | | 3 |
| | 4 (1,0) | | 10 | 0 | | | | | |
| 1) | 1 | | 9 | 1 | | | | | 1 |
| 1) | 14 (1,0) | 0 | 74 | 3 | 2 | 2 | | | 5 |

associated with high-grade CIN II–III for HPV 16 than for other types. Thirty-four of 49 (69%) persistent HPV 16 lesions showed CIN II–III, compared to only 1 of 6 transient lesions. Qualitatively similar results were seen for the other types, but the results were not so strong quantitatively: 59% of high-level HPV 18 lesions were persistent and another 24% were weakly persistent. Of high-level HPV 31 lesions 58% were persistent and 78% of high-level HPV 33 lesions were persistent. Persistent HPV 33 lesions showed a weaker relationship to CIN II–III than the other types.

## References

1 Hildesheim A, Schiffman MH, Gravitt PE *et al.* Persistence of type-specific human papillomavirus infection among cytologically normal women. *J Infect Dis* 1994; **169**: 235–240.

2 Remmink AJ, Walboomers JMM, Helmerhorst TJM *et al.* The presence of persistent high-risk HPV genotypes in dysplastic cervical lesions is associated with progressive disease: natural history up to 36 months. *Int J Cancer* 1995; **61**: 306–311.

3 Ho GYE, Burk RD, Klein S *et al.* Persistent genital human papillomavirus infection as a risk for persistent cervical dysplasia. *J Natl Cancer Inst* 1995; **87**: 1365–1371.

4 Londesborough P, Ho L, Terry G *et al.* Human papillomavirus (HPV) genotype as a predictor of persistence and development of high grade lesions in women with minor cervical abnormalities. *Int J Cancer* 1996; **69**: 364–368.

5 zur Hausen H. Disrupted dichotomous intracellular control of human papillomavirus infection in cancer of the cervix. *Lancet* 1994; **343**: 955–957.

6 Odunsi K, Terry G, Ho L *et al.* Association between HLA DQB1*03 and cervical intra-epithelial neoplasia. *Mol Med* 1995; **1**: 161–171.

7 Barton SE, Jenkins D, Cuzick J *et al.* Effect of cigarette smoking on cervical epithelial immunity: a mechanism for neoplastic change? *Lancet* 1988; **ii**: 652–654.

8 Lacey CJN. Assessment of exposure to sexually transmitted agents other than human papillomavirus. In: Munox N, Bosch FX, Shah KV, Meheus A (eds) *The Epidemiology of Cervical Cancer and Human Papillomavirus*. Lyon: IARC, 1992, pp 93–105.

9 Terry G, Ho L, Jenkins D *et al.* Definition of human papillomavirus type 16 DNA levels in low and high grade cervical lesions by a simple polymerase chain reaction technique. *Arch Virol* 1993; **128**: 123–133.

10 Cuzick J, Terry G, Ho L, Hollingworth T, Anderson M. Human papillomavirus type 16 DNA in cervical smears as predictor of high-grade cervical intraepithelial neoplasia. *Lancet* 1992; **339**: 959–960.

11 Cuzick J, Terry G, Ho L, Hollingworth T, Anderson M. Type-specific human papillomavirus DNA in abnormal smears as a predictor of high-grade cervical intraepithelial neoplasia. *Br J Cancer* 1994; **69**: 167–171.

12 Bavin PJ, Giles JA, Deery A *et al.* Use of semi-quantitative PCR for human papillomavirus DNA type 16 to identify women with high grade cervical disease in a population presenting with a mildly dyskaryotic smear report. *Br J Cancer* 1993; **67**: 602–605.

13 Cox JT, Lorincz AT, Schiffman MH *et al.* Human papillomavirus testing by hybrid capture appears to be useful in triaging women with a cytologic diagnosis of atypical squamous cells of undetermined significance. *Am J Obstet Gynecol* 1995; **172**: 946–954.

14 Cuzick J, Szarewski A, Terry G *et al.* Human papillomavirus testing in primary cervical screening. *Lancet* 1995; **345**: 1533–1537.

# 44: Molecular Variant Analysis as a Tool in Natural History Studies of Human Papillomavirus Infection and Cervical Neoplasia

L. L. Villa,[1] P. Rahal[1] & E. L. Franco[2]

## Summary

Recent evidence from epidemiological studies has indicated that when a woman is persistently infected with oncogenic types of human papillomavirus (HPV), she is more likely to develop cervical neoplastic lesions than when she is only transiently infected with HPV. In consequence, a number of cohort studies have begun in different populations examining the predictive value of persistence of HPV infection with respect to the subsequent occurrence of cervical neoplasia. Persistence can be defined as the repeated detection of the same HPV type on subsequent cervical specimens. But how would one interpret cases with concordance of types during follow-up, particularly for HPV 16, the most common genital type? Could they represent consecutive transient infections with HPV 16? The solution is to augment the typing data with additional taxonomic detail using DNA sequencing techniques to detect molecular variants of HPV. These variants are identified on the basis of mutational patterns in the DNA, thus allowing interpretation of persistence on firmer grounds.

We are currently conducting a cohort study of persistent cervical HPV infection in a high-risk area in Brazil using sequencing of the long control region of the viral genome to probe for molecular variants. On the basis of the first 453 specimens analysed, five distinct variants of HPV 16 and one of HPV 18 have been associated with persistent infections with these oncogenic types.

*Correspondence*: Professor E.L. Franco, Department of Oncology, McGill University, 546 Pine Avenue West, Montreal, QC, Canada H2W 1S6.
[1]Virology Unit, Ludwig Institute for Cancer Research, São Paulo, Brazil; [2]Division of Epidemiology, Department of Oncology, McGill University, Montreal, Canada.

## Introduction

Cervical HPV infection detected by polymerase chain reaction (PCR) techniques is found in 5–50% of asymptomatic women of reproductive age presenting for Papanicolaou (Pap) smear screening in different countries [1]. When additional cervical specimens are taken from these women in follow-up surveys the majority of the infections are found to be transient, and only a small proportion of the women tend to harbour the same HPV type in specimens collected during subsequent visits [2–4]. Prospective epidemiological studies have indicated that the risk of subsequent cervical neoplasia seems to be proportional to the number of specimens testing positive for HPV [5]. More recently, Ho *et al.* [6] have shown that HPV infection detected in previous visits and persisting during follow-up was highly predictive of a woman's short-term risk for developing squamous intraepithelial lesions. Taken together, these findings suggest that only persistent infections of the cervical epithelium may be the ones eventually triggering development of lesions.

In theory, the difference between persistent infection and periodic reacquisition of transient infections from the same sexual partners cannot be satisfactorily established without resorting to detailed follow-up studies of transmission between the woman and her partners. Practically speaking, however, the difference may be more of scientific interest than of public health value since, regardless of the origin of the infection, the risk for development of lesions is elevated in persistent cases.

Another difficulty is the level of detail in defining persistence. Viral typing provides a first screen of multiple specimens from the same woman, thus indicating which cases can be safely ruled out as being transient infections because different HPV types were found in consecutive specimens. But how would one interpret cases with concordance of types during follow-up? For instance, would two HPV 16 (the most common genital type)-positive specimens taken a few months apart from the same woman indicate persistent infection or could they represent two consecutive transient infections with HPV 16?

The solution is to augment the typing data with additional taxonomic detail. We [7] and others [8] have recently proposed a solution to this problem by demonstrating the applicability of DNA sequencing techniques to detect molecular variants of the HPV in epidemiological studies of the natural history of cervical neoplasia. These variants are identified on the basis of mutational patterns in the DNA, thus allowing interpretation of persistence on firmer grounds.

## Brazilian cohort study of persistent HPV infection and CIN

In 1993 we began an epidemiological study (Ludwig–McGill cohort) of the natural history of HPV infection and cervical neoplasia in a population of low-income women in São Paulo, Brazil, one of the highest-risk areas world-wide for cervical cancer. This study is testing the hypothesis that persistent infections with oncogenic HPV types are more likely to be the true precursor events leading to cervical carcinogenesis. Persistence of HPV infection is being assessed by molecular variant analysis [7] and measurement of viral burden by quantitative PCR [9], which provides a much finer level of detail than simple HPV testing.

The study will accrue 3000 female subjects through January 1997. Subjects are being followed up over a 5-year period in scheduled returns every 4 months, in the first year, and once yearly thereafter, for a total of eight visits as follows: initial, 4, 8, 12, 24, 36, 48 and 60 months. In each of these visits, subjects are submitted to a questionnaire-based interview, have a cervical specimen taken for Pap cytology and HPV testing, and a blood sample drawn for serological testing for HPV antibodies. A cervicography is performed once in the first year and at 24 and 48 months.

Specimens are tested for the presence of HPV DNA by the L1 PCR protocol with consensus primers MY09/11 [4,10]. Typing of the amplified products is performed by hybridization with individual oligonucleotide probes specific for all 27 HPV genital types whose nucleotide sequences for probes within the MY09/11 fragment have been published in the literature. Twenty-three of these have received a taxonomic entry as HPV types: 6/11, 16, 18, 26, 31, 33, 35, 39, 40, 42, 45, 51–59, 66, 68 and 73; whereas three additional genital types still await taxonomic classification: PAP155, PAP291, and W13B [4].

Amplified products that hybridize with the generic probe but with none of the type-specific probes are considered positive for HPV of unknown types. As a quality control verification of the specificity of the hybridizations, the PCR amplification products are further tested by restriction fragment length poly-morphism (RFLP) analysis of the L1 fragment [11] to confirm the results from the dot blot hybridization and to distinguish among unknown HPVs. Use of the RFLP analysis extends the range of identifiable HPV types in our study to more than 30 genital types, e.g. by allowing detection of HPVs 61, 70, 72, CP8304 and CP8061.

## Molecular variant analysis

For the analysis of persistence, whenever the same HPV type is detected in two or more specimens from the same woman we analyse the isolates to character-ize molecular variants. For HPVs 16 and 18, we use a PCR sequencing method with primers flanking a 364 bp segment (nucleotide positions 7478–7841 for HPV 16; 7585–7805 for HPV 18) within the long control region (LCR), a hypervariable genomic segment of HPV [12,13]. The amplified products are cloned using the SureClone plasmid cloning kit (Pharmacia Biotech) according to the manufacturer's instructions and introduced into *Escherichia coli* XL1-Blue. Recombinant plasmid DNAs are isolated from positive clones and submitted to DNA sequencing by the dideoxy method. Due to possible misincorporation of bases by the Taq polymerase and the possibility of multiple coexisting variants, a minimum of five clones are sequenced for each isolate (see rationale below). For types other than HPVs 16 or 18 the same procedure will be used to sequence nucleotides in the L1 segment amplified by primers MY09/11.

## Results and discussion

We have thus far completed HPV typing and molecular variant analyses for HPVs 16 and 18 in specimens from the first three or four visits for the initial 453 participants. Only a third of the subjects in whom HPV infection had been detected at least once were cases of persistent infection on the basis of the same viral type being found in multiple specimens. The LCR sequence analyses completed so far indicate that the same molecular variants were present in all isolates, bolstering the interpretation of persistence. We have found five different molecular variants of HPV 16 in those showing presumably persistent HPV 16 infection (Table 44.1). These were variants S21A, B2, B12 the HPV 16 prototype variant and a new, as yet undescribed variant. Similarly, for HPV 18 all isolates tested thus far from cases of presumably persistent

**Table 44.1** Ludwig–McGill cohort study: human papillomavirus (HPV) 16 variants in cases of presumably persistent HPV 16 infections.

| | HPV 16 variants found in each visit | | | |
| Case ID | First visit (admission) | Second visit (4th month) | Third visit (8th month) | Fourth visit (12th month) |
| --- | --- | --- | --- | --- |
| 132 | Prototype | Prototype | Other type | HPV-negative |
| 202 | Prototype | Prototype, CP8061 | CP8061 | NT |
| 340 | S-21A | S-21A | S-21A | HPV-negative |
| 372 | B2 | B2 | B2 | NT |
| 393 | Other type | B12 | B12 | NT |
| 453 | B2 | B2 | B2 | B2 |
| 491 | HPV-negative | New variant | New variant | New variant |
| 652 | Prototype | Prototype | Prototype | Prototype |
| 793 | NT | B12 | B12 | HPV-negative |
| 819 | Prototype | Prototype | Prototype | Prototype |
| 845 | B2 | B2 | NT | HPV-negative |
| 969 | Prototype | Prototype | NT | NT |
| 1277 | Prototype | Prototype | NT | NT |

NT, Not tested.

infection had the same variant (Table 44.2). Two HPV 18 variants have been found so far in these persistent cases, B18-2 and B18-6. These data indicate that there is appreciable diversity of variants within the two main HPV types in this population, at least in the cases with persistent HPV detection.

A criticism about molecular variants is the concern that mutational patterns may not reflect infections by distinct variants but, rather, they may represent recent mutations contributing to augment falsely the taxonomic variability [14]. Such concern is not justified in the case of HPVs. Mutation rates for DNA viruses are much lower than those for RNA viruses and in-depth studies of the molecular genetics of HPVs have indicated that variants have coevolved with human races over several millennia [15]. It has been suggested that fixation of single-point mutations in the HPV genome have occurred every $10^4$ to $10^5$ years [16,17].

A concern with PCR-based sequencing methods is the possibility of having errors introduced by the DNA polymerase. In general, however, the rate at which point mutations are introduced by PCR is much lower than that of naturally occurring mutations in HPV and they would be expected to occur randomly. Such errors are easily detected by replicate testing. The molecular variants of HPV detected by the LCR sequencing technique are defined on the basis of mutations in about 50 fixed, non-random nucleotide positions [16].

A woman could harbour more than one variant of the same HPV type. Polyclonality of HPV 16 lesions is not uncommon, at least in carcinomas [14,16]. Multiple concurrent HPV 16 infections by different variants can be detected sequencing a sufficiently large number of bacterial colonies expressing the cloned plasmids containing the HPV inserts. An important assumption in this regard is that the relative proportions of the different variants remain unaltered after amplification. The confidence that one would have in detecting a variant present in a polyclonal isolate is also a function of the relative proportion represented by that variant in the mixture. After consecutively

Table 44.2 Ludwig–McGill cohort study: human papillomavirus (HPV) 18 variants in cases of presumably persistent HPV 18 infections.

| Case ID | HPV 18 variants found in each visit | | | |
| | First visit (admission) | Second visit (4th month) | Third visit (8th month) | Fourth visit (12th month) |
| --- | --- | --- | --- | --- |
| 314 | B18-2 | B18-2 | NT | NT |
| 452 | B18-2 | B18-2 | NT | NT |
| 510 | HPV-negative | B18-2 | B18-2 | NT |
| 658 | HPV-negative | HPV-negative | B18-2 | B18-2 |
| 779 | HPV-negative | HPV-negative | B18-6 | B18-6 |
| 793 | B18-2 | B18-2 | B18-2 | HPV-negative |

NT, Not tested.

testing a given number of clones and failing to identify a discrepant variant, one could say with a fixed level of statistical confidence that a sample would be unlikely to contain another or additional variants representing more than a given proportion of all HPV copies of that type in the specimen. For instance, by sampling five clones and finding that they all contained exactly the same sequence, we will have 83% confidence that a variant representing not less than 30% of the HPV 16 copies would be detected in the specimen, i.e. $1 - (1 - 0.3)^5$. It is to be expected that the level of confidence decreases as a variant becomes less represented in the post-amplification mixture. One would have 67% confidence that the same strategy of selecting five clones would not miss a variant with not less than 20% representation, i.e. $1 - (1 - 0.2)^5$.

Alternative techniques to sequencing, such as the single-strand conformation polymorphism [14] and RFLP [11] are somewhat less laborious but do not produce the same level of detail that can be achieved with sequence analysis, since there is no assurance that all mutations will cause differences in fragment size and mobility.

The choice of HPV gene is also an important consideration. The LCR method [12] targets a hypervariable region of the viral genome, thus theoretically enabling the detection of a greater diversity of variants than when conserved genes are analysed, which maximizes the probability that isolates can be distinguished. Sequencing of defined segments of other genes, such as E6 and L2, has also been shown to indicate substantial diversity in molecular variants of HPV 16 [18].

As we ask more refined questions relating to the natural history of HPV infection and the role of the virus in the genesis of cervical cancer, it is befitting that we enhance our methods of viral detection in epidemiological studies. Issues such as polyclonality of lesions and frequency of particular HPV variants may be critical to our understanding of viral infectivity and pathogenicity. We can only advance our knowledge in this regard if we employ a much greater level of detail in measuring the diversity of HPV in the target tissue.

## Acknowledgements

E. Franco is recipient of a Senior Scholar Award from the *Fonds de la recherche en santé du Québec*. P. Rahal is supported by a graduate fellowship from the Conselho Nacional para o Desenvolvimento Científico e Tecnológico (CNPq).

## References

1 IARC Working Group. *Human Papillomaviruses*, vol. 64. IARC monographs on the evaluation of carcinogenic risks to humans. Lyon: International Agency for Research on Cancer, 1995.

2 Moscicki AB, Palefsky J, Gonzales J, Smith G, Schoolnik GK. Colposcopic and histologic findings and human papillomavirus (HPV) DNA test variability in young women positive for HPV DNA, *J Infect Dis* 1992; **166**: 951–957.

3 Moscicki AB, Palefsky J, Smith G, Siboshski S, Schoolnik G. Variability of human papillomavirus DNA testing in a longitudinal cohort of young women. *Obstet Gynecol* 1993; **82**: 578–585.

4 Hildesheim A, Schiffman MH, Gravitt PE *et al*. Persistence of type-specific human papillomavirus infection among cytologically normal women. *J Infect Dis* 1994; **169**: 235–240.

5 Koutsky LA, Holmes KK, Critchlow CW *et al*. A cohort study of the risk of cervical intraepithelial neoplasia grade 2 or 3 in relation to papillomavirus infection. *N Engl J Med* 1992; **327**: 1272–1278.

6 Ho GYF, Burk RD, Klein S *et al*. Persistent genital human papillomavirus infection as a risk factor for persistent cervical dysplasia. *J Natl Cancer Inst* 1995; **87**: 1365–1371.

7 Franco EL, Villa LL, Rahal P, Ruiz A. Molecular variant analysis as an epidemiological tool to study persistence of cervical human papillomavirus infection. *J Natl Cancer Inst* 1994; **86**: 1558–1559.

8 Xi LF, Demers GW, Koutsky LA *et al*. Analysis of human papillomavirus type 16 variants indicates establishment of persistent infection. *J Infect Dis* 1995; **172**: 747–755.

9 Caballero OL, Villa LL, Simpson AJG. Low stringency-PCR (LS-PCR) allows entirely internally standardized DNA quantitation. *Nucleic Acid Res* 1995; **23**: 193–203.

10 Bauer HM, Ting Y, Greer CE *et al*. Genital human papillomavirus infection in female university students as determined by a PCR-based method. *JAMA* 1991; **265**: 472–477.

11 Bernard HU, Chan SY, Manos MM *et al*. Identification and assessment of known and novel human papillomaviruses by polymerase chain reaction amplification, restriction fragment length polymorphisms, nucleotide sequence, and phylogenetic algorithms. *J Infect Dis* 1994; **170**: 1077–1085.

12 Ho L, Chan S-Y, Chow V *et al*. Sequence variants of human papillomavirus type 16 in clinical samples permit verification and extension of epidemiological studies and construction of a phylogenetic tree. *J Clin Microbiol* 1991; **29**: 1765–1772.

13 Ong CK, Chan SY, Campo MS *et al*. Evolution of human papillomavirus type-18: an ancient phylogenetic root in Africa and intratype diversity reflect coevolution with human ethnic groups. *J Virol* 1993; **67**: 6424–6431.

14 Xi LF, Demers GW, Kiviat NB, Kuypers J, Beckmann AM, Galloway DA. Sequence variation in the non-coding region of human papillomavirus type 16 detected by single-strand conformation polymorphism analysis. *J Infect Dis* 1993; **168**: 610–617.

15 Chan S-Y, Ho L, Ong C-K *et al*. Molecular variants of human papillomavirus-16 from four continents suggest ancient pandemic spread of the virus and its coevolution with humankind. *J Virol* 1992; **66**: 2057–2066.

16 Ho L, Chan SY, Burk RD *et al*. The genetic drift of human papillomavirus type-16 is a means of reconstructing prehistoric viral spread and the movement of ancient human populations. *J Virol* 1993; **67**: 6413–6423.

17 Bernard HU, Chan SY, Delius H. Evolution of papillomaviruses. *Curr Top Microbiol Immunol* 1994; **186**: 33–53.

18 Yamada T, Wheeler CM, Halpern AL, Stewart ACM, Hildesheim A, Jenison SA. Human papillomavirus type 16 variant lineages in United States populations characterized by nucleotide sequence analysis of the E6, L2, and L1 coding segments. *J Virol* 1995; **69**: 7743–7753.

# Section 7
# Adjunct Screening Tests

# 45: Evaluation of Multiple Screening Techniques in a High-risk Area: The Guanacaste Project

R. Herrero,[1] M. H. Schiffman,[2] C. Bratti,[3] A. Hildesheim,[2]
M. E. Sherman,[2,4] J. Morales,[5] S. Mekbel,[5] M. Alfaro,[5] I. Balmaceda,[3]
M. Greenberg[6] & A. Lorincz[7]

## Summary

To investigate the potential of conventional cytology, cervicography, human papillomavirus (HPV) DNA testing and their combinations as primary screening techniques for cervical neoplasia, we conducted a screening of a large random sample of women in Guanacaste, a high-risk province of Costa Rica. Of the women considered eligible to participate, 94% were interviewed, and of those eligible for a pelvic examination, 97% ($n = 9175$) were examined. The sensitivity of each technique was evaluated by calculating the proportion of confirmed cases of cancer or cervical intraepithelial neoplasia (CIN) that would have been referred to colposcopy with different referral thresholds or combinations of diagnoses. Conventional cytology alone detected 91% of the invasive cancers, 78% of high-grade CIN and 61% of low-grade CIN, requiring colposcopic referral of 7% of the women. When referral based on cervicography was restricted to diagnoses potentially associated with high-grade CIN or cancer, sensitivity for cancer was 100% (based on small numbers), but only 15% for high-grade CIN and 5% for low-grade CIN, requiring referral of 2% of the patients. When other positive diagnoses were included, sensitivity for high-grade CIN increased to 45% and that for low-grade CIN to 35%, with

*Correspondence*: Dr Rolando Herrero, Unit of Field and Intervention Studies, International Agency for Research on Cancer, 150 Cours Albert Thomas, 69372 Lyon Cedex 08, France. [1]Unit of Field and Intervention Studies, International Agency for Research on Cancer, 150 Cours Albert Thomas, 69372 Lyon Cedex 08, France; [2]Environmental Epidemiology Branch, National Cancer Institute, Bethesda, MD, USA; [3]Guanacaste Project, FU-CODOCSA, Caja Costarricense de Seguro Social, Costa Rica; [4]Department of Pathology, John Hopkins Hospital, 600 N Wolfe St, Baltimore, MD 21287, USA; [5]Caja Costarricense de Seguro Social, Costa Rica; [6]Department of Gynecology, Graduate Hospital, Pennsylvania, USA; [7]Digene Diagnostics Inc., Silver Spring, MD, USA.

referral of 6% of the women. HPV testing with the Hybrid Capture tube technique detected 64% of cancers, 77% of high-grade CIN and 61% of low-grade CIN, requiring referral of 9%. The combination of conventional cytology and cervicography, conventional cytology and HPV testing, and even cervicography and HPV testing, increased substantially the sensitivity of any single technique, but required referral to colposcopy of large numbers of subjects. Modifications of referral thresholds of different combinations of techniques could provide cost-effective alternatives for improving screening programmes.

## Introduction

Cytological screening for cervical cancer and its precursor, CIN, has been successful at reducing incidence and mortality from cervical cancer in developed countries [1]. However, the applicability of cytological screening in developing countries has been hampered by the considerable expense and organization required for the establishment of successful programmes.

It is necessary to develop more effective screening strategies that would ideally be more accurate than conventional Papanicolaou (Pap), easier to implement and less expensive. Some of the new techniques under investigation consist of improvements of cytology (e.g. monolayer cytology, semi-, or fully automated screening and diagnosis). Other techniques under study rely on the evaluation of the macroscopic aspect of the cervix with or without acetic acid and with or without the aid of special equipment or training (e.g. visual inspection of the cervix, speculoscopy, cervicography). In addition, the vast amount of knowledge recently accumulated on the role of certain types of HPV in cervical carcinogenesis promises to offer clinical applicability in the near future. However, it is not yet clear what the specific role of HPV DNA or serological testing will be in the context of cervical cancer screening programmes.

We are conducting a population-based study in a rural province of Costa Rica with the purpose of evaluating a variety of new screening techniques. In this report, we present preliminary data on the performance of conventional cytology, cervicography and the Hybrid Capture tube HPV DNA test for detection of cervical cancer and CIN.

## Materials and methods

Methodological aspects of the study are reported elsewhere [2]. Briefly, a random sample of 11 742 adult women residing in Guanacaste, Costa Rica was selected and invited to participate in the study. After signing informed consent, eligible women (excluding pregnant and ill) were administered an interview and, on those reporting sexual activity, pelvic exams were performed by study nurses with the following protocol: the vulva, vagina and cervix were inspected for obvious lesions and patients with abnormalities were referred immediately for colposcopic evaluation. When clinical signs of severe candidiasis, trichomoniasis or severe atrophy were present, the rest of the exam was postponed until treatment was completed. Exfoliated cervical cells were collected by firmly rotating a Cervex brush (Unimar, CT) five times (180°) in the ecto- and endocervical area [3]. A conventional smear was prepared and the sample immediately spray-fixed. After the smear was made, the Cervex brush was swirled in 20 ml of PreservCyt solution and then discarded (see below). Next, cervical cells were collected for virological assays with a dacron swab which was swabbed over the ectocervix and rotated in the endocervical canal. The swab was stored in Virapap DNA standard transport medium tubes and frozen initially at −30°C and then at −70°C until tested. After collection of the materials mentioned above, the cervix was rinsed with 5% acetic acid and two photographic images (Cervigrams) were taken with a cerviscope. The film was processed and evaluated at the National Testing Laboratories in Missouri, USA.

The conventional smears were stained and interpreted at a cytopathology laboratory in Costa Rica with technical support from our collaborating departments of pathology at Johns Hopkins and Tufts universities. Additional cytological reports were obtained at Johns Hopkins University after processing the conventional smears with the semiautomated PAPNET system [4]. In addition, monolayer smears were prepared from the cells stored in PreservCyt solution and interpreted at Tufts University. Thus, one cytology report corresponding to each technique was obtained for the majority of women and classified using the Bethesda system [5].

Cervigrams were interpreted at Graduate Hospital in Philadelphia. The categories of evaluation were negative (no lesion seen), atypical (a lesion was seen, but the site and/or morphology of the lesion was such that colposcopy was not recommended), positive (colposcopy recommended) and technically defective (not positive and unable to be properly evaluated). The positive category has four classifications as follows: P0, probable normal variant, but colposcopy preferable to rule out serious neoplasia; P1–P1A, compatible with trivial disease but colposcopy recommended because part of the lesion extends into the canal; P1B, compatible with CIN I; P2, compatible with high-grade disease; P3, compatible with cancer. Reports were sent back to the field with a colour photograph including a mark in the most significant area, which was available at the time of colposcopy, as a recommendation of biopsy site.

All patients with abnormal result (atypical cells of undetermined significance (ASCUS) or worse) in any of the three cytologic tests (conventional, PAPNET/JHU, ThinPrep/Tufts) or positive Cervigrams (P0–P3) were referred for colposcopy and biopsy of any visible lesions. In addition, any patients considered for urgent evaluation on the basis of visual inspection and approximately a random 1 in every 50 women (controls) were referred. HPV DNA detection was not a criterion for referral to colposcopy.

Colposcopic examination was performed and biopsies taken of visible lesions. Final diagnoses were defined after review of all available materials for each patient. Diagnoses of CIN I and koilocytotic atypia (KA) were combined (low-grade CIN), as well as those of CIN II–III (high-grade CIN).

HPV testing was performed with first generation Hybrid Capture tube method (Digene) [6]. Briefly, with this technique, the specimens are first hybridized with full-length genomic HPV DNA probes for 16 HPV types. The resultant RNA–DNA hybrid is captured on to the surface of a tube coated with an anti-RNA–DNA hybrid antibody. Immobilized hybrids are then reacted with an antihybrid antibody conjugated to alkaline phosphatase. When a chemiluminiscent substrate is added, light is emitted, which is measured as relative light units (RLUs) on a luminometer. The intensity of the light emitted is proportional to the amount of target RNA in the specimen. Viral types were grouped into cancer-associated types (16, 18, 31, 33, 35, 39, 45, 51, 52, 56, 58) and not cancer-associated types (6, 11, 42, 43, 44).

We calculated the sensitivity of each technique by dividing the number of cases that would have been referred to colposcopy on the basis of the results of that technique (or a combination of techniques) by the total number of cases with a specific diagnosis. We also present the proportions of women who would have been referred to colposcopy with different thresholds of colposcopic referral.

## Results

The study enrolment was conducted from June 1993 to December 1994. Of the 11 742 women in the sample, 10 738 were considered eligible. A total of 10 049 women were interviewed, corresponding to 93.6% of the eligibles. Of the 10 049 women interviewed, 9466 reported previous sexual experience and were eligible for a pelvic examination. Such an exam was performed on 9175 women. The 298 women on which the pelvic exam was not performed either refused that specific component ($n$ = 213) or had medical problems precluding the examination, most of them associated with extreme old age.

The population included in the survey had a median age of 37 years, low educational levels (with only 32% having gone beyond elementary school) and low income (with the majority reporting family incomes under US$ 4100 per year). Fifty-four per cent reported having had only one life-time sexual partner, and only 12% reported four or more. The population was also characterized by high parity, with almost 40% reporting more than five pregnancies. In addition, smoking was uncommon (11% ever) and 60% of the women had used oral contraceptives. Almost 90% of the women reported having had at least one Pap and 6.8% reported having had a hysterectomy.

Hysterectomized women were excluded from this analysis for a final total number of 8554 evaluable women.

Results of conventional cytology were obtained for virtually all subjects examined and fewer than 1% were considered inadequate. Cervigram results were available for 98.9%, with 1.6% technically defective, and HPV results were available for 99.8%. Table 45.1 presents the frequencies of cytological diagnoses, cervicography diagnosis and results of HPV testing. Seven per cent of women had an abnormal conventional cytology, 5.7% had positive Cervigrams and 8.6% were HPV-positive.

A total of 1948 patients (23.2%) were referred to colposcopy because of abnormal results (ASCUS+) in any of the three cytological techniques, positive Cervigrams (P0+), abnormal clinical findings or as colposcopy controls. The controls were selected randomly from the whole cohort, regardless

**Table 45.1** Prevalence of results of different screening techniques.*

| Diagnosis | n | (%) |
|---|---|---|
| *Conventional cytology* | | |
| Normal | 4853 | 57.2 |
| Reactive changes | 3038 | 35.8 |
| ASCUS | 163 | 1.9 |
| LSIL | 270 | 3.2 |
| HSIL | 135 | 1.6 |
| Cancer | 25 | 0.3 |
| | | |
| *Cervicography* | | |
| Negative | 7123 | 84.2 |
| Atypical | 853 | 10.1 |
| P0 | 144 | 1.7 |
| P1 | 290 | 3.4 |
| P2 | 32 | 0.4 |
| P3 | 18 | 0.2 |
| | | |
| *HPV testing* | | |
| Negative | 7807 | 91.4 |
| Non-cancer-associated types† | 77 | 0.9 |
| Cancer-associated types‡ | 655 | 7.7 |

* Excluding hysterectomized women and rare inadequate results for each technique.
† Includes types 6, 11, 42, 43, 44.
‡ Includes types 16, 18, 31, 33, 35, 39, 45, 51, 52, 56 and 58.
ASCUS, Atypical squamous cells of undetermined significance; LSIL, low-grade squamous intraepithelial lesion; HSIL, high-grade squamous intraepithelial lesion; HPV, human papillomavirus.

of screening diagnosis, to verify the sensitivity of the screening. As expected, no CIN or cancer was diagnosed among the 128 controls referred only by this mechanism.

Table 45.2 presents the prevalence of final diagnoses in the population. A total of 12 cases were diagnosed with invasive cervical cancer for a prevalence of 0.1% (one of the cancers did not have results of screening tests because it was too obviously advanced at diagnosis). An additional 128 had high-grade CIN (prevalence = 1.5%) and 189 had low-grade CIN (prevalence = 2.2%). All cancers were histologically confirmed, compared to 92% of the high-grade CIN and 39% of the low-grade CIN. The lesions that were not confirmed histologically were included in the specific diagnostic group after extensive review of the cytologic materials available. The equivocal category indicates lesions suggested by different techniques that were not definitely confirmed or ruled out by the diagnostic algorithm or pathologist's review.

The sensitivity of the different techniques and the proportions of women who would require referral using different combinations of referring diagnoses are presented in Table 45.3. Conventional cytology detected 91% of the cancers, 78% of the high-grade CIN and 61% of the low-grade CIN, requiring referral of 7% of the women when referring those with ASCUS or worse. Sensitivity of this technique decreased to 82%, 75%, and 57% when restricting referral to women with cytological LSIL, reducing the proportion requiring referral to 5%.

Cervicography detected 100% of the cancers when referring diagnoses of P0, and P2 and P3, but this combination of diagnoses, although requiring referral of only 2% of the patients, detected only 15% of the high-grade CIN and 5% of the low-grade CIN. If P1 diagnoses are included, these proportions increase to 45% and 35% respectively, and would imply referral of 6% of women.

Considering all HPV types, Hybrid Capture detected 64% of the cancers, 77% of high-grade CIN and 61% of low-grade CIN, with a referral of 9% of the population to colposcopy. When the referral is restricted to cancer-associated

**Table 45.2** Prevalence of final diagnosis, Guanacaste.

| Diagnosis | $n$ | (%) |
|---|---|---|
| Normal | 7626 | 89.2 |
| Equivocal diagnoses* | 599 | 7.0 |
| Low-grade CIN† | 189 | 2.2 |
| High-grade CIN‡ | 128 | 1.5 |
| Cancer | 12 | 0.1 |

* Conflicting results not resolved by the diagnostic algorithm or pathologist's review.
† Includes cervical intraepithelial neoplasia (CIN) I and koilocytotic atypia.
‡ Includes CIN II and CIN III.

**Table 45.3** Sensitivity of different screening techniques and proportions of women referred to colposcopy with different referral diagnoses.

| Referring diagnoses | Sensitivity (%) | | | Referred (%) |
|---|---|---|---|---|
| | Low-grade CIN | High-grade CIN | Cancer | |
| *Conventional cytology** | | | | |
| ASCUS+ | 60.8 | 77.8 | 90.9 | 7.0 |
| LSIL+ | 57.1 | 74.6 | 81.8 | 5.1 |
| HSIL+ | 17.5 | 62.7 | 81.8 | 1.9 |
| | | | | |
| *Cervicography†* | | | | |
| P0–P2–P3 | 4.8 | 15.2 | 100.0 | 2.3 |
| P0–P1–P2–P3 | 35.4 | 44.8 | 100.0 | 5.7 |
| P2–P3 | 2.6 | 13.6 | 72.7 | 0.6 |
| P3 | 0.0 | 4.0 | 45.5 | 0.2 |
| | | | | |
| *HPV testing‡* | | | | |
| Any HPV | 61.2 | 77.3 | 63.6 | 8.6 |
| Cancer-associated HPV§ | 55.3 | 75.8 | 63.6 | 7.7 |

* 8484 women evaluable, 11 cancers, 126 CIN II–III and 189 CIN I koilocytotic atypia (KA).
† 8460 women evaluable, 11 cancers, 125 CIN II–III and 189 CIN I/KA.
‡ 8539 women evaluable, 11 cancers, 128 CIN II–III and 188 CIN I/KA.
§ Includes types 16, 18, 31, 33, 35, 39, 45, 51, 52, 56 and 58.
CIN, cervical intraepithelial neoplasia; ASCUS, atypical squamous cells of undetermined significance; LSIL, low-grade squamous intraepithelial lesion; HSIL, high-grade squamous intraepithelial lesion; HPV, human papillomavirus.

types, corresponding percentages are 64%, 76% and 55%, with referral of 8%.

Table 45.4 presents the sensitivity of different combinations of techniques. The combination of conventional cytology with the nurses' referral based on clinical findings, which in this case could be based on the aspect of the cervix before or after application of acetic acid, added very little to cytology alone but would increase referral rates to 10%.

The combination of conventional cytology and cervicography, when referring diagnoses of ASCUS or worse and P0–P2–P3, obviously increases the sensitivity of cytology alone for cancer to 100%, but does not modify it substantially for CIN, and would imply referral of 9% of women. The inclusion of P1 in the referral groups increases detection of high-grade CIN to 90% and that of low-grade CIN to 84% but requires referral of 12% of women. With this combination, increasing the cytological referral threshold to LSIL, similar sensitivity is achieved with referral of 10% of subjects.

The combination of conventional cytology with HPV testing achieved sensitivity of 100% for cancer, 90% for high-grade CIN and 80% for low-grade CIN, maintaining similar proportions if the threshold was increased to refer

**Table 45.4** Proportions of lesions detected by combinations of screening techniques and proportions of women referred to colposcopy with different combinations of referral diagnoses.

| Referring diagnoses | Sensitivity (%) | | | Referred (%) |
|---|---|---|---|---|
| | Cancer | Low-grade CIN | High-grade CIN | |
| *Conventional + visual inspection* | | | | |
| ASCUS | 61.9 | 80.2 | 91.7 | 9.9 |
| *Conventional + cervicography* | | | | |
| ASCUS+/P0–P2–P3 | 64.0 | 82.5 | 100.0 | 8.9 |
| LSIL+/P0–P2–P3 | 60.8 | 80.2 | 100.0 | 7.1 |
| HSIL+/P0–P2–P3 | 22.2 | 68.3 | 100.0 | 3.9 |
| ASCUS+/P0–P1–P2–P3 | 83.6 | 89.8 | 100.0 | 11.7 |
| LSIL+/P0–P1–P2–P3 | 81.0 | 88.2 | 100.0 | 9.9 |
| HSIL+/P0–P1–P2–P3 | 50.3 | 78.7 | 100.0 | 7.0 |
| ASCUS+/P2–P3 | 62.4 | 82.5 | 100.0 | 7.3 |
| LSIL+/P2–P3 | 58.7 | 80.2 | 100.0 | 5.4 |
| HSIL+/P2–P3 | 20.1 | 68.3 | 100.0 | 2.3 |
| ASCUS+/P3 | 60.8 | 78.6 | 90.9 | 7.1 |
| LSIL+/P3 | 57.1 | 76.2 | 90.9 | 5.2 |
| HSIL+/P3 | 17.5 | 64.3 | 90.9 | 2.0 |
| *Conventional + HPV testing* | | | | |
| ASCUS+/any HPV | 79.9 | 89.0 | 100.0 | 12.9 |
| LSIL+/any HPV | 78.3 | 88.2 | 100.0 | 11.3 |
| HSIL+/any HPV | 65.6 | 86.6 | 100.0 | 9.2 |
| ASCUS+/cancer-associated HPV | 76.7 | 89.0 | 100.0 | 12.1 |
| LSIL+/cancer-associated HPV | 74.6 | 88.2 | 100.0 | 10.5 |
| HSIL+/cancer-associated HPV | 59.8 | 86.6 | 100.0 | 8.3 |
| *Cervicography + HPV testing* | | | | |
| P0–P2–P3/any HPV | 63.0 | 81.9 | 100.0 | 10.5 |
| P0–P1–P2–P3/any HPV | 76.7 | 89.0 | 100.0 | 13.2 |
| P2–P3/any HPV | 62.4 | 81.9 | 72.7 | 9.0 |
| P3/any HPV | 60.8 | 79.5 | 63.6 | 8.7 |
| P0–P2–P3/cancer-associated HPV | 57.7 | 80.3 | 100.0 | 9.7 |
| P0–P1–P2–P3/cancer-associated HPV | 74.1 | 87.4 | 100.0 | 12.3 |
| P2–P3/cancer associated HPV | 57.1 | 80.3 | 72.7 | 8.1 |
| P3/cancer-associated HPV | 55.0 | 78.0 | 63.6 | 7.8 |

CIN, cervical intraepithelial neoplasia; ASCUS, atypical squamous cells of undetermined significance; LSIL, low-grade squamous intraepithelial lesion; HSIL, high-grade squamous intraepithelial lesion; HPV, human papillomavirus.

LSIL cytological diagnosis or worse or if referring only women with cancer-associated HPV types. However, this required the referral of 11% of the women. Additional analysis is warranted to determine the efficacy of this approach with certain age restrictions.

The combination of cervicography and HPV DNA testing, when referring P0–P2–P3 and all HPV types, was associated with a sensitivity of 100% for cancer, 82% for high-grade CIN and 63% for low-grade CIN, and would imply referral of 11% of the women. Similar percentages are obtained restricting to cancer-associated types. When including P1 as a referral diagnosis and restricting referral to cancer-associated types, sensitivity for high-grade CIN is 87% and for low-grade CIN 74%, but also requires referral of 12% of the women to colposcopy.

## Discussion

In this report, we present results of the evaluation of three different screening techniques in a sample of women participating in a population-based screening conducted in a rural area of Costa Rica. Participation rates were over 90% for all the components of the study. Women were screened with conventional cytology, semiautomated cytology, monolayer smears and cervicography, and referred to colposcopy if results of any of those tests presented an abnormality. After colpobiopsy and review of all the material a final diagnosis was established. We compared the results of conventional cytology, cervicography and HPV testing and their combinations with the final diagnosis to determine the sensitivity of these screening tools in this setting.

Conventional cytology was an effective technique for detection of lesions along the whole spectrum of cervical neoplasia, and would imply the referral to colposcopy of a relatively small number of those screened (7%). If should be kept in mind that this conventional cytology was carried out in the setting of a research project, in which the nurses who collected and fixed the samples received special training, and the fixation and staining processes were optimized with the collaboration of international experts. Therefore, it is not comparable to the usual conventional cytology available in developing countries. However, the interpretation of the smears was made by local cytotechnologists and cytopathologists, selected from amongst the most experienced in the country, but who received only limited feedback during the course of the screening.

When referring to colposcopy only women with P0, P2 and P3, which are the cervicographic diagnoses considered to have the highest probability of high-grade CIN and cancer, cervicography alone was able to detect 100% of the 11 invasive cancers, with referral of only 2% of women to colposcopy, a finding that can be of special interest in certain screening settings, but requires confirmation with a larger number of cases. Cervicography was available for almost all the participants and the proportion of technically inadequate images was minimal, partly as a result of the careful training of the nurses who had no previous experience with the technique. However, this approach would detect only 15% of high-grade CIN and 5% of low-grade CIN, suggesting that it is not an appropriate technique for primary screening aimed at the detection of precursor lesions. If P1 is also included, detection of CIN increases, but still to only 45% and 35% respectively, and would require referral of 6%. This is in concordance with the findings of other investigators [7,8].

HPV testing with Hybrid Capture as a primary screening tool detected, in our study, similar numbers of CIN as conventional cytology, but surprisingly, only 64% of the invasive cancers. In addition, it required the referral of more women to colposcopy (9%). It is likely that referral could be restricted to women in certain age groups without affecting detection of abnormalities. The low detection of invasive cancers requires confirmation in larger series. Amplification techniques like polymerase chain reaction are likely to increase sensitivity, and their evaluation as potential screening tools is warranted.

The first combination of techniques that we explored was conventional Pap and visual inspection by the nurses, which in this case included the application of acetic acid performed before the cervicography. Visual inspection appeared to add little to detection of lesions but increased referral to an important extent.

As expected, the combination of conventional cytology and cervicography (with P0, P1, P2, P3 referral), conventional cytology and HPV testing, and even cervicography and HPV testing, achieved an important improvement in sensitivity, in the order of 100% for invasive cancer, 90% for high-grade CIN and 80% for low-grade CIN. This gain in sensitivity was obtained with a corresponding loss in specificity, substantially increasing the proportion of women requiring referral to colposcopy.

Modification of the referral thresholds of the different combinations could provide interesting alternatives suitable for the capabilities and expectations of particular screening programmes.

## Acknowledgement

This study was supported by contract N01-CP-21081 and N01-CP-31061 of the National Cancer Institute, National Institutes of Health, USA.

## References

1 Beral V, Hermon C, Muñoz N, Devesa SS. Cervical cancer. *Cancer Surv* 1994; **19–20**: 265–285.

2 Herrero R, Schiffman MH, Bratti C *et al*. Design and methods of a population-based natural history study of cervical neoplasia in a rural province of Costa Rica: the Guanacaste Project. *Bull PAHO* (in press).

3 Ferris DG, Berrey MM, Ellis KE, Petry LJ, Voxnaes J, Beatie RT. The optimal technique for obtaining a Papanicolaou smear with the Cervex Brush. *J Fam Pract* 1992; **34**: 276–280.

4 Mango LJ. Neuromedical Systems Inc. *Acta Cytol* 1996; **40**: 53–59.

5 National Cancer Institute Workshop. The 1988 Bethesda system for reporting cervical/vaginal cytologic diagnoses. *JAMA* 1989; **262**: 931–934.

6 Schiffman MH, Kiviat N, Burk RD *et al*. Accuracy and interlaboratory reliability of HPV DNA testing by Hybrid Capture. *J Clin Microbiol* 1995; **33**: 545–550.

7 Coibion M, Autier P, Vandam P *et al*. Is there a role for cervicography in the detection of premalignant lesions of the cervix? *Br J Cancer* 1994; **70**: 125–128.

8 Greenberg M, Sedlacek TV, Campion MS. Cervical neoplasia: are adjunctive tests to cervical cytology worthwhile? *Clin Obst Gynecol* 1995; **38**: 600–609.

# 46: Colposcopy as a Screening Tool for Cervical Cancer Detection: A Review

## R. Barrasso

Diagnosis of intraepithelial lesions of the cervix uteri presents specific problems. Histological features of human papillomavirus (HPV) infection are tightly intermingled with features of preneoplastic and neoplastic lesions and a clear-cut distinction between viral infection and cancer precursors cannot yet be drawn. Moreover, morphological identification of HPV-associated and precancerous lesions is rendered difficult by the fact that some physiological modifications of cervical epithelium, i.e. squamous metaplasia, may colposcopically and even histologically mimic HPV-associated changes. Thus, only a careful diagnostic approach may avoid overdiagnosis and overtreatment. The third problem is the low specificity of diagnostic procedures as for the identification of HPV-associated lesions of the cervix.

As for screening, cytology is considered the best cost-effective method. However, its sensitivity for intraepithelial neoplasia and even for cancer has been discussed [1]. Moreover, its specificity for the identification of low-grade intraepithelial lesions is low, since various physiological conditions may mimic the existence of HPV-associated lesions [2]. This is why other procedures (cervicography, viral testing) have been proposed as a complement to cytology [3], in order better to identify those cervices which need further examination. Colposcopy has often been proposed in association with cytology, in order to increase the sensitivity of the screening [2]. We will discuss this proposal and detail the reasons why colposcopy has too low a specificity in distinguishing metaplasia from intraepithelial lesions. When used as a screening method, the risk of overdiagnosis and consequent overtreatment of benign conditions would be too high.

Colposcopic features of the normal transformation zone are well known.

*Correspondence*: R. Barrasso, Chief of the Colposcopy Unit, Obstetrics/Gynaecology Department, Bichat University Hospital, Paris, France.

During the metaplastic process, thin, white areas are detected by the colposcopist around glandular tissue. However, the maturation of metaplastic tissue is usually fast, this allowing its easy colposcopic identification: the metaplastic tissue progressively loses the white reaction to the acetic acid and becomes iodine-positive. In some cases, the maturation of metaplastic tissue is not as fast as described. In this case, large parts and even the entire metaplastic tissue remain immature long enough to be detected by cytology and colposcopy [4,5]. On the same cervix, immature areas may be intermingled with more mature portions of the process.

The colposcopist detects abnormal findings within the transformation zone: a mostly red area (thinner epithelium and stromal hyperaemia), strongly reacting to the acetic acid test (high cellular and nuclear activity) with the possible presence of punctation and mosaic (stromal projections centred by capillaries within the epithelium), uniformly iodine-negative (lack of glycogen) [5]. Thus, colposcopic features of immature metaplasia recall, as we will see, those of intraepithelial lesions. In some cases, this immature metaplasia is thought to be congenital and to persist until the beginning of sexual life, as shown by the study of fetal cervices and of virgin women [4].

Can abnormal colposcopic findings due to the immature (congenital) T zone be distinguished from intraepithelial lesions? The experienced colposcopist may guess in most cases whether he or she is observing immature metaplasia or CIN [6,7]. The atypical findings detected in cases of immature metaplasia present as a smooth or papillary, markedly but homogeneously white area: punctation and mosaic are regularly distributed and the size and shape of capillaries are uniform; the area is homogeneously iodine-negative, without any partial Lugol's uptake. However, some early intraepithelial lesions present with the same features, rendering incomplete specific criteria for differential diagnosis. And how could it be otherwise, if even the pathologist may have problems distinguishing immature metaplasia from carcinoma *in situ*? Thus, the colposcopist will not be surprised or disappointed if biopsies on markedly acetowhite epithelium show immature metaplasia.

The maturation of the metaplastic process may also be arrested at almost terminal stages. If the finding of immature metaplasia is occasional, arrested metaplasia is frequently encountered and it is at the heart of the most controversial subject in colposcopy [2,8]. In these cases, histology shows a well-differentiated but not fully mature metaplastic epithelium, without cytological atypia but lacking glycogen. Its main morphological character is the sharp and totally flat caudal border with normal squamous epithelium [2].

Consecutive colposcopic observations have shown that the process may originate any time during the metaplastic process and that the arrested metaplasia progresses toward the os, as the normal one. This is why the caudal border is always sharp, while the cephalic border is indistinguishable from that of normal metaplasia, until at terminal stages, it shows the lack of glycogen.

The explanation for arrested metaplasia is unknown. It has been thought that this subtle change could represent minor degrees of HPV infection [9], since histology of these areas shows mild degrees of acanthosis and parakeratosis, but this hypothesis has not been confirmed [10].

Arrested metaplasia may be infected by HPVs but it may also be detected in the absence of HPV infection, confirming that the phenomenon is not related to papillomaviruses [10]. Colposcopically, the cervix looks normal on direct observation (normal height of the epithelium, normal amount of stromal vascularization). A flat acetowhite area, mostly tiny (mild degrees of cellular and nuclear activity), will appear after the acetic acid test. It may contain various degrees of punctation and mosaic, due to the stromal arrangement during metaplasia: capillaries are regular in size and shape and the intercapillary distance is uniform. Those areas remain homogeneously iodine-negative (lack of glycogen) after the Schiller test.

The most characteristic colposcopic feature is the very sharp and flat border between the caudal part of this normal squamous epithelium. The stereoscopic vision of the colposcope clearly shows the difference with the elevated border of intraepithelial lesions as well as with the progressively iodine-positive external border of normal metaplasia. Histology illustrates the sharp demarcation between the peripheral border of arrested metaplasia and normal epithelium. The external border of the area may be located at the original junction, showing that the maturation of the entire metaplastic epithelium may be arrested at this stage. Arrested metaplasia may also originate during the metaplastic process. In those cases, a caudal area of normal transformation will be observed.

Arrested metaplasia may appear as a circumferential area or it may coexist with normal metaplasia, covering only one or more sections of the T zone. In this case, it may have a geographic map-like appearance. Since areas of normal metaplasia progress faster toward the os, they may become isolated on the ectocervix areas of arrested metaplasia.

Most cervical intraepithelial lesions appear during the metaplastic process within the transformation zone. At the colposcopic examination [5], intraepithelial lesions will appear as abnormal findings within the transformation zone: a normally pink or, most often, red area (stromal hyperaemia) reacting to the acetic acid test (increased cellular and nuclear activity) and mostly showing areas of punctation and mosaic (stromal finger-like projections or ridges within the epithelium and/or angiogenesis), homogeneously iodine-negative (absence of glycogen) or irregularly taking up the iodine solution (focal maturation). Areas of keratosis may also be present.

The progression line toward the os (SCJ) will be much better demarcated than that of normal metaplasia, since the morphological transition between atypical and columnar cells is sharp. The caudal limit will mostly appear well defined; atypical epithelium is thicker than the normal one. However, as compared to arrested metaplasia, atypical tissue towers over the normal one, translating the progressive mechanical replacement. Thus, the stereoscopic vision by the colposcope will clearly show the difference between the two processes. However, arrested metaplasia may be infected by HPV, further complicating the colposcopic distinction between normal and pathological tissues.

As we have seen, immature metaplasia, arrested metaplasia and intraepithelial lesions appear to the colposcopist as abnormal findings within the transformation zone. The differential diagnosis may be difficult without a biopsy. This is the main cause of the low specificity of colposcopy when used as a screening tool.

When colposcopy was introduced by Hinselmann [11], he thought that leukoplasia and acetowhitening were features specific for neoplasia and that colposcopy could provide a screening method for early cervical cancer. Further studies showed, as already discussed, that arrested or immature metaplasia could colposcopically mimic intraepithelial lesions. Cytology replaced colposcopy as a screening method, since it was easier to perform and more specific for the detection of cervical cancer precursors.

Colposcopy was reintroduced in English-speaking countries at the beginning of the 1960s as a topographic procedure, allowing the identification of atypical tissue and the localization of its limits in women presenting an abnormal smear [4]. Colposcopy was mostly performed in women with disease, and thus the differential diagnosis with immature and arrested metaplasia did not present a major problem, since their observation was rare. The colposcopic classification adopted thus comprises two groups of features, detected within the normal and the atypical T zone, as they are almost synonymous for normal and atypical.

In most European countries, colposcopy was proposed from the early 1950s as a screening technique, complementary to cytology, to be used by each gynaecologist in order to improve the detection rate of intraepithelial lesions [2,12,13]. Thus, the differential diagnosis with immature and, mostly, arrested metaplasia represented a major problem: using the dual classification, only 20% of ATZs would correspond to an intraepithelial lesion. Arrested metaplasia is detected in 30% of women of child-bearing age [2]!

Several studies were performed in order to search for colposcopic changes specific for intraepithelial lesions. Differences in colour, angioarchitecture, surface characters and contours of lesions were analysed, but no fully specific reproducible sign was identified [6,7]. Most colposcopic classification comprised three instead of two groups of features; this emphasized the need for an intermediate category of minor abnormal changes, not necessarily pathological [2,12–14]. Arrested metaplasia was particularly studied and described as several different terms [2,12–14].

Colposcopy is still currently performed as a topographic tool or as a screening technique. The terminology and classification proposed by the International Federation of Cervical Pathology and Colposcopy in 1990 [15] represents the result of a common effort of both schools in order to offer to colposcopists all over the world a terminology suitable for both approaches.

The new terminology renders the colposcopist familiar with the existence of non-pathological colposcopic changes, for two reasons. First of all, the term atypical transformation zone is suppressed, and acetowhite areas are defined as abnormal colposcopic findings within the transformation zone. This dedramatizes the abnormal colposcopy and introduces the concept that an abnormal finding is not necessarily histologically atypical. Second, the colposcopist is invited to identify minor and major changes among these abnormal findings. Minor changes mostly correspond to arrested metaplasia or low-grade intraepithelial lesions, while major changes mostly correspond to high-grade intraepithelial lesions, even if the immature metaplasia may be encountered.

Our study [10] clearly shows that, using this terminology, the specificity of colposcopy in identifying intraepithelial neoplasia as typical findings with major changes is 82%. It also clearly shows that, when colposcopy is used as a routine technique, 60% of abnormal findings with minor changes correspond to metaplasia.

Even if not fully specific and reproducible, these distinctions contribute to educating the colposcopist in the concept that a white area is not necessarily a cancer precursor.

Colposcopy is frequently used as a complement of a gynaecological examination in most Latin countries and in Germany. The colposcopist is thus faced with the observation of several whitening immature and arrested metaplasias.

In English-speaking countries, the enormous increase in mildly abnormal smears and low-grade intraepithelial lesions also brings to the colposcopy clinic several cases of immature and arrested metaplasia.

We personally discourage the use of colposcopy as a screening technique, since the number of useless biopsies would be too high. When colposcopy is used as part of the routine gynaecological visit, we recommend that abnormal colposcopic findings showing minor changes should not be biopsied unless the smear shows dyskaryotic cells.

## References

1 International Agency for Research on Cancer working group on evaluation of cervical screening programmes. Screening for squamous cervical cancer: duration of low risk

after negative results of cervical cytology and its implication for screening policies. *Lancet* 1986; **239**: 659–664.

2 Oupez F, Carrera JM, Dexeus S. *Trait et Atlas de Colposcopie*. Paris: Masson, 1974.

3 Richart RM. Screening. The next century. *Cancer* 1995; **76**: 1919–1927.

4 Coppleson M, Pixley E, Reid B. Colposcopic appearances of the atypical transformation zone. In: Coppleson, Pixley, Reid (eds) *Colposcopy*. Springfield: Thomas, 1986, pp 254–286.

5 Barrasso R, Guillemotonia A. Cervix and vagina: diagnosis. In: Gross, Barrasso (eds) *Papillomaviruses in Human Pathology: A Clinical Atlas* Wiesbaden: Mosby, 1996 (in press).

6 Barrasso R, Coupez F, Ionesco M, De Brux J. Human papillomaviruses and cervical intraepithelial neoplasia: the role of colposcopy. *Gynecol Oncol* 1987; **27**: 197–207.

7 Reid R, Stanhope CR, Herschmann BR, Crum CP, Agronow SJ. Genital warts and cervical cancer. IV. A colposcopic index for differentiating subclinical papillomavirus infection from cervical intraepithelial neoplasia. *Am J Obstet Gynecol* 1984; **149**: 815–823.

8 Jordan J, Singer A. *The Cervix*. Philadelphia: WB Saunders, 1976.

9 Schneider A, Sterzik K, Buck G, De Villiers EM. Colposcopy is superior to cytology for the detection of early genital human papillomavirus infection. *Obstet Gynecol* 1988; **71**: 236–241.

10 Barrasso R. Human papillomavirus infection of the uterine cervix: the role of colposcopy. *Cervix* 1992; **10**: 95–99.

11 Hinselmann H. Verbesserung der Inspektionsmöglichkeiten von Vulva, Vagina und Portion. *Munch Med Wschr* 1925; 1733–1737.

12 Wespi HJ. Colposcopic–histologic correlations in the benign acanthotic non glycogenated squamous epithelium. *Colposc Gynecol Laser Surg* 1986; **2**: 147–158.

13 Burghardt E. *Colposcopy, Cervical Pathological, Textbook and Atlas*. Stuttgart: Georg Thieme Verlag, 1991.

14 De Palo G. *Manuale de Colposcopia e Pathologia del Tratto Genitale Inferiore*. Milan: Masson, 1990.

15 Stafl A, Wilbanks GD. An international terminology of colposcopy: report of the nomenclature committee of the International Federation of Cervical Pathology and Colposcopy. *Obstet Gynecol* 1991; **77**: 313–314.

# 47: Adjuvant Tests to Cytology: Cervicography and the Polarprobe

T. A. J. Mould[1] & A. Singer

## Summary

The high false-negative rates associated with the Papanicolaou (Pap) smear and the increasing number of minor cytological abnormalities have prompted gynaecologists to look for an adjuvant test either to improve primary screening or to act as a triage for minor abnormalities. Two of the candidates for this test are cervicography and the Polarprobe™. Cervicography has been extensively tested since its introduction in 1981. It has been shown to be a sensitive method of detecting cervical lesions with a lower false-negative rate than cytology. However, it has been criticized for poor specificity and lack of cost-effectiveness. Both of these factors are less important in a high-risk population such as women with minor Pap smear abnormalities and cervicography has been shown to be an effective triage technique for this population. Outside the USA, its uptake has been limited by the initial cost of the equipment, the need for lithotomy in the general practitioner's surgery and the lack of evaluation centres.

The Polarprobe is a new electronic method of detecting cervical precancer and cancer. It relies on the different response to light and electrical stimuli between normal and abnormal cervical tissue. It gives an immediate and objective diagnostic assessment of the cervix. It is also extremely portable and potentially not expensive due to its low labour needs, and thus could be used in developing countries. A preliminary study showed accuracy to be between 90 and 95% for high-grade lesions and this has been confirmed for invasive cancer. Further studies on the efficacy in precancerous lesions in low- and high-risk populations are awaited.

*Correspondence*: Professor A. Singer, Department of Women's Health, F Block, Whittington Hospital, Highgate Hill, London N19 5NF, UK.
[1] Department of Gynaecology, Whittington Hospital, Highgate Hill, London N19 5NF, UK.

## Introduction

The traditional Pap smear for cervical screening has been the subject of adverse criticism in the literature [1]. Further improvements to the screening process may not be possible without the addition of another test to augment the smear [2]. Furthermore, an additional test may be able to resolve the dilemma of the increasing number of mildly abnormal smears in young women. Two candidates for this additional test are cervicography and the Polarprobe.

## Cervicography

The technique of cervicography, in which a photograph of the cervix obtained after application of 5% acetic acid, was developed in 1981 [3]. It was soon proposed as a new or adjunctive screening method for cervical precancer and cancer [4]. Studies showed it to be a more sensitive screening method than the smear test [5] and to be cost-effective [6]. However, its major problem was the high false-positive rate of 26% when a reporting system in which any abnormality resulted in a referral to colposcopy was used [7]. A later study showed a specificity comparable to cytology, 0.92 versus 0.94, with a significantly better sensitivity, 0.89 versus 0.52 [8]. This study was performed in an area which was previously unscreened and this may be the reason for the higher specificity.

Cervicography has not been widely taken up as a primary screening method in the UK and this may be due to the higher false-positive rate. Also, the need for the lithotomy position and the expense of the cerviscope may have discouraged the use of cervicography in general practitioners' surgeries, and the lack of centres providing analysis facilities is a practical obstacle in the UK.

Studies have reported the use of cervicography as a triage method for the increasing numbers of atypical squamous cells of undetermined significance (ASCUS) smears and again the sensitivity of the technique was high, with cervicography detecting 88% of cervical intraepithelial neoplasia (CIN) II and 75% of CIN III [9]. Thus, women with a normal cervicography result could be kept under cytological surveillance rather than referred on to colposcopy. As the cervicography clinic is nurse-led, there was also adequate time for counselling and thus a potential reduction in anxiety levels, although this was not measured.

Cervicography has been found to be more effective than repeat smears [10] or human papillomavirus testing for the purpose of triaging mildly abnormal Pap smears [11]. High false-positive rates have again been a criticism but this is not so critical in women who would have been sent to colposcopy anyway. Poor cost-effectiveness has also been reported, principally because even with an additional test, a large proportion of the women will still be referred on to colposcopy [12,13].

In a retrospective review of the figures for our own clinic where cervicography has been used to triage 1436 women referred with minor cytological abnormalities since 1988, the sensitivity to detect CIN II or above was 91%, with a specificity of 51%. The cases missed were all of small-volume disease. The low specificity was offset by the fact that this was a very high-risk population, with 21% of women having CIN II or above.

## Polarprobe

We are evaluating a new electronic method of cervical screening, known as the Polarprobe, which uses electrical and optical techniques to distinguish between malignant and non-malignant tissues [14].

The Polarprobe comprises a 25-cm-long case with a 5-mm tip which is fitted with elements for optical and electrical stimulation of the tissue. It relays response signals to a notebook-sized computer.

Low-voltage electrical impulses and four different wavelengths of light are applied to the surface of the cervix. Normal, precancerous and cancerous cervical tissue reflect the light and the voltage in different and characteristic ways. The responses are picked up by the tip of the probe and relayed to the computer. The computer contains a pattern recognition system which compares the returned signal from the women to a catalogue of preprogrammed signal patterns held in the computer's memory. There are patterns in the computer for normal tissues, low- and high-grade abnormalities and invasive cancer. An immediate decision is made as to the tissue type and this is indicated to the operator via the display panel and an optical or acoustic signaller.

The probe is used similarly to a conventional Pap smear test. The cervix is visualized with a cuscoe's speculum and then the tip of the probe is gently passed over the surface of the cervix. This process takes approximately 20 s. The technique is simple and can be done by anyone who has previously taken a smear, with a minimum of instruction. Thus it could be used at the general practitioner's surgery by either the practice nurse or the doctor. The device is very safe and no side-effects have been reported by doctors or patients in well over 5000 episodes of its use. Furthermore, studies at the Whittington Hospital show it is extremely acceptable to the women being tested. The instant diagnosis is very attractive to women, and the examination by the probe is less painful than the traditional cytology spatula being passed over the cervix (Mould, unpublished data).

Initial studies using an early prototype show that on a tissue observation basis, the concordance between colposcopy/histology and the Polarprobe diagnoses ranges from 85% for low-grade lesion to 90% for CIN II and III and 99% for invasive cancer [15]. An extrapolation of these results suggests that false-positive/negative rates in the order of 10% may be achievable.

The latest prototype has just been tested in a trial on women with invasive cervical cancer in Recife, Northern Brazil (Singer, unpublished data). The probe was used on 41 women with invasive cervical cancer which was confirmed histologically on colposcopically directed punch biopsy specimens. The probe was also used on 45 women with a colposcopically normal cervix. The probe correctly detected 40 out of 41 cancers. There were 4 false positives in the normal control group. The sensitivity to predict invasive cancer correctly was 97% whilst the specificity was 94%. The next stage of the trials is to evaluate the efficacy of the probe to detect precancers.

This device exhibits significant potential as an adjunct to cytological screening. It is aimed at being used in general practitioners' surgeries as part of the National Health Service screening programme. It could be used at the same time as the initial smear to reduce the rate of false negatives associated with cytological screening, which have been reported to be as high as 48% [8]. Alternatively, the probe could be used on women who have had a borderline or mildly dyskaryotic smear. Up to 49% of women with these low-grade smears will actually have CIN II or III [16]. Thus, a triage test could be used to select these women for immediate colposcopy, whilst the remaining women could be safely left under cytological surveillance.

The device is still in research at the moment as its efficacy is fully assessed, and thus its cost has not been set. However, after an initial capital outlay for the device, the cost per examination should be minimal, as no laboratory investigation will be involved.

The computer used by the probe is the size of a conventional notebook computer and the device is extremely portable. This fact, combined with the ease of use and the relatively low cost compared to setting up a conventional cytology programme, makes the device ideal for use in developing countries where no screening exists.

In summary, the Polarprobe is an electronic device for detecting cervical precancer and cancer, designed for use in the general practitioner's surgery by either the nurse or doctor. Its potential advantages are its instant diagnosis capacity, high patient acceptability, the objectivity of the reading and the relatively low patient assessment costs, which will enhance the community benefit of the screening programme. It is extremely portable, and thus could be used in developing countries, where three-quarters of the deaths from cervical cancer occur. At present, trials are underway to confirm initial studies on its accuracy. Cervicography is a sensitive method of cervical screening, but low specificity has limited its use as a primary screening technique. It has been shown to be an effective technique for triage of minor cytological abnormalities but its uptake outside the USA has not been widespread as yet.

## References

1 Raffle AE, Alden B, Mackenzie EFD. Detection rates for abnormal cervical smears: what are we screening for? *Lancet* 1995; **345**: 1469–1473.

2 Reid R, Greenburg MD, Lorincz A *et al*. Should cervical cytological testing be augmented by cervicography or human papillomavirus deoxyribonucleic acid detection? *Am J Obstet Gynecol* 1991; **164**: 1461–1471.

3 Stafl A. Cervicography: a new method for cervical cancer detection. *Am J Obstet Gynecol* 1981; **139**: 815–821.

4 Blythe JG. Cervicography: a preliminary report. *Am J Obstet Gynecol* 1985; **152**: 192–197.

5 Ferris DG, Payne P, Frisch LE, Milner H, DiPaola FM, Petry LJ. Cervicography: adjunctive cervical cancer screening by primary care physicians. *J Fam Pract* 1993; **37**: 158–164.

6 Tawa K, Forsythe A, Cove JK, Saltz A, Peters HW, Watring WG. A comparison of the Papanicolaou smear and the cervigram: sensitivity, specificity, and cost analysis. *Obstet Gynecol* 1988; **71**: 229–234.

7 Szarewski A, Cusick J, Edwards R, Singer A. The use of cervicography in a primary screening service. *Br J Obstet Gynaecol* 1991; **98**: 313–317.

8 Kesic VI, Soutter WP, Sulovic V, Juznic N, Alesic M, Ljubic A. A comparison of cytology and cervicography in cervical screening. *Int J Gynecol Cancer* 1993; **3**: 395–398.

9 Ferris FG, Payne MD, Lawrence E, Frisch MD. Cervicography: an intermediate triage test for the evaluation of cervical atypia. *J Fam Pract* 1993; **37** 463–468.

10 Jones DE, Creasman WT, Dombroski RA, Lentz SS, Waeltz JL. Evaluation of the atypical smear. *Am J Obstet Gynecol* 1987; **157**: 544–549.

11 August N. Cervicography for evaluating the 'atypical' Papanicolaou smear. *J Reprod Med* 1991; **36**: 89–94.

12 Spitzer M, Krumholtz BA, Cherynys AE, Seltzer V, Lightman AR. Comparative utility of repeat Papanicolaou smears, cervicography, and colposcopy in the evaluation of atypical Papanicolaou smears. *Obstet Gynecol* 1987; **69**: 731–735.

13 Solomen D, Wied GL. Cervicography: an assessment. *J Reprod Med* 1989; **34**: 321–332.

14 Wunderman I, Coppleson M, Skladnev VN, Reid BL. Polarprobe: a precancer detection instrument. *J Gynecol Technique* 1995; **1**: 105–109.

15 Coppleson M, Reid BL, Skladnev VN, Dalrymple JC. An electronic approach to the detection of precancer and cancer of the uterine cervix: a preliminary evaluation of the Polarprobe. *Int J Gynecol Cancer* 1994; **4**: 79–83.

16 Soutter WP, Wisdom S, Brough AK, Monagham JM. Should patients with mild atypia in a cervical smear be referred for colposcopy? *Br J Obstet Gynaecol* 1986; **93**: 70–74.

# 48: Visual Inspection as a Screening Test for Cervical Cancer Control in Developing Countries

R. Sankaranarayanan,[1] B. Syamalakumari,[2] R. Wesley,[3] Thara Somanathan,[4] B. Chandralekha,[5] N. Sreedevi Amma[5] & D. M. Parkin[1]

## Summary

Visual-inspection-based screening tests are considered in the context of general approaches to cervical cancer prevention in developing countries. Unaided visual inspection involving naked-eye speculum examination of the uterine cervix under adequate light has been promoted as a screening test in India. Depending on the criteria used to define abnormalities, 6–70% of women in these studies were found to have an abnormal cervix. Approximately half of the women with cancers detected by the reference test (cytology and/or biopsy) revealed an abnormal cervix on visual screening. Hence, half the women with clinical disease are likely to be missed by the test. The sensitivity to detect clinical invasive cancer varied from 39 to 94% in different population groups; it varied from 29 to 89% to detect moderate dysplasia lesions and the specificity varied from 38 to 96%. If the intention of unaided visual inspection is to detect clinical cancer, both the sensitivity and specificity should be sufficiently high to ensure that only few cases are missed and the false-negative and false-positive rates are low.

The performance of this test is not satisfactory to detect preinvasive lesions. The test is unlikely to result in much cost savings, as the costs of locating and motivating women, the need to repeat at frequent intervals, and the load of women requiring further investigations (cytology/colposcopy/biopsy/

*Correspondence*: Dr R. Sankaranarayanan, Unit of Descriptive Epidemiology, International Agency for Research on Cancer, 150 cours Albert Thomas, 69372 Lyon Cedex 08, France. [1]Unit of Descriptive Epidemiology, International Agency for Research on Cancer, Lyon, France; [2]Early Cancer Detection Centre, Kallor, Ernakulam, India; [3]Division of Community Oncology, Regional Cancer Centre, Trivandrum 695011, India; [4]Department of Pathology, Armed Forces Medical College, Poona, India; [5]Division of Cytopathology, Regional Cancer Centre, Trivandrum 695011, India.

follow-up) would offset the cost savings achieved by offering cytology/gynaeco-logical examination to those with an abnormal cervix. It is likely that the magnitude of stage shift aimed for by active case finding by unaided visual inspection may be achieved by a programme of health education and improv-ing professional awareness.

Aided visual inspection with (gynoscopy) or without magnification (cervi-coscopy), after 3–4% freshly prepared acetic acid impregnation of uterine cervix to detect acetowhite areas, is still an experimental procedure. Cervicos-copy, in preliminary studies, was more sensitive than Papanicolaou (Pap) smear in detecting preinvasive lesions, though the specificity is lower. The test characteristics need to be established in well-conducted studies with adequate reference tests to establish true positive lesions before considering aided visual inspection for further evaluation.

## Introduction

Cervical cancer is the most frequent cancer and the leading cause of cancer mortality among women in developing countries. In 1985, four-fifths of the estimated 437 000 incident cases and 203 000 deaths from uterine cervical cancer in the world occurred in developing countries [1,2]. Despite being one of the few cancers amenable to effective prevention measures based on currently available knowledge, it continues to be a major cause of ill health among women in their most productive period in developing countries, as a result of a lack of planned control measures and research.

Though considerable progress in the prevention and control of cervical cancers has been achieved in developed countries with cervical cytology programmes [3], such models of disease prevention are not considered to be feasible in developing countries, in view of competing health priorities and limited resources. Hence, there has been some interest in evaluating low-cost alternatives to organized cytology programmes, suitable for implementation in developing countries. A strategy based on visual inspection of the uterine cervix is one of the approaches considered [4–7]. In this chapter, we briefly review and discuss the visual-inspection-based screening tests in the control of cervical cancer.

## Unaided visual inspection

Unaided visual inspection, referred to frequently as downstaging, involves naked-eye speculum examination of the appearance of the uterine cervix under adequate light by health workers and designating the findings as normal or abnormal [4–7]. Those with abnormal findings need to be further investigated, which would entail cytology (in situations where some cytology facilities are available) or examination by gynaecologists (where no cytology services are available).

To our knowledge, all the studies involving unaided visual inspection (both published and unpublished) in the early detection of cervix cancer have been conducted in India [8–15]. These studies indicate that 6–70% of the women subjected to visual inspection are found to have an abnormal-looking cervix, depending upon the criteria used to define a positive visual inspection.

If any abnormal finding (ranging from excessive discharge up to growth/ulcer) is used to define a positive visual inspection (lower threshold), 41–70% of the women have been found to have an abnormal cervix. On the other hand, if more limited criteria (one or more of the following: bleeding on touch, bleeding erosions, hypertrophied elongated oedematous cervix, growth/ulcer) are used to define abnormalities, 6–11% of women have a positive test. All the reported studies have used findings from cytology and/or biopsy as a reference test ('gold standard') to study the performance of unaided visual inspection.

Approximately half of the cancers detected by the reference test (cytology and/or biopsy) among women subjected to unaided visual inspection revealed abnormal cervix on visual screening (Table 48.1). This means that half of the women with clinical disease are likely to be missed by the test and left alone. The performance of unaided visual inspection to detect carcinoma-*in-situ* and/or invasive cervical cancer is given in Table 48.2. If the intention of unaided visual inspection is to detect clinical cancer, then both the sensitivity

**Table 48.1** Proportion of subjects with clinically detected cervical cancer revealing abnormal visual inspection findings.

| Author (year) | Subjects examined | Subjects with abnormality | Total cervical cancers detected | Cervical cancer patients with abnormal findings |
|---|---|---|---|---|
| Seghal *et al.* (1991) [9] | 11 760 | | 215 | 88 (41%) |
| | 1107 | | 63 | 33 (52%) |
| Singh *et al.* (1992) [11] | 44 970 | 31 330 (70%)* | 238 | |
| | | 5135 (11%)† | | |
| Das *et al.* (1992) [10] | 117 471 | | 213 | 88 (41%) |
| Bhargava *et al.* (1993) [8] | 3608 | 2065 (63%)* | 59 | 50 (85%) |
| Sujathan *et al.* (1995) [12] | 3602 | 2267 (63%)* | 51 | 46 (90%) |
| Rao *et al.* (1995) [15] | 1956 | 801 (41%) | 4 | 2 (50%) |
| Nene *et al.* (1997) [13] | 1954 | 1120 (57%)* | 7 | 6 (86%) |
| | | 118 (6%)† | | 5 (71%) |
| Wesley *et al.* (1997) [14] | 2843 | 1279 (45%)* | 13 | 12 (92%) |
| | | 179 (6%)† | | 7 (54%) |

* A low threshold was used to define a positive test.
† A high threshold was used to define a positive test.

**Table 48.2** Performance of visual inspection in detecting carcinoma-*in-situ* and/or invasive cervical cancer.

| Author (year) | Visual inspection findings | Cytology/biopsy findings | | Sensitivity (%) | Specificity (%) |
|---|---|---|---|---|---|
| | | + ve | –ve | | |
| Singh *et al.* (1992) [11] | + ve | 149 | 4986 | 63 | 89 |
| | – ve | 89 | 39 746 | | |
| Bhargava *et al.* (1993) [8] | + ve | 50 | 125 | 85 | 96 |
| | – ve | 9 | 3424 | | |
| Sujathan *et al.* (1995) [12] | + ve | 68‡ | 2199 | 89 | 38 |
| | – ve | 5‡ | 1330 | | |
| | + ve | 60 | 2207 | 94 | 38 |
| | – ve | 4 | 1331 | | |
| Rao *et al.* (1995) [15] | + ve | 2 | 811 | 50 | 59 |
| | – ve | 2 | 1170 | | |
| Nene *et al.* (1997) [13] | + ve* | 9 | 1111 | 90 | 43 |
| | – ve | 1 | 833 | | |
| | + ve† | 6 | 112 | 60 | 94 |
| | – ve | 4 | 1832 | | |
| Wesley *et al.* (1997) [14] | + ve* | 17‡ | 1262 | 74 | 55 |
| | – ve | 6‡ | 1558 | | |
| | + ve† | 9‡ | 170 | 39 | 94 |
| | – ve | 14‡ | 2650 | | |

\* A low threshold was used to define a positive test.
† A high threshold was used to define a positive test.
‡ Includes carcinoma-*in-situ* and invasive cancers.

(> 90%) and specificity (> 90%) should be sufficiently high to ensure that only a few cases are missed and the false-negative as well as the false-positive rates are low. This has not been consistently observed in reported studies (Table 48.2): the sensitivity to detect invasive cancer varied from 39 to 94% in different populations, using different providers and different criteria to define a positive visual inspection. Attempts to increase the specificity by using a high threshold to define a positive test resulted in unacceptably low sensitivity.

The sensitivity and specificity of visual inspection in detecting preinvasive (moderate dysplasia and above) as well as clinical cancer are given in Table 48.3. The values for these parameters are unacceptably low. In studies involving patients attending gynaecology outpatient clinics or early cancer detection centres, the sensitivity to detect these lesions was higher compared to studies involving subjects recruited in community-based settings.

**Table 48.3** Performance of visual inspection in detecting moderate dysplasia plus lesions.

| Author (year) | Visual inspection findings | Cytology/biopsy findings | | Sensitivity (%) | Specificity (%) |
|---|---|---|---|---|---|
| | | + ve | −ve | | |
| Sujathan et al. (1995) [12] | + ve | 90 | 2177 | 89 | 38 |
| | − ve | 11 | 1324 | | |
| Rao et al. (1995) [15] | + ve | 12 | 801 | 41 | 59 |
| | − ve | 17 | 1155 | | |
| Wesley et al. (1997) [14] | + ve* | 25 | 1254 | 66 | 55 |
| | − ve | 13 | 1551 | | |
| | + ve† | 11 | 168 | 29 | 94 |
| | − ve | 27 | 2637 | | |

* A low threshold was used to define a positive test.
† A high threshold was used to define a positive test.

If cost savings are a major concern, unaided visual inspection is unlikely to achieve this objective, as at least half of the women need to be subjected to further investigations. The costs of locating and motivating women, the need to repeat visual inspection at frequent intervals to improve the programme effectiveness, and the number of women requiring further investigations (cytology/colposcopy/biopsy/follow-up) would offset the cost savings achieved by limiting cytology/gynaecological examination to those with an abnormal cervix.

If the range of aberrant normal cervices is considered responsible for the insensitivity and non-specificity of detecting lesions, the attempts to improve the specificity of unaided visual inspection by using a high threshold to define a positive visual inspection (thereby reducing the number of women subjected to further investigations) resulted in an unacceptably low sensitivity (Tables 48.2 and 48.3), with many serious lesions missed. A high rate of false-positive referrals may cause undue anxiety and a false-negative rate gives a feeling of false safety.

If the major intention of unaided visual inspection is the detection of diseases in an earlier stage when still curable, this amounts to active case finding. Visual inspection is quite unlikely to achieve a stage shift as soon as it is introduced. A significant proportion of invasive cancers detected through unaided visual inspection in the initial rounds are likely to be relatively advanced lesions. The findings on stage distribution of cancers detected in two studies of visual detection in India reveal that less than one-quarter of cancers were detected in localized (stage I) stage (Table 48.4). The necessary facilities (surgical and radiotherapeutic) required to treat more advanced cases may not be available in some developing countries: one of the accepted criteria

**Table 48.4** Stage distribution of invasive cervical cancers detected in downstaging studies.

| Author (year) | Stages | | Total |
|---|---|---|---|
| | I | II–IV | |
| Bhargava *et al.* (1993) [8] | 12 (20%) | 47 (80%) | 59 |
| Wesley *et al.* (1997) [14] | 2 (15%) | 11 (85%) | 13 |

underlying a programme of early detection is that facilities for diagnosis and treatment should be available [16]. Moreover, the treatment for invasive cervical cancer is not very effective, particularly for stage II and above (5-year survival < 50%), as evidenced by results from developing countries [17,18].

It may take several years to achieve an improvement in stage distribution by a programme of visual screening. The available evidence suggests that a shift towards early stages at detection could be achieved at considerably lower costs by health education and improved awareness, as revealed by the findings from Sweden and Barsi, India [19,20].

## Aided visual inspection

The naked-eye visualization of the cervix after impregnation with 3–4% acetic acid is termed *cervicoscopy*. The results are reported as negative (no acetowhite areas) and positive (evidence of acetowhite) areas. It has been shown in western countries that cervicoscopy could detect lesions missed by cervical cytology and could augment the detection rates of CIN II–III lesions, when used as an adjunct to Pap smear [21,22]. It was found to be more sensitive than Pap smear in detecting preinvasive cervical lesions, though its specificity was lower. To our knowledge, there are no published studies on this technique for the early detection and prevention of cervical cancers in developing countries. We now report some preliminary results from one of our ongoing studies evaluating cervicoscopy in India.

Women reporting for opportunistic cervical cytology at an early cancer detection centre in Ernakulam, central Kerala, India are currently being recruited for a study evaluating unaided visual inspection, cervicoscopy and low-intensity cytology. Women who are found to be positive on one or more of the above tests (high-threshold findings on unaided visual inspection; acetowhite areas on cervicoscopy; dysplasia and cancer on Pap smear) are further subjected to colposcopy and biopsy. Thus the reference test colposcopy/biopsy was not applied to women who were found to be negative for the three screening tests and hence direct estimation of sensitivity and specificity is not possible. The following parameters are used to compare the outcome of cervicoscopy and Pap smear [23,24]:

1   The detection rate of each test: the number of screened women with a true positive lesion divided by the total number of screened women.

2   The ratio of sensitivities between the two tests: the detection rate of the first test divided by the detection rate of the second. A ratio of greater than unity indicates that the first test is more sensitive; McNemar's test is used for significance testing of the differences in sensitivities.

3   The approximated specificity: the number of negative screening tests divided by the total number of screened subjects less the number of true positive cases detected by the test. McNemar statistics applied to the discordant women assess the statistical significance.

The following result are based on 868 women recruited from April to December 1995. Those positive on unaided visual inspection, cervicoscopy and Pap smear were 78 (9%), 160 (18%) and 45 (5%) respectively. In all, 193 (22%) were eligible for colposcopy, of whom 127 had been subjected to it, at the time of this report.

Table 48.5 displays the results of cytology and cervicoscopy contrasted with colposcopy results. Among the 127 women who underwent colposcopy, 87 were classified as negative, 13 as having atypia, 6 as having mild dysplasia, 9 as having moderate dysplasia, 8 as having severe dysplasia and carcinoma-*in-situ* and 4 as having invasive cancer. Cervicoscopy resulted in the diagnosis of 23 of 27 (85.2%) mild dysplasia and above lesions, 11 of 12 (91.2%) severe dysplasia plus lesions. Pap smear identified 69.6% (*n* = 16) and 75.0% (*n* = 9) of these lesions respectively.

If all dysplasias and carcinoma were considered as true positives (Table 48.6), 14 of 27 (54%) lesions were detected by both tests; 9 (35%) lesions were missed by Pap smear and 2 (7%) lesions by cervicoscopy. There are more false-positive results with cervicoscopy (73) when compared to false-positive Pap smears (8). If moderate dysplasia and cancer were considered as true

**Table 48.5** Results of colposcopy.

| Screening | Colposcopy findings* | | | | | | |
|---|---|---|---|---|---|---|---|
| | Atypia | Mild dysplasia | Moderate dysplasia | Severe dysplasia | Invasive carcinoma | Normal | Total |
| Cervicoscopy | | | | | | | |
| + | 11 | 5 | 7 | 7 | 4 | 74 | 108 |
| – | 2 | 1 | 2 | 1 | 0 | 702 | 708 |
| Papanicolaou smear | | | | | | | |
| + | 3 | 1 | 6 | 6 | 3 | 18 | 37 |
| – | 10 | 5 | 3 | 2 | 1 | 758 | 779 |
| Total | 13 | 6 | 9 | 8 | 4 | 776 | 816 |

*Only 127 subjects underwent colposcopy.

**Table 48.6** Comparison of cervicoscopy and Pap smear findings.

| Pap smear | True positives | | True negatives on colposcopy or with a negative Pap smear | |
|---|---|---|---|---|
| | Cervicoscopy | | Cervicoscopy | |
| | Positive | Negative | Positive | Negative |
| All dysplasia + carcinoma | | | | |
| Positive | 14 | 2 | 13 | 8 |
| Negative | 9 | 2 | 73 | 695 |
| | | | | |
| Moderate and severe dysplasia + carcinoma | | | | |
| Positive | 13 | 2 | 14 | 8 |
| Negative | 5 | 1 | 77 | 696 |

Pap, Papanicolaou.

positive (Table 48.6), 13 of 21 (62%) lesions were detected by both tests; Pap smear missed 5 of 21 (24%) lesions and cervicoscopy missed 2 (10%) lesions. Cervicoscopy detected 33 of 38 (87%) lesions as compared to 19 (50%) lesions by Pap smear.

Table 48.7 summarizes the detection rate, ratio of sensitivities, approximated specificities and the positive predictive value of both the tests in detecting lesions. Cervicoscopy was more sensitive in detecting lesions as compared to cytology, though the difference did not reach statistical significance. However, the specificity of cytology was significantly higher when compared to that of cervicoscopy.

**Table 48.7** Comparison of performance of cervicoscopy and Pap smears.

| | Cervicoscopy | Pap smear |
|---|---|---|
| *Detection rate for dysplasia + carcinoma* | 28.2/1000 | 23.0/1000 |
| Ratio of sensitivities | 23/16 = 1.44 | |
| McNemar's test for sensitivity | $\chi^2 = 3.3, P > 0.05 < 0.10$ | |
| Approximated specificity | 89.3 | 97.4 |
| McNemar's test for specificity | $\chi^2 = 50.6, P < 0.001$ | |
| Positive predictive value | 21.3% | 43.2% |
| | | |
| *Detection rate for moderate, severe dysplasia and carcinoma* | 22.1/1000 | 18.4/1000 |
| Ratio of sensitivities | 18/15 = 1.2 | |
| McNemar's test for sensitivity | $\chi^2 = 0.57, P$ NS | |
| Approximated specificity | 88.7 | 96.2 |
| McNemar's test for specificity | $\chi^2 = 54.4, P < 0.001$ | |
| Positive predictive value | 16.7% | 40.5% |

Pap, Papanicolaou; NS, not significant.

In a study reported by Cecchini *et al.* [22], cervicoscopy was positive for 25.4% of 2105 subjects, as opposed to positive cytology findings in 3.8%. It was found to be more sensitive in detecting CIN II–III lesions, but its specificity was lower than that of the Pap smear. Even though its low specificity is of concern, its value in triaging subjects for further investigations and diagnosis of preinvasive/early invasive lesions of cervix needs to be further evaluated. It seems to be a more objective test than unaided visual inspection. The test may emerge more specific and may reduce the false-positive referrals if those with acetowhite areas wholly or partially within the transformation zone are scored positive for the test. This aspect needs to be investigated and we are currently evaluating the performance of cervicoscopy in three different locations in India in order to validate this test in different populations by different providers.

A second approach to aided visual inspection involves the use of a small, light-weight monocular telescope called a *gynoscope* to visualize the acetic acid-impregnated cervical tissue, which has a magnification of two and a half times [7]. Aided visual inspection using gynoscope was evaluated in a preliminary study involving 920 women in Indonesia [25]. The sensitivity and specificity to detect cytologically proven CIN I plus lesions were reportedly 95.8% and 96.4% respectively, the reference test being Pap smear. It is still not clear whether low-power magnification offers any real benefits over cervicoscopy, which involves unmagnified visual inspection after acetic acid lavage.

## Conclusion

It is doubtful that an active attempt to detect disease in early clinical stages by unaided visual inspection in settings without facilities for cytology will be cost-effective in the control of cervical cancer. The assumed benefits of such an approach may be attained by public health education to improve the awareness of the general public and by efforts to improve referral practices among physicians. If the objective of unaided visual inspection is to preselect women for the detection of both preinvasive and invasive lesions by limited cytology, the test characteristics are not very promising for such a task. In summary, the performance of unaided visual inspection is not satisfactory to consider this as an approach for cervical cancer control in developing countries.

Aided visual inspection using acetic acid impregnation with (gynoscopy) or without magnification (cervicoscopy) is still an experimental procedure, the test characteristic and the accuracy of which need to be established in well-conducted studies. This information is important when taking them into consideration for further evaluation in randomized controlled trials.

## References

1 Parkin DM, Pisani P, Ferlay J. Estimates of the worldwide incidence of 18 major cancers in 1985. *Int J Cancer* 1993; **54**: 594–606.

2 Pisani P, Parkin DM, Ferlay J. Estimates of the world-wide mortality from 18 major cancers in 1985. *Int J Cancer* 1993; **55**: 891–903.

3 Hakama M, Miller AB, Day NE. *Screening for Cancer of the Uterine Cervix*. IARC Scientific Publications no. 76. Lyon: International Agency for Research on Cancer, 1986.

4 World Health Organization. Control of cancer cervix, a WHO meeting. *Bull WHO* 1986; **64**: 607–618.

5 Stjernsward J, Eddy D, Luthra UK, Stanley K. Plotting a new course for cervical cancer screening in developing countries. *World Health Forum* 1987; **8**: 42–45.

6 Miller AB. *Cervical Cancer Screening Programmes. Managerial Guidelines*. Geneva: World Health Organization, 1992.

7 Sherris J, Wells ES, Tsu VD, Bishop A. *Cervical Cancer in Developing Countries: A Situation Analysis*. Women's Health and Nutrition working paper. Washington: The World Bank, 1993.

8 Bhargava VL, Verma K, Sharma R, Batra S, Anandalakshmy PN. A hospital based study on the use of paramedical personnel for clinical downstaging of cancer cervix. *Indian J Med Res* 1993; **98**: 65–68.

9 Seghal A, Singh V, Bhampani S, Luthra UK. Screening for cervical cancer by direct inspection. *Lancet* 1991; **i**: 282.

10 Das DK, Murthy NS, Bhatnager P *et al.* Efficacy of a hospital based cytology screening program. *Neoplasma* 1992; **39**: 381–384.

11 Singh V, Seghal A, Luthra UK. Screening for cervical cancer by direct inspection. *BMJ* 1992; **304**: 534–535.

12 Sujathan K, Kannan S, Pillai KR *et al.* Implications of gynaecological abnormalities in pre-selection criteria for cervical cancer screening: preliminary evaluation of 3602 subjects in south India. *Cytopathology* 1995; **6**: 75–87.

13 Nene BM, Deshpande S, Jayant K *et al.* Early detection of cervical cancer by visual inspection: a population based study in rural India. *Int J Cancer* 1997 (in press).

14 Wesley R, Sankaranarayanan R, Mathew B *et al.* Evaluation of visual inspection as a screening test for cervical cancer. *Br J Cancer* 1997 (in press).

15 Rao SR, Revathy S, Malvi SG, Taskar V, Rao RS. Pitfalls in the visual inspection of the cervix, as a method of downstaging cancer of the cervix in developing countries. *Indian J Obstet Gynaecol* 1995; **28** 659–665.

16 Wilson JMG, Jungner G. *Principles and Practice of Screening for Disease*. Public Health papers no. 34. Geneva: World Health Organization, 1968.

17 Sankaranarayanan R, Nair MK, Jayaprakash PG *et al.* Cervical cancer in Kerala: a hospital registry-based study on survival and prognostic factors. *Br J Cancer* 1995; **72**: 1039–1042.

18 Nandakumar A, Anantha N, Venugopal TC. Incidence, mortality and survival in cancer of the cervix in Bangalore, India. *Br J Cancer* 1995; **71**: 1348–1352.

19 Ponten J, Adami HO, Bergstorm R *et al.* Strategies for control of cervical cancer. *Int J Cancer* 1995; **60**: 1–26.

20 Jayant K, Rao RS, Nene BM, Dale PS. Improved stage at diagnosis of cervical cancer with increased cancer awareness in a rural Indian population. *Int J Cancer* 1995; **63**: 161–163.

21 Van Le L, Broekhuizen FF, Janzer-Steele R, Behar M, Samter T. Acetic acid visualization of the cervix to detect cervical dysplasia. *Obstet Gynecol* 1993; **81**: 293–295.

22 Cecchini S, Bonardi R, Mazzotta A, Grazinni G, Iossa A, Ciatto S. Testing cervicography and cervicoscopy as screening tests for cervical cancer. *Tumori* 1993; **79**: 22–25.

23 Schatzkin A, Connor RJ, Taylor PR, Bunnag B. Comparing new and old screening tests when a reference procedure cannot be performed on all screenees. *Am J Epidemiol* 1987; **125**: 672–678.

24 Verbeek ALM, van den Ban MC, Hendricks JHCL. A proposal for short-term quality control in breast cancer screening. *Br J Cancer* 1991; **63**: 261–264.

25 Sjamsuddin S, Prihartono J, Nuranna L *et al*. Aided visual inspection: preliminary results of the Indonesian gynoscope assessment. In: *Proceedings from a Working Meeting on Cervical Cancer Prevention, Screening, and Treatment*. Montreal, Quebec: PATH, 1994.

# Section 8
# Prevention and Therapy
# by Immunization

# 49: Human Papillomavirus Vaccines and their Potential Use in the Prevention and Treatment of Cervical Neoplasia

## N. Muñoz

The potential use of human papillomavirus (HPV) vaccines in the prevention and treatment of cervical cancer was the theme of the workshop organized by the International Agency for Research on Cancer (IARC) and the Fondation Marcel Mérieux at Veyrier du Lac, near Annecy, on 12–14 December 1994. This international workshop was attended by 38 scientists from nine countries. Short reports of the meeting proceedings, including a list of participants, have been published elsewhere [1,2]. A more detailed report is given below.

## Session I: Epidemiology of cervical cancer and HPV infection

During the first part of this session, the public health importance of cervical cancer was highlighted. This tumour is the second most frequent cancer of women worldwide, and the most common cancer of women in developing countries, where 17% of cancer cases are cervical cancer, corresponding to a life-time risk (0–75 years) of almost 3%, in comparison to developed countries, where it represents only 5% of all cancers and a risk to age 75 of about 1%.

The time trend studies indicate that, although cervical cancer rates have been declining in many countries, they remain high in developing countries, where well-organized screening programmes are lacking. In addition, in women under 40 years of age, incidence and mortality rates are levelling off or increasing in several developed countries and these increases would probably have been more marked in the absence of screening programmes.

The epidemiology of HPV infections and their association with cervical cancer were then reviewed.

*Correspondence*: Dr N. Muñoz, Unit of Field and Intervention Studies, International Agency for Research on Cancer, 150 Cours Albert Thomas, F-69372 Lyon Cédex 08, France.

The best methods to assess exposure to HPV are currently hybridization tests aimed at detecting HPV DNA and especially the polymerase chain reaction (PCR)-based methods. The PCR-based assay using elongated general primers and an enzyme-linked immunosorbent assay (ELISA) format that is being developed were described in detail. The prevalence of HPV DNA is highly dependent on the hybridization method used. Higher prevalences are obtained with PCR-based assays than with non-amplified methods. The HPV DNA prevalence also varies with age — in most populations a peak is observed at 15–25 years of age after initiation of sexual intercourse, reaching prevalence rates of 30–50% and thereafter declining sharply with age to 2–15%. Most infections in women under 25 years appear to be transient, while those in older women tend to be persistent. HPV DNA becomes undetectable in most HPV-infected cytologically normal women within 1–2 years but the immunological determinants of viral suppression or persistence are not well understood.

Observations from a number of studies suggest that after HPV genital infection, most individuals do not develop clinical signs or symptoms, and those who develop these signs will do it within 3 years of infection. The morphological changes occurring in the cervix during productive HPV infection are referred to as low-grade cervical intraepithelial neoplasia (CIN I). Most of these lesions will regress spontaneously but a small proportion will progress to high-grade CIN (CIN II–III) and eventually to invasive cancer.

Although the geographical distribution in the general population of HPV types associated with cervical cancer is not well known, available evidence indicates that their prevalence is 3–5 times higher in developing countries than in developed countries, whereas the incidence of cervical cancer is up to 10 times higher in developing countries. This, in addition to the fact that only a fraction of women with persistent HPV infections eventually develop cervical cancer, suggests the existence of cofactors that will enhance the risk of cervical cancer in HPV DNA-positive women.

The epidemiological evidence for the association includes an impressive and largely consistent set of case series, case-control studies and some cohort studies.

The available epidemiological data indicate that the association between certain HPV types and cervical cancer fulfil the accepted criteria of causality proposed by Sir Bradford Hill:

1　It is very strong, with odds ratios over 15 in all methodologically sound case-control studies using reliable methods for HPV DNA detection. The strength of the association rules out the possibility that it can be explained by chance, bias or confounding.

2　It is consistent, as equally strong associations have been found both in high- and low-risk countries for cervical cancer. Results from case-control studies and the international prevalence survey of HPV DNA in invasive cervical cancer coordinated by the IARC indicate that over 90% of these tumours can be attributed to certain HPV types.

**3**  There is a dose–response relationship between viral load and the risk of developing cervical neoplasia.

**4**  Results form a few cohort studies indicate that infection with certain HPV types precedes the development of CIN II–III lesions.

**5**  The association is specific for certain HPV types, called high-risk HPV types. Out of the 30 HPV types that infect the uterine cervix, HPV 16, 18, 31 and 45 account for 80% of the HPV infections associated with cervical cancer.

**6**  The epidemiological evidence is supported by a great number of laboratory investigations indicating a carcinogenic potential of the HPV types implicated in cervical neoplasia.

The first session was closed with a review of the current preventive strategies for cervical cancer and their efficacy.

## Session II: Humoral immune response

Several advances have recently been made in understanding the immune response to HPVs with the use of genetically engineered viral proteins and synthetic peptides. Sero-reactive and T-cell epitopes of HPV proteins have been identified using a variety of techniques. In most instances, it is unclear if these epitopes are recognized in the course of natural infection. Antibodies to early HPV proteins and to virus-like particles (VLPs) have also been detected in patients with HPV-associated diseases as well as in healthy individuals. Antibodies to E6 and E7 proteins are the most consistent serological response in patients with invasive cervical cancer. However, it remains to be seen whether accurate and reliable immunological assays that measures exposure to HPVs can be developed.

## Session III: Cell-mediated immune responses

Regression of HPV-induced warts is accompanied histologically by a response characteristic of a CD4$^+$-cell-dependent delayed-type hypersensitivity reaction; animal models support this observation. The increased prevalence of HPV infections in immunosuppressed individuals (such as those undergoing organ transplantation, those with HIV infection or those with inherited T-cell immunodeficiencies) further supports a role for CD4$^+$ cells in the control of HPV infection. In HPV-associated cancers the E6/E7 genes are expressed and theoretically are targets for cytotoxic T lymphocyte (CTL) response. An antibody response to these proteins is found in at least 50% of cervical cancers, indicating that these proteins are potential targets for immunotherapy. However, the down-regulation of class I major histocompatibility complex (MHC) expression observed in cervical cancer may interfere with T-cell recognition of these target antigens.

## Session IV: Lesson from animal models

Bovine papillomavirus (BPV) 2 and BPV4 induce benign lesions that might progress to cancer under natural conditions. Effective prophylactic and therapeutic vaccines for BPV2 and BPV4 have been produced. The first general prophylactic vaccines used tumour extracts or purified viral particles. The second-generation vaccines using recombinant L1 and L2 proteins induced protection mediated through the production of neutralizing antibodies. The third-generation vaccines, VLPs of BPV4 L1 or L2 administered in alum, protected calves from experimental BPV4 infection of the soft palate up to 2 years.

The demonstration of effective BPV4 vaccines is highly relevant to the development of HPV vaccines, because BPV4 is a mucosotropic virus that induces papillomas of the upper alimentary canal that evolve to cancer under certain conditions. This situation could be considered similar to that of genital HPV types inducing CIN lesions, a proportion of which, under the influence of certain cofactors, will eventually progress to cancer.

The successful experience with canine oral papillomavirus (COPV) vaccines is also highly relevant to the development of HPV vaccines. COPV is a mucosotropic virus that causes endemic oral papillomatosis among young beagles. Two types of COPV vaccines have been developed: formalin-inactivated papilloma extracts and recombinant COPV-L1 VLPs. Both have been shown to be highly protective against experimental and natural infections of the oral mucosa by COPV, through the induction of neutralizing antibodies.

The cottontail rabbit papillomavirus (CRPV) induces skin papillomas that can regress spontaneously or persist or progress to carcinomas. Three generations of effective CRPV vaccines have been produced: first-generation or crude wart extracts, second-generation or recombinant L1 or L2 proteins and third-generation or CRPV L1 or L2 VLPs. All vaccines have been shown to be effective in protecting rabbits against experimental infection with CRPV. Protection is type-specific, requires intact VLPs and it is probably mediated through the production of neutralizing antibodies. In addition to the reasons mentioned for the BPV and the COPV models, the rabbit model could have special relevance to the development of HPV vaccines because it has been shown that the risk of regression or of malignant progression is linked to MHC class II gene DR-DQ haplotypes.

Therapeutic vaccines based on recombinant E6 or E7 proteins have also been shown to be effective in inducing regression of lesions produced by BPV4 and CRPV.

## Session V: Prophylactic HPV vaccines

The overall results presented at the meeting showing how effective papillomavirus vaccines are in preventing and treating tumours associated with these viruses provided further encouragement for the development of equivalent vaccines against HPV.

In the rationale for development of prophylactic HPV vaccines the following considerations should be made:

1   Does natural infection with HPV protect against subsequent infection with the same type?

2   If not, why not? Is the amount of virus too small to elicit an antibody response? Is the route of infection non-optimal? Does the infection elicit only a local response?

3   Since little is known on the role of humoral response in HPV infection, minimal deviations from procedures used for vaccines that work (vaccinia, yellow fever, polio, hepatitis B virus), should be allowed.

4   An HPV vaccine should be safe, cheap and stable to be able to used in developing countries where 80% of the cervical cancers occur.

There was consensus that the immunogens of choice are the VLPs synthesized *in vitro*. These DNA-free particles seem to have the same conformation as authentic viral particles, as shown by their ability to induce neutralizing antibodies. Since genital HPV genotypes probably represent distinct serotypes, various HPV type-specific vaccines or a polyvalent VLP vaccine would have to be produced.

The recent development of an animal xenograph model for HPV replication has made possible the identification of neutralizing antibodies and antigens. The development of surrogate assays for neutralizing antibodies such as VLP cell-surface binding inhibition and haemagglutination inhibition assays were also reported.

The development of a vaccine based on VLPs of HPV 16-L1 was described. This vaccine was shown to be immunogenic in mice with good antibody response and induction of T-cell response at doses ranging from 0.25 to 10 µg. Several laboratories and companies are now proceeding to the development and production of VLPs at the standards required for human trials.

The production of chimeric VLPs incorporating full-length or truncated E7 proteins is also underway.

## Session VI: Therapeutic vaccines

The rationale for the development of HPV therapeutic vaccines against cervical neoplasia relies on the fact that E6 and E7 proteins are present in the majority of tumour cells. Since neither protein is in the cell surface, the most effective mechanism for the destruction of tumour cells is likely to be CTL which recognizes intracellularly processed peptides in complex with host MHC antigens. Experimental studies using E6 or E7-expressing tumour cells suggest that each of these oncoproteins can act as tumour-rejection markers. However, there is little evidence of CTL response in natural HPV infections.

Preliminary results from two small ongoing phase I trials were reported. In the one being carried out in the UK, a vaccine based on a recombinant vaccinia vector expressing mutated E6 and E7 from both HPV 16 and 18 is being given to 8 patients with late-stage cervical cancer. No side-effects of vaccination have been observed after 9 months.

In the other trial, a vaccine based on bacterial fusion proteins for HPV 16 E7 with algammulin adjuvant has been administered to 5 patients with advanced cervical cancer. These patients made antibodies to E7 and no adverse effects of vaccination were observed, but at 32 weeks all women have died.

A similar trial employing peptides related to HPV 16 E7 for use in HPV 16+ and human leukocyte antigen (HLA)-A*0201-cervical cancer patients was soon to start in the Netherlands.

## Session VII: Validation of vaccine efficacy

Both oncogenic and low-risk HPV types are of interest. Evaluation of the vaccines against low-risk types should be easier and quicker than those against the oncogenic types since the benign tumours develop more quickly than the malignant ones. Emphasis was put on the importance of the end-points for assessing vaccine efficacy and on the necessity for developing adequate tests for cell-mediated and humoral responses induced by vaccines. End-points for viral replication could be HPV DNA detection by PCR-based assays or by serological tests to be developed. These end-points for disease development will be colposcopical, cytological and histological abnormalities of the uterine cervix.

For prophylactic vaccines, there were lengthy discussions on how severe the cervical lesions would have to be to provide convincing evidence of protection against cancer.

Demonstration of prevention of low- and high-grade squamous intraepithelial lesions would probably require follow-up periods of 5–10 years.

For therapeutic vaccines designed to improve survival, the end-point studies would be death.

## Session VIII: Practical and ethical issues on HPV vaccine trials

The importance of careful design and ethical considerations was emphasized for large-scale trials having as an end-point the reduction in cervical cancer, in view of the many years they will take to complete.

## References

1 Muñoz N, Crawford L, Coursaget P. HPV vaccines for cervical neoplasia. *Lancet* 1995; **345**: 249.
2 Muñoz N, Crawford L, Coursaget P. HPV vaccines and their potential use in the prevention and treatment of cervical neoplasia. *Papillomavirus Rep* 1995; **2**: 54–55.

# 50: Animal Models for Evaluation of Human Papillomavirus Vaccines

## F. Breitburd, J. Salmon & G. Orth

## Summary

Vaccines against infection with oncogenic human papillomaviruses cannot be evaluated in the usual animal models owing to the strict species-specificity of papillomaviruses. Some papillomavirus-associated diseases of rabbits, cattle and dogs involve potential oncogenic papillomaviruses with a tropism for skin or for mucous membranes: the cottontail rabbit papillomavirus (CRPV), the bovine papillomaviruses types 2 and 4 (BPV2, BPV4) and the canine oral papillomavirus (COPV). In domestic rabbits, CRPV induces skin warts converting into carcinomas. BPV2 causes benign fibropapillomas of the skin, rumen and oesophagus but has been found to be associated with cancer of the urinary bladder in cattle. BPV4 induces alimentary tract papillomas evolving into carcinoma upon feeding with bracken. COPV causes oral papillomas that most frequently regress but may convert into carcinoma. Protection against infection by live or inactivated virus or papilloma extracts warranted trials with subunit vaccines composed of structural viral proteins. The major L1 capsid protein, used as various fusion proteins (β-galactosidase, glutathione-*S*-transferase (GST) or TrpE), as self-assembled into virus-like particles, as expressed *in vivo* by a recombinant vaccinia virus or from a plasmid vector, confers long-term protection and induces neutralizing antibodies against conformational epitopes. Antibody titres can be monitored by enzyme-linked immunosorbent assay (ELISA) or haemagglutination inhibition tests using

*Correspondence* : Dr Françoise Breitburd, Unité des Papillomavirus, Institut Pasteur, 25 rue du Dr Roux, 75015 Paris, France.
Unité Mixte Institut Pasteur – INSERM (U.190), Unité des Papillomavirus, Institut Pasteur, 25 rue du Dr Roux, 75015 Paris, France.

intact virus-like particles as antigen. Protection is type-specific, indicating that, so far, human vaccines against oncogenic human papillomavirus (HPV) types will have to include several L1 proteins. The minor L2 capsid protein shows a lesser extent of protection, except for BPV2 L2, which, surprisingly, induces wart regression associated with infiltrates of lymphocytes and macrophages, typical of a cell-mediated immune response. Non-structural proteins, like the E6 and E7 viral oncogenes or the E1 and E2 viral replication and regulatory proteins, are expressed in proliferating cells of papillomas and emerging malignant tumour cells. They were considered as potential targets for both prophylactic and therapeutic vaccines, in as much as cell-mediated immune responses against some of them have been characterized in infected animals showing spontaneous regression. When given before challenge, either as fusion proteins or as expressed from recombinant vaccinia viruses, E6, E1 and E2 vaccines were efficient in promoting enhanced regression rates of CRPV-induced rabbit warts early after outgrowth, whereas E7 vaccine was not. This was in contrast with the regression of BPV4-induced alimentary tract papillomas induced by an E7 fusion protein vaccine, given before or after challenge, and resulting in an E7-specific cell-mediated immune response. Thus, virus-encoded tumour rejection antigens may differ among papillomaviruses, possibly according to their tissue tropism (skin or mucous membranes). As yet, there is no evidence for a therapeutic vaccine curing long-term persistent warts or malignant tumours in animals but trials are currently being performed in rabbits with DR-DQ haplotypes associated with a high risk of persistence and malignant conversion of CRPV-induced warts.

## Introduction

The potential use of HPV vaccines in the prevention and treatment of human cervical cancer has prompted much effort to develop prophylactic and therapeutic vaccines [1]. The evaluation of HPV vaccines had to overcome two major difficulties – the lack of an abundant *in vivo* or *in vitro* source of infectious viruses and the strict species-specificity of HPV [2] that precludes the development of simple animal models. Diseases caused by animal papillomaviruses in their natural hosts provide good experimental models to test the efficacy of both prophylactic and therapeutic vaccines. Protection against challenge with infectious virus may be monitored, as well as any beneficial effects on the course of lesions at risk of malignant progression. Furthermore, immune responses to infection and vaccination are expected to reflect the natural responses and should help to design reliable tests and define end-points to assess infection and immunization in humans. In addition, some of these animal vaccines would be of interest in veterinary medicine.

## Models for vaccine studies

### Papillomavirus-associated animal diseases

Three models have been used, involving four animal papillomaviruses with an oncogenic potential. Although none of them infect the genital tract, it is known that, in spite of differences reflecting their specific interactions with host, tissue and cofactors, the molecular mechanisms involved in tumour progression among oncogenic papillomaviruses share very conserved features [3,4].

### *The rabbit model*

CRPV induces cutaneous warts in both cottontail and domestic rabbits [5]. Warts may regress or persist and, in at least half of the animals with persistent warts, carcinomas develop within 6–12 months following infection. The mechanisms involved in wart regression have not yet been elucidated. Evidence has been obtained for the involvement of a delayed-type hypersensitivity reaction rather than a cytotoxic T-cell-mediated reaction [6,7]. It has been shown that wart regression and the risk for malignant transformation of persistent warts were linked to specific major histocompatibility class II gene DR-DQ haplotypes, as identified by a restriction fragment length polymorphism [8]. Extended rabbit families with defined DR-DQ haplotypes have been obtained in which about 75% of the rabbits show the expected wart evolution towards either prompt regression or prolonged persistence, according to the haplotype (Salmon *et al.*, submitted). In view of the HPV type-specific human leukocyte antigen (HLA) DR-DQ disease associations with cervical carcinoma found in Hispanic women [9], such rabbit families should provide the possibility of testing the efficacy of vaccines in individuals prone to lesion persistence and malignant conversion. This adds interest to the rabbit model, already rather amenable by the easy monitoring of lesions, the reasonable animal size and the development of a high rate of cancers over a 1-year period. Furthermore, the rabbit model has been well characterized as regard to the molecular mechanisms of CRPV-associated carcinogenesis [5,10].

### *The bovine model*

Cattle, like humans, are infected by several types of BPV. Of the six types characterized so far, two are associated with cancer in natural conditions, BPV2 and BPV4. The molecular mechanisms of the papilloma-to-carcinoma sequence have been thoroughly investigated in these models [11,12].

BPV2 induces skin fibropapillomas in cattle, like BPV1, but it also infects the oesophagus and the rumen. Skin and alimentary tract fibropapillomas never evolve into carcinomas but the cell-transforming capacity of BPV1 and BPV2 is illustrated both by the proliferation of the dermal component of fibropapillomas *in vivo* and by rodent cell transformation *in vivo* and *in vitro*. Furthermore, the presence of BPV2 DNA sequences in cancers of the urinary bladder of animals fed on bracken supports a causative role of this virus, together with the immunosuppressive and mutagenic substances contained in bracken.

BPV4 is a mucosotropic papillomavirus, like genital oncogenic HPVs, that induces papillomas of the upper alimentary tract in calves. Papillomas usually start regressing about 8 months following infection. However, under the influence of dietary factors, such as feeding on bracken, papillomas persist and convert into carcinomas.

The natural history of the BPV4 papilloma-to-carcinoma sequence compares well with that of the cervical lesions induced by oncogenic HPV which become malignant under the influence of additional cofactors. It is worth stressing that, unlike cancers of the urinary bladder, carcinomas derived from BPV4-associated papillomas do not retain detectable viral genomes, a model for cervical carcinomas with undetectable HPV DNA sequences.

### The canine model

COPV is a mucosotropic papillomavirus responsible for endemic papillomatosis of the oral mucosa among young beagles in kennels. Oral papillomas usually regress rather rapidly (about 3–5 weeks after papilloma outgrowth) but transformation into carcinoma has been described [13,14].

### Rodent models

Rat or mouse cells transformed *in vitro* by oncogenic genital HPVs or cotransformed with E6, E7 oncoproteins and EJ-*ras* develop into tumours when grafted into syngeneic hosts. The role of helper and cytotoxic T-cell responses in the defence against papillomavirus-associated tumour cells, the identification of E6 and E7 cytotoxic T lymphocyte (CTL) epitopes and their efficiency as peptide-based vaccines to prevent tumour growth have been studied [15] in rodent models presented elsewhere.

## Vaccine studies

### Rationale

Early immunization experiments with virus, live or inactivated tumour extracts had shown either effective protection or papilloma regression in rabbit [16,17], cattle [18,19] and dog [13,14] models, warranting immunoprophylactic and immunotherapeutic approaches in the control of papillomavirus-associated human diseases. Prophylactic vaccines have been designed to elicit neutralizing antibodies directed against the L1 and L2 viral proteins, the structural components of the viral capsid, in order to prevent infection. Therapeutic vaccines were aimed at stimulating cell-mediated immune responses capable of interfering with disease development or recurrence by eradicating proliferating cells of benign, premalignant or malignant tumours. In that respect, the viral E6 and E7 oncoproteins expressed in tumour cells at all stages of tumour progression and, most probably, the viral replication and regulatory E1 and E2 proteins, represented quite relevant targets [4]. It was thought that such therapeutic vaccines given before challenge could also be protective, since emerging infected cells expressing non-structural viral proteins should be eliminated by primed cell-mediated immunity.

## Methodological approaches

### Obtention of vaccines

The different forms of vaccines studied in the different models are summarized in Table 50.1, together with the main references. Structural (L1, L2 and subfragments) and non-structural (E1, E2, E6 and E7) proteins have been produced in bacteria, generally as fused to bacterial proteins like β-galactosidase, GST or TrpE and used as subunit vaccines after purification. Recombinant

**Table 50.1** Vaccine studies in animal models.

| Vaccine | Animal species (PV type) | References |
| --- | --- | --- |
| Virions, tissue extract | Rabbit (CRPV), catttle (BPV1, 2, 4), dog (COPV) | 13, 14, 16–19 |
| L1 protein (fusion protein) | Rabbit (CRPV), cattle (BPV1, 2) | 24, 37–40 |
| L1 protein (vaccinia virus) | Rabbit (CRPV) | 39 |
| L2 protein (fusion protein) | Rabbit (CRPV), cattle (BPV1, 2, 4) | 37–40 |
| L1 virus-like particles (VLPs) | Rabbit (CRPV), dog (COPV), cattle (BPV4) | 22 23, 25, 27, 28 |
| L1/L2 VLPs | Rabbit (CRPV), cattle (BPV4) | 25, 27, 28 |
| L1 DNA (plasmid) | Rabbit (CRPV) | 20 |
| E6 protein (vaccinia virus) | Rabbit (CRPV), rodent (HPV16, BPV1) | 31, 41 |
| E7 protein (vaccinia virus) | Rabbit (CRPV), rodent (HPV16, BPV1) | 31,41 |
| E7 protein (fusion protein) | Cattle (BPV4) | 40 |
| E7 peptide (CTL epitope) | Mouse (HPV16) | 15 |
| E1 protein (fusion protein) | Rabbit (CRPV) | 32 |
| E2 protein (fusion protein) | Rabbit (CRPV) | 32 |

CRPV, cottontail rabbit papillomavirus; BPV, bovine papillomavirus; COPV, canine oral papillomavirus; HPV, human papillomavirus; CTL, cytotoxic T lymphocyte.

vaccinia viruses expressing non-structural proteins (E6, E7) were used as live vaccines. The CRPV L1 DNA sequence inserted in an expression vector downstream of the cytomegalovirus enhancer and promoter was used *in vivo* as a polynucleotide vaccine in a DNA-based immunization protocol [20]. Interestingly, when expressed in high amounts from recombinant vaccinia viruses, baculoviruses or yeast expression vectors, L1 protein or L1 plus L2 proteins self-assemble into virus-like particles (VLPs). The structural morphology of VLPs closely resembles that of empty viral capsids and VLPs present the conformational epitopes recognized by neutralizing antibodies of hyperimmune sera and infected individuals [21]. VLPs purified from mammalian, insect or yeast cells were used as immunogens in vaccination trials in rabbits, dogs and cattle.

## *Immunization and challenge*

The most frequent immunization protocol includes 2–3 inoculations (at 2-week intervals) of about 20–50 µg of proteins or VLPs, $10^8$ plaque forming units (PFU) of recombinant vaccines or 60 µg of plasmid DNA. When tested for VLPs [22] and polynucleotide vaccine [20] lower doses proved to be protective. Adjuvants used with subunit vaccines were Freund's adjuvant or alum. VLPs, however, proved efficient without adjuvant [23]. Challenges were performed 2–3 weeks after the last injection by applying dilutions of the stock virus to scarified or abraded areas of skin or mucous membranes since natural infection occurs by virus entry through minor epithelial abrasions [2]. For therapeutic vaccines in cattle, immunization took place 4–5 weeks after wart outgrowth [24,25].

Stock virus was recovered from warts of the natural host and used as centrifuged wart homogenates. As an alternative to cottontail rabbit warts, CRPV could be obtained from cysts formed under the renal capsules of athymic mice after implantation of cottontail rabbit skin fragments infected *in vitro* with CRPV, a method allowing production of an HPV11 strain and used for the assay of neutralizing antibodies against HPV11, CRPV and BPV1 [26].

## Results of vaccine studies

Most, if not all, vaccine studies performed in animal papillomavirus-associated diseases have been done in two animal models, at least, and the same immunogens have often been administered under two different forms, e.g. L1 fusion proteins and VLPs (Table 50.1). This strengthens the data and should help to extrapolate the results to HPV vaccines. The vaccination trials performed in the rabbit and cattle models are presented in Tables 50.2 and 50.3. The results, together with the data obtained with COPV [14,22], may be summarized as follows.

**Table 50.2** Vaccination trials in the rabbit model.

| Vaccines | Protection | Neutralizing antibodies | Enhanced regression rate | References |
|---|---|---|---|---|
| Virions, wart extracts | + | + | | 16, 17 |
| L1 fusion protein | | | | |
|   Full-length (TrpE) | + | + | | 39 |
|   C-term two-thirds (λCII) | − | − | | 38 |
|   Epitopes (TrpE) | − | − | | 42 |
| L1 vaccinia virus | + | | | 39 |
| L1 VLPs (baculovirus, yeast) | + | + | | 24, 27, 28 |
| L1 DNA (pCMV) | + | + | | 20 |
| L2 fusion proteins | | | | |
|   C-term half (λCII) | +/− | + | | 38 |
|   C-term 86% (TrpE) | + | −/+ | | 39 |
| L1/L2 VLPs (baculovirus, yeast) | + | + | | 27, 28 |
| E6 protein (vaccinia virus) | − | | + | 31 |
| E7 protein (vaccinia virus) | − | | ? | 31 |
| E1 fusion protein (TrpE) | − | | + | 32 |
| E2 fusion protein (TrpE) | − | | + | 32 |

VLPs, Virus-like particles; pCMV, expression vector containing cytomegalovirus (CMV) promoter and enhancer.

## L1 vaccines

The L1 protein, whether given as a fusion protein, as expressed from a vaccinia virus recombinant or from a plasmid DNA or as assembled into VLPs, is protective. This has been found for CRPV and BPV1, 2 and 4 (Tables 50.2 and 50.3) and for COPV [14,22]. It was shown that vaccination induced neutral-

**Table 50.3** Vaccination trials in the bovine model.

| Vaccines | BPV type | Protection | Neutralizing antibodies | Regression | CMI response | References |
|---|---|---|---|---|---|---|
| Virions | 1, 2, 4 | type-specific | + | | | 18, 19, 43 |
| L1 fusion protein (βgal) | 1, 2 | + | + | | | 24, 37 |
|   C-terminal | 2 | − | | | | 24 |
|   N-terminal | 2 | + | | | | 24 |
| L2 fusion protein (βgal) | 2 | − | − | + * | + | 12, 24, 37 |
| L2 fusion protein (GST) | 4 | + | | | | 40 |
|   N-terminal | 4 | + | + | | | 40, 30 |
|   Mid-portion | 4 | − | | | | 40 |
|   C-terminal | 4 | − | | | | 40 |
| L1 or L1/L2 VLPs | 4 | + | + | − * | +/− (L2) | 25 |
| E7 fusion protein (βgal, GST) | 4 | − | − | + | + | 33, 40 |

\* By prophylactic or therapeutic administration.
BPV, Bovine papillomavirus; CMI, cell-mediated immunity; βgal, β-galactosidase; GST, glutathione-S-transferase.

**Table 50.4** Protection against cottontail rabbit papillomavirus (CRPV) infection by virus-like particle (VLP) vaccines.

| VLP vaccines | Total number of rabbits | Disease after challenge* | | | |
|---|---|---|---|---|---|
| | | None | Abortive | Expected | Cancer |
| CRPV L1/L2<br>CRPV L1 | 29 | 17 (5) | 11 (23) | 1 (1) | None |
| Disrupted CRPV L1/L2<br>Disrupted or intact BPV1 L1/L2<br>Adjuvant alone | 40 | 1 (1) | 2 (1) | 37 (38) | 20 |

* Number of rabbits responding to challenge with $5 \times 10^{10}$ particles or $2 \times 10^{11}$ particles (in parentheses).
See Fig. 50.1 and Breitburd *et al.* [27].
BPV, Bovine papillomavirus.

izing antibodies. Protection required a full-length protein (Tables 50.2 and 50.3) or intact VLPs since disrupted VLPs were not protective (Table 50.4). Protection was found to be type-specific both with fusion proteins exposing linear epitopes or, possibly, conformational capsomer epitopes and with VLPs presenting conformational capsid epitopes. As shown in Table 50.4, there was no cross-protection between BPV and CRPV, confirming that group-specific epitopes shared by all papillomaviruses are not neutralizing. It is worth stressing that there was no cross-protection either between two different types of BPV, BPV2 and BPV4 (Table 50.3). Passive transfer experiments of sera or purified immunoglobulin G (IgG) from VLP-vaccinated rabbits or dogs protected naive animals against challenge [22,27,28] indicating that protection involved neutralizing antibodies. VLP vaccines induced long-term protection [23].

It was found that VLPs could be used in an ELISA assay or a haemagglutination inhibition test to titre antibodies against intact VLPs and that the titres determined by the latter test correlated well with the extent of protection (no or abortive, transient disease) that was observed in rabbits challenged with high CRPV doses yielding semiconfluent to confluent papillomatosis (Fig. 50.1; Table 50.4) [29].

### L2 vaccines

The L2 protein was found to be protective in the rabbit model and induced neutralizing antibodies, but to somewhat lesser extent than the L1 protein (Table 50.2). Protection was greater with a near full-length protein (Table 50.2). Incorporation of L2 into L1 VLPs seemed to result in a better protection against massive infection with CRPV [27]. Similarly, BPV4 L2 protein was protective and induced neutralizing antibodies. Epitopes were

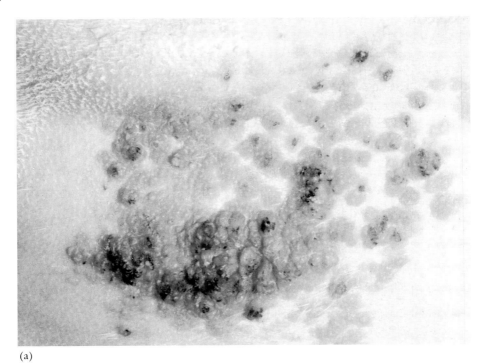

(a)

(b)

**Fig. 50.1** (a) Semiconfluent and (b) confluent cutaneous papillomatosis induced in rabbits by application of (a) $5 \times 10^{10}$ and (b) $2 \times 10^{11}$ particles of cottontail rabbit papillomavirus.

mapped within the *N*-terminal portion of the protein, which was sufficient for protection [30] (Table 50.3). Incorporation of L2 into BPV4 L1 VLPs did not increase protection, however, and antibodies elicited did not recognize the same epitopes [25]. Intriguingly, however, the L2 protein of BPV2 was not found to be protective and induced antibodies that were not neutralizing. Strikingly, the L2 vaccination stimulated wart regression whether administered before or after challenge (Table 50.3). Regression was accompanied by a massive cellular infiltration of warts, indicative of a cell-mediated immune response. It was suggested that the L2 protein in the configuration of the fusion protein produced was exposing T-cell epitopes masked in the intact BPV2 particles [12]. When tested as therapeutic vaccine in calves with established BPV4-induced papillomas, L1/L2 VLPs were not found significantly efficient although vaccinated animals appeared to undergo tumour regression more rapidly than nonvaccinated animals [25].

### *Non-structural protein vaccines*

E1 and E2 fusion proteins and E6 protein expressed from a recombinant vaccinia virus, all given prior challenge, enhanced significantly the regression rate of CRPV-induced rabbit papillomas (Table 50.2), whereas no clear effect on regression was observed with the E7 vaccine [31,32]. In contrast, vaccination against BPV4 E7 protein resulted in wart rejection (Table 50.3). A BPV4 E7 specific cell-mediated immune response was demonstrated and E7-specific T-cell epitopes were mapped [33]. It must be stressed that BPV4 E7 protein shows many similarities with the E7 protein of HPV16 [11]. The E7 gene of oncogenic HPVs is more abundantly expressed than the E6 gene in tumours and derived cell lines. This is in contrast to the CRPV-associated rabbit tumours and cell lines in which the E6 gene is abundantly expressed [10]. Interestingly, a cell-mediated immune response to E2 was found to be more frequently detected in non-vaccinated regressor rabbits [34]. Thus, altogether wart regression appears to be stimulated by vaccination against different non-structural viral proteins depending on the animal model. It may suggest that virus-encoded tumour rejection antigen may differ among papillomaviruses, in particular those with different tissue tropism (skin or mucous membranes). It remains to be determined whether vaccination against such antigens could result in efficient cure of established persistent premalignant or malignant lesions or prevent recurrence of surgically removed cancers.

## Conclusion

From vaccine studies in the different animal models available, it is clear that prophylactic vaccines are within reach. Two types of vaccines, recombinant vaccinia viruses expressing L1 protein and self-assembled L1 VLPs devoid of infectious or oncogenic viral genetic material, are relevant to vaccination in humans. Vaccination against the major structural L1 protein of papillomaviruses provides long-term protection against challenge. Protection correlates with the production of neutralizing antibodies that can be monitored by either an ELISA or a haemagglutination inhibition test, using VLPs produced *in vitro* as an antigen. Protection, however, is virus-type-specific, implying that human vaccines will have to incorporate several type-specific L1 proteins. It might be worth exploring, thus, the possibility of obtaining multiple type specificities by vaccinating with anti-idiotypic antibodies, since some papillomavirus-neutralizing antibodies that recognize unrelated papillomavirus types, like BPV1 and HPV11, have been shown to share cross-reactive idiotopes [35]. As yet, no data are available in animal models that would demonstrate the efficiency of a therapeutic vaccine on the regression of long-term persistent warts or malignant tumours. Enhanced regression rate of warts early after outgrowth has been observed after vaccination before or after challenge, using different non-structural (E1, E2, E6 or E7) or structural (L2) viral proteins, depending on the virus.

The efficacy of E6 vaccines in the eradication of long-standing warts in rabbits with DR-DQ haplotypes associated with a higher risk for wart persistence and malignant conversion is currently being evaluated. It may be necessary in such individuals to introduce modifications that reroute nuclear/cytoplasmic tumour antigens to the endosomal/lysosomal compartment in order to enhance their presentation to major histocompatibility class II-restricted T cells that are instrumental in generating potent antitumour immune responses [36].

Another approach to incorporate multiple specificities in a cost-effective and innocuous manner would be to develop in animal models investigations aimed at designing peptide-based vaccines, as currently done for HPV in rodent models.

## Acknowledgements

The help of Danielle Senlecques in the preparation of the manuscript is gratefully acknowledged.

## References

1 Muñoz N, Crawford L, Coursaget P. HPV vaccines for cervical neoplasia. *Lancet* 1995; **345**: 249.
2 Orth G. Human papillomaviruses: general features. In: Webster RG, Granhoff A (eds) *Encyclopedia of Virology*. London: Academic Press, 1994; pp 1013–1021.

3 Galloway DA. Human papillomavirus vaccines: a warty problem. *Infect Agent Dis* 1994; **3**: 187–193.

4 Brandsma JL. Animal models of human-papillomavirus-associated oncogenesis. *Intervirology* 1994; **37**: 189–200.

5 Wettstein FO. Papillomaviruses and carcinogenic progression: cottontail rabbit (Shope) papillomavirus. In: Howley PM, Salzman NP (eds) *The Papovaviridae*. New York: Plenum, 1987, pp 167–186.

6 Okabayashi M, Angell MG, Christensen ND, Kreider JW. Morphometric analysis and identification of infiltrating leucocytes in regressing and progressing Shope rabbit papillomas. *Int J Cancer* 1991; **49**: 919–923.

7 Hagari Y, Budgeon LR, Pickel MD, Kreider JW. Association of tumor necrosis factor-α gene expression and apoptotic cell death with regression of Shope papillomas. *J Invest Dermatol* 1995; **104**: 526–529.

8 Han R, Breitburd F, Marche PN, Orth G. Linkage of regression and malignant conversion of rabbit viral papillomas to MHC class II genes. *Nature* 1992; **356**: 66–68.

9 Apple RJ, Erlich HA, Klitz W, Manos MM, Becker TM, Wheeler CM. HLA DR-DQ associations with cervical carcinoma show papillomavirus-type specificity. *Nature Genet* 1994; **6**: 157–162.

10 Harry JB, Wettstein FO. Transforming properties of the cottontail rabbit papillomavirus oncoproteins LE6 and SE6 and of the E8 protein. *J Virol* 1996; **70**: 3355–3362.

11 Campo MS. Infection by bovine papillomavirus and prospects for vaccination. *Trends Microbiol* 1995; **3**: 92–97.

12 Campo MS. Vaccination against papillomavirus in cattle. *Curr Top Microbiol Immunol* 1994; **186**: 255–266.

13 Bell JA, Sundberg JP, Ghim S, Newsome J, Jenson AN, Schlegel R. A formalin-inactivated vaccine protects against mucosal papillomavirus infection: a canine model. *Pathobiology* 1994; **62**: 194–198.

14 Ghim S-J, Newsome J, Jenson AB *et al*. Formalin-inactivated oral papilloma extracts and recombinant L1 vaccines protect completely against mucosal papillomavirus infection: a canine model. In: Chanock RM *et al*. (eds) *Vaccines 95*. Cold Spring Harbor: Cold Spring Harbor Lab Press, 1995, pp 375–379.

15 Kast WM, Feltkamp MCW, Ressing ME, Vierboom MPM, Brandt RMP, Melief CJM. Cellular immunity against human papillomavirus associated cervical cancer. *Semin Virol* 1996; **7**: 117–123.

16 Shope RE. Infectious papillomatosis of rabbits (with a note on the histopathology by E.W. Hurst) *J Exp Med* 1993; **58**: 607–624;

17 Evans CA, Gorman LR, Ito Y, Weiser RS. Antitumor immunity in the Shope papilloma–carcinoma complex of rabbits. I. Papilloma regression induced by homologous and autologous tissue vaccines. *J Natl Cancer Inst* 1962; **29**: 277–285.

18 Olson C, Skidmore LV. Therapy of experimentally produced bovine cutaneous papillomatosis with vaccines and excision. *J Am Vet Med Assoc* 1959; **135**: 339–343.

19 Jarrett WFH, O'Neill BW, Gaukroger JM, Laird HM, Smith KT, Campo MS. Studies on vaccination against papillomaviruses: a comparison of purified virus, tumour extract and transformed cells in prophylactic vaccination. *Vet Rec* 1990; **126**: 449–452.

20 Donnelly JJ, Martinez D, Jansen KU, Ellis RW, Montgomery DL, Liu MA. Protection against papillomavirus with a polynucleotide vaccine. *J Infect Dis* 1996; **173**: 314–320.

21 Schiller JT, Roden RBS. Papillomavirus-like particles. *Papillomavirus Rep* 1995; **6**: 121–128.

22 Suzich JA, Ghim S-J, Palmer-Hill FJ *et al*. Systemic immunization with papillomavirus L1 protein completely prevents the development of viral mucosal papillomas. *Proc Natl Acad Sci USA* 1995; **92**: 11553–11557.

23 Christensen ND, Reed CA, Cladel NM, Han R, Kreider JW. Immunization with viruslike particles induces long-term protection of rabbits against challenge with cottontail rabbit papillomavirus. *J Virol* 1996; **70**: 960–965.

24 Jarrett WFH, Smith KT, O'Neill BW *et al.* Studies on vaccination against papillomaviruses: prophylactic and therapeutic vaccination with recombinant structural proteins. *Virology* 1991; **184**: 33–42.

25 Kirnbauer R, Chandrachud LM, O'Neil BW *et al.* Virus-like particles of bovine papillomavirus type 4 in prophylactic and therapeutic immunization. *Virology* 1996; **219**: 37–44.

26 Christensen ND, Kreider JW. Antibody-mediated neutralization *in vivo* of infectious papillomavirus. *J Virol* 1990; **64**: 3151–3156.

27 Breitburd F, Kirnbauer R, Hubbert NL *et al.* Immunization with viruslike particles from cottontail rabbit papillomavirus (CRPV) can protect against experimental CRPV infection. *J Virol* 1995; **69**: 3959–3963.

28 Jansen KU, Rosolowsky M, Schultz LD *et al.* Vaccination with yeast-expressed cottontail rabbit papillomavirus (CRPV) virus-like particles protects rabbits from CRPV-induced papilloma formation. *Vaccine* 1995; **13**: 1509–1514.

29 Roden RBS, Hubbert NL, Kirnbauer R, Breitburd F, Lowy DR, Schiller JT. Papillomavirus L1 capsids agglutinate mouse erythrocytes through a proteinaceous receptor. *J Virol* 1995; **69**: 5147–5151.

30 Chandrachud LM, Grindlay GJ, McGarvie GM *et al.* Vaccination of cattle with the N-terminus of L2 is necessary and sufficient for preventing infection by bovine papillomavirus-4. *Virology* 1995; **211**: 204–208.

31 Lathe R, Kieny MP, Dott K *et al.* Vaccination against polyoma- and papillomavirus-induced tumors using vaccinia recombinants expressing non-structural proteins. In: Meheus A, Spier RE (eds) *Vaccines for Sexually Transmitted Diseases*. London: Butterworths, 1989, pp 166–174.

32 Selvakumar R, Borenstein LA, Lin Y-L, Ahmed R, Wettstein FO. Immunization with nonstructural proteins E1 and E2 of cottontail rabbit papillomavirus stimulates regression of virus-induced papillomas. *J Virol* 1995; **69**: 602–605.

33 McGarvie GM, Grindlay GJ, Chandrachud LM, O'Neil BW, Jarrett WFH, Campo MS. T cell responses to BPV-4 E7 during infection and mapping of T cell epitopes. *Virology* 1995; **206**: 504–510.

34 Selvakumar R, Ahmed R, Wettstein FO. Tumor regression is associated with a specific immune response to the E2 protein of cottontail rabbit papillomavirus. *Virology* 1995; **208**: 298–302.

35 Christensen ND, Reed CA, Cladel NM. Induction of neutralizing antibodies to papillomaviruses by anti-idiotypic antibodies. *Virology* 1995; **210**: 292–301.

36 Lin K-Y, Guarnieri FG, Staveley-O'Carroll KF *et al.* Treatment of established tumors with a novel vaccine that enhances major histocompatibility class II presentation of tumor antigen. *Cancer Res* 1996; **56**: 21–26.

37 Pilacinski WP, Glassman DL, Glassman KF *et al.* Immunization against bovine papillomavirus infection. *Ciba Found Symp* 1986; **120**: 136–156.

38 Christensen ND, Kreider JW, Kan NC, DiAngelo SL. The open reading frame L2 of cottontail rabbit papillomavirus contains antibody-inducing neutralizing epitopes. *Virology* 1991; **181**: 572–578.

39 Lin Y-L, Borenstein LA, Selvakumar R, Ahmed R, Wettstein FO. Effective vaccination against papilloma development by immunization with L1 or L2 structural protein of cottontail rabbit papillomavirus. *Virology* 1992; **187**: 612–619.

40 Campo MS, Grindlay GJ, O'Neil BW, Chandrachud LM, McGarvie GM, Jarrett WFH. Prophylactic and therapeutic vaccination against a mucosal papillomavirus. *J Gen Virol*

1993; **74**: 945–953. (Erratum published in *J Gen Virol* 1993; **74**: 2038.)

41  Meneguzzi G, Gerni C, Kieny MP, Lathe R. Immunization against human papillomavirus type 16 tumor cells with recombinant vaccinia viruses expressing E6 and E7. *Virology* 1991; **181**: 62–69.

42  Lin Y-L, Borenstein LA, Ahmed R, Wettstein FO. Cottontail rabbit papillomavirus L1 protein-based vaccines: protection is achieved only with a full-length, nondenatured product. *J Virol* 1993; **67**: 4154–4162.

43  Jarrett WFH, O'Neill BW, Gaukroger JM, Smith KT, Laird HM, Campo MS. Studies on vaccination against papillomaviruses: the immunity after infection and vaccination with bovine papillomaviruses of different types. *Vet Rec* 1990; **126**: 473–475.

# 51: Induction of Human Papillomavirus-Specific Immune Response

L. Qiao,[1] A. M. Kaufmann,[1] G. Maass,[2] C. Schreckenberger,[1] M. Hunter,[1] P. Heinrich[2] & L. Gissmann[1]

## Summary

Infection by human papillomaviruses (HPV), especially type 16 and 18, plays an important role in the pathogenesis of cervical cancer. HPV early proteins, such as E7 of HPV 16, are constantly expressed in cervical cancers. Thus, induction of HPV-specific antibodies or cytotoxic T lymphocyte (CTL) responses will prevent HPV infection or eliminate HPV-containing premalignant cells or malignant cervical cancer cells. Recent advances in virology, immunology and molecular biology have allowed the development of novel vaccines, such as genetic vaccines and genetically modified tumour cells. We have explored these approaches to induce HPV-specific immune responses (antibody and CTL responses). In this study, we will review some of the data obtained from our laboratory and discuss their potential use in humans.

## Introduction

HPV types 16 and 18 infect cervical epithelium and play an important role in the pathogenesis of cervical cancer [1,2]. In order to interfere with the development of this disease, it is necessary either to prevent the entry of the viruses or to kill the infected cells. These strategies require the production of cervicovaginal mucosal antibodies to neutralize the infectious viruses or, alternatively, the generation of CTLs to eliminate the infected cells. The target antigens for neutralizing antibodies are conformational epitopes of the virus

*Correspondence*: Dr Liang Qiao, Department of Microbiology and Immunology, Stritch School of Medicine, Loyola University Medical Center, Maywood, IL 60153, USA.
[1]Departments of Obstetrics and Gynecology, Microbiology and Immunology, Stritch School of Medicine, Loyola University Medical Center, Maywood, IL 60153, USA;
[2]MediGene, Inc., Martinsried, Germany.

capsid proteins. The potential antigenic epitopes for CTLs are most likely early viral proteins such as E7. To treat cervical cancer, it is important to induce CTL responses against HPV E7 because it is constantly expressed by cervical cancer cells.

## Genetic vaccines

Genetic vaccines are also called DNA or polynucleotide vaccines consisting of plasmids containing the respective gene under the control of a suitable promoter. The DNA is injected into the muscle or skin of an experimental animal or DNA coated onto gold beads is introduced by gene gun [3,4]. Genetic immunization induces both antibody and CTL responses to the expressed proteins [3–6].

To prevent genital HPV infection, production of cervicovaginal mucosal neutralizing immunoglobulin G (IgG) and IgA is required. We tested whether a genetic vaccine can be used to induce an HPV 6b L1-specific antibody response at the vaginal mucosa. Using DNA of an expression vector containing the HPV 6b L1 gene under the control of the cytomegalovirus (CMV) promoter, we immunized BALB/c mice either systemically (i.m.) or locally (in vagina). As expected, we obtained a HPV 6b L1-specific IgG and IgA response in the serum after either route of immunization. The antibodies recognize the conformational epitopes as well as linear epitopes because they bind to HPV 6b L1 VLPs and proteins. However, no specific antibodies against HPV 6b L1 were detected in vaginal secretions of the immunized mice (Schreckenberger *et al.* unpublished data). Currently, we are exploring different adjuvants to induce a mucosal HPV-specific antibody response.

DNA vaccines have a number of advantages as compared to other vaccines:
**1** The vectors can be easily prepared. Genes inserted into the vector can be modified in a short period of time, allowing convenient removal or insertion of certain sequences.
**2** DNA vaccines are temperature-stable. The feature is particularly important for use in countries where cold chains are difficult to maintain.
**3** The immune responses induced by genetic vaccines are long-lasting [6].

On the other hand, genetic vaccines may not induce a local immune response (see above), and the DNA may integrate into the genome of a multiplying cell, generating the risk for transformation. These questions need to be addressed in future investigations before DNA vaccines can be used in humans.

## Genetically modified tumour cells

Although cervical cancer cells express HPV gene products, for example, the HPV 16 E7 protein, no HPV (i.e. cervical cancer)-specific CTL response is induced. This is evidenced by the fact that lymphocytes infiltrating cervical cancers are not activated (CD25-negative) [7]. Based on the two-signal theory of T-cell activation [8–10], T cells, in order to proliferate, need to recognize antigens (peptides) in the context of major histocompatibility complex (MHC) and to receive costimulatory signals (e.g. through the interaction of CD28 on T cells and CD80 on antigen-presenting cells [11–14]). However, cervical cancer cells do not express CD80, although most of the cells do express MHC class I [15]. This suggests that cervical cancer cells themselves are not immunogenic, i.e. they cannot stimulate tumour-specific T lymphocytes to proliferate and no HPV (cervical cancer)-specific CTL response can be induced.

To develop therapeutic vaccines, it is important to define the conditions for the activation of HPV/tumour-specific CTLs. We tested whether it is possible to use tumour cells themselves as a therapeutic vaccine. Because tumour cells have a whole variety of different antigens shared by all tumour cells, variants are unlikely to develop that become resistant to the lysis by tumour-specific CTLs during the therapy. We wanted to determine whether introduction of the CD80 gene into cervical cancer cells would render the cell immunogenic. We first used established cervical cancer cell lines (CaSki and HeLa) as stimulators and allogeneic peripheral blood T cells as responders. An expression vector containing the CD80 gene under the control of the SV40/HTLV1 (SRα) promoter was used to transfect cells of cervical carcinoma lines. The cells were shown to express high amounts of CD80 on their surface as determined by flow cytometric analysis. In contrast to the (untransfected) parental cervical cancer cells, the CD80-expressing tumour cells induced a strong proliferative response of the allogeneic T cells. The proliferating T cells were able to kill the stimulator, i.e. the CD80-expressing tumour cells and, importantly, also the parental tumour cells (determined by a 4-h standard $^{51}$Cr-release assay) [15].

We further determined whether HPV-containing tumour cells can activate HPV-specific CTLs. As CaSki cells (HLA-A*0201-positive) express the HPV 16 E7 protein, and the HPV 16 E7 peptides binding to HLA-A2 are known [16], we used CaSki cells as stimulators and peripheral blood T cells from HLA-A2-positive donors as responders. We found that the T cells activated by CD80-expressing CaSki cells were able to kill autologous Epstein–Barr virus (EBV)-transformed B cells pulsed with different HLA-A*0201-restricted HPV 16 E7 peptides (#11-20, 82-89, 86-94). The lysis is HPV-specific because the T cells did not kill the B cells pulsed with HLA-A*0201-binding peptides derived from the human immunodeficiency virus (HIV) reverse transcriptase [15]. The data indicate that the CD80-expressing and HPV-containing tumour cells are able to activate tumour/HPV-specific CTLs.

To analyse whether generation of CTLs by CD80-expressing tumour cells will be further enhanced by cytokines, we tested the effects of interleukin

(IL)-2, IL-7, IL-12 and combinations thereof on the proliferation of allogeneic peripheral blood T cells stimulated by CD80-expressing cervical tumour cell lines. Our data indicate that all cytokines tested enhanced the proliferation. However, stimulation in the presence of IL-2 or IL-12 greatly enhanced the generation of T cells with natural killer (NK)-like activity because these cells lysed the stimulators as well as K562 cells (NK-sensitive target cells). In contrast, the T cells activated by CD80-expressing tumour cells in the presence of IL-7 generated CTLs specific for the tumour cells with minimal NK-like activities (Kaufmann *et al.*, unpublished data).

Our data indicate that tumour cells after modification, i.e. expressing CD80 in the presence of IL-7 may be used as therapeutic vaccines. However, introduction of the genes into freshly isolated tumour cells by electroporation is not practically feasible due to a low efficiency. Adeno-associated virus (AAV) infects both dividing and non-dividing cells in culture and *in vivo* [17–20], and its DNA was shown to integrate stably into the cellular genome. Recombinant AAV is able to transduce foreign genes and maintain high levels of their expression [21]. A recombinant AAV containing the CD86 gene was used to infect a human lymphoid cell line and the percentage of the cells expressing CD86 yielded up to 78% [22].

Our data show that the CD86AAV infects cervical carcinoma cell lines which subsequently expressed CD86. In addition, a recombinant AAV containing the β-galactosidase gene was able to infect freshly isolated cervical carcinoma cells with high efficiency (>70%). This evidence strongly suggests that AAV can be used as a vector to deliver the CD80 and IL-7 genes into freshly isolated cervical cancer cells. These autologous tumour cells can eventually be used as a therapeutic vaccine.

## Acknowledgement

We thank Dr L.L. Lanier, DNAX, CA, USA for providing the CD80 expression vector. We also thank Dr S.C. Meuer for providing us with monoclonal antibodies. The work was aided by grant number 96-34 from the American Cancer Society, Illinois Division, Inc.

## References

1 Durst M, Gissmann L, Ikenberg H, zur Hausen H. A new type of papillomavirus DNA from a cervical carcinoma and its prevalence in cancer biopsies from different geographic regions. *Proc Natl Acad Sci USA* 1983; **60**: 3812–3815.
2 Boshart M, Gissmann L, Ikenberg H, Kleinheinz A, Scheurlen W, zur Hausen H. A new type of papillomavirus DNA, its presence in genital cancer biopsies and in cell lines derived from cervical cancer. *EMBO J* 1984; **3**: 1151–1157.
3 Tang D, DeVit M, Johnston SA. Genetic immunization is a simple method for eliciting an immune response. *Nature* 1992; **356**: 152–155.

4 Fynan EF, Webster RG, Fuller DH, Haynes JR, Santoro JC, Robinson HL. DNA vaccines, protective immunization by parenteral, mucosal and gene gun inoculations. *Proc Natl Acad Sci USA* 1993; **90**: 11478–11482.

5 Wang B, Ugen KL, Srikantan V *et al.* Gene-inoculation generates immune responses against immunodeficiency virus type I. *Proc Natl Acad Sci USA* 1993; **90**: 4156–4160.

6 Davis HL, Michel NL, Whalen RG. DNA based immunization for hepatitis B induces continuous secretion of antigen and high levels of circulating antibody. *Hum Mol Genet* 1993; **2**: 1847–1851.

7 Hilders CGJM, Ras L, van Eendenburg JDH, Nooyen Y, Fleuren GJ. Isolation and characterization of tumour-infiltrating lymphocytes from cervical carcinoma. *Int J Cancer* 1994; **57**: 805–813.

8 Janeway CA. Approaching the asymptote? Evolution and revolution in immunology. *Cold Spring Harbor Symp Quant Biol* 1989; **54**: 1–13.

9 Nossal GJ. Immunologic tolerance: collaboration between antigen and lymphokines. *Science* 1989; **245**: 147–153.

10 Schwartz RH. Acquisition of immunologic self-tolerance. *Cell* 1989; **57**: 1073–1081.

11 Schwartz RH. Costimulation of T lymphocytes: the role of CD28, CTLA-4, and B7/BB1 in interleukin-2 production and immunotherapy. *Cell* 1992; **71**: 1065–1068.

12 Jenkins MK, Taylor PS, Norton SD, Urdhl KB. CD28 delivers a costimulatory signal involved in antigen-specific IL-2 production by human T cells. *J Immunol* 1991; **147**: 2461–2466.

13 Harding FA, McArthur JG, Gross JA, Raulet DH, Allison JP. CD28-mediated signalling co-stimulates murine T cells and prevents induction of anergy in T-cell clones. *Nature* 1992; **356**: 607–609.

14 Azuma M, Cayabyab M, Buch M, Phillips D, Lanier LL. CD28 interaction with B7 costimulates primary allogeneic proliferative responses and cytotoxicity mediated by small resting T lymphocytes. *J Exp Med* 1992; **175**: 353–360.

15 Kaufmann AM, Gissmann L, Street D, Schreckenberger C, Hunter M, Qiao L. Expression of CD80 enhances immunogenicity of cervical carcinoma cells *in vitro*. *Cell Immunol* 1996; **169**: 246–291.

16 Kast WM, Brandt RMP, Sidney JH *et al.* Role of HLA-A motif in identification of potential CTL epitopes in human papillomavirus type 16 E6 and E7 proteins. *J Immunol* 1994; **152**: 3904–3912.

17 Flotte TR, Afione SA, Conrad C *et al.* Stable *in vivo* expression of the cystic fibrosis transmembrane regulator with an adeno-associated virus vector. *Proc Natl Acad Sci USA* 1993; **90**: 10163–10617.

18 Russell DW, Miller AD, Alexander IE. Adeno-associated virus vectors preferentially transduce cells in S phase. *Proc Natl Acad Sci USA* 1994; **91**: 8915–8919.

19 Kaplitt MG, Leone PS, Samulski RJ *et al.* Long term gene expression and phenotype correction using adeno-associated virus vectors in the mammalian brain. *Nature Genet* 1994; **8**:148–154.

20 Podsakof G, Wong KKJ, Chartterjee S. Efficient gene transfer into non-dividing cells by adeno-associated virus based vectors. *J Virol* 1994; **68**: 5656–5666.

21 Walsh CE, Liu JM, Xiao X, Young NS, Nienhuis AW, Samulski RJ. Regulated high level expression of a human gamma-globulin gene introduced into erythroid cells by an adeno-associated virus vector. *Proc Natl Acad Sci USA* 1992; **89**: 7257–7261.

22 Chiorini JA, Wendtner CM, Urceley E, Safer B, Hallek M, Kotin RM. High-efficiency transfer of the T cell co-stimulatory molecule B7-2 to lymphoid cells using high-titer recombinant adeno-associated virus vectors. *Human Gene Ther* 1995; **6**: 1531–1541.

# Section 9
# Summary of
# Presentations and Consensus

# 52: Rapporteurs' Summary of Presentations

E. L. Franco (general rapporteur), on behalf of F. X. Bosch, C. De Wolf,
A. Ferenczy, E. L. Franco, E. McGoogan, A. Meheus, N. Muñoz
J. Patnick, A. Singer and K. Syrjänen (session rapporteurs)

The preceding chapters represent state-of-the-art overviews of the more active areas in cervical cancer screening and prevention. The present report supplements the information given in the authors' chapters with the summaries of all presentations and relevant discussions during the June 1996 World Health Organization (WHO)–European Research Organization on Genital Infection and Neoplasia (EUROGIN) Geneva meeting.

In the epidemiology session, N. Muñoz showed that there is now ample evidence to implicate infection by certain human papillomavirus (HPV) types as the main cause of cervical neoplasia. HPV infection by types 16 and 18 fits the International Agency for Research on Cancer (IARC) definition of human carcinogens. Some other HPV types are considered probable carcinogens. The association between HPV and cervical cancer satisfies all of Hill's criteria for causality. It is now clear that over 90% of cervical cancers worldwide are attributable to HPV infection.

E.L. Franco reviewed the methodological developments in molecular epidemiology studies of HPV and cervical neoplasia. Earlier studies using assays of insufficient specificity and sensitivity failed to show unequivocally that HPV was sexually transmitted and that HPV infection was the biological precursor of cervical neoplasia. The continuous improvement of amplified and non-amplified DNA hybridization protocols has enabled the demonstration of the sexual transmissibility of HPV infection, making a coherent case for HPV in the aetiology of cervical cancer.

F.X. Bosch showed how detection of penile HPV DNA among male partners was not a uniformly strong predictor of risk of cervical cancer in the IARC study in Spain and Colombia. Proper understanding of the role of men as vectors in cervical cancer may be limited by geographical differences in HPV endemicity among males. Research on the natural history of genital HPV infection in males is likely to contribute to our understanding of the

453

role of the virus in the genesis of cervical neoplasia.

M. Hakama reviewed the historical trends of declining rates of invasive cervical cancer due to mass screening by cytology in Scandinavian countries. D.M. Parkin discussed the value of time series data before and after implementation of screening. The reduction in rates is generally correlated with the extent of coverage. Studies examining individual changes in cancer risk due to screening are less prone to difficulties in interpretation than historical trends in whole populations. These studies show reductions in cancer risk among screened women as compared to unscreened women and complement historical trends in providing evidence for the effectiveness of cytology screening in western populations.

In the session devoted to presentations on the natural history of cervical cancer and its implications for screening policy, H. Zur Hausen reviewed the molecular pathogenesis of HPV infection, describing the correlation between the morphological spectrum of cervical lesions and specific genetic modifications due to persistent HPV infection interfering in cellular functions. Recent evidence from molecular biology studies shows that HPV infection can be considered a sufficient cervical carcinogen.

A. Ferenczy described the problems associated with diagnosing glandular lesions and preinvasive adenocarcinoma. These lesions are on the rise in women younger than 35 years and are primarily associated with HPV 18.

R. Richart reviewed the common aspects of virally induced cancers and presented evidence for the similarity in natural histories of HPV infection and cervical intraepithelial neoplasia (CIN). All studies conducted so far show that women with persistently abnormal smears have a high probability of developing high-grade lesions and eventually invasive cancer. The notion that some lesions may arise as high-grade without a detectable low-grade phase has gained acceptance following the results from some recent cohort studies.

K. Syrjänen presented evidence from the Finnish cohort for predicting likelihood of lesion progression as a function of morphological severity and HPV type. In immunocompromised hosts, such as human immunodeficiency virus (HIV)-infected women, there is a substantially increased risk of cervical HPV infection that eventually progresses rapidly to high-grade lesions (reviewed by T.C. Wright).

In the session about cervical cancer screening programmes, F.X. Bosch showed the correlation between prevalence of risk factors and cervical cancer incidence worldwide, making the case for the role of screening, sexual behaviour and socioeconomic status.

M. Hakama showed that, when properly organized and maintained, cytology screening is effective in reducing the risk of invasive cervical cancer. The differences in national health care systems across Europe have not permitted a uniform reproduction of the Scandinavian experience. European guidelines on quality assurance have been published to indicate minimal and optimal standards to be achieved in ongoing model screening projects in the European Union (reviewed by C. De Wolf). J. Patnick showed how population screening in the UK has begun to have an impact after extensive assessment of outcome indicators and of the reasons for the poor performance of previous policies and procedures. J. Monsonego discussed the reasons for failure of opportunistic screening in general and the potential impact of policy recommendations in France. Presenters agreed that insufficient coverage, long interval between smears, low-quality cytology, inadequate management guidelines and lack of follow-up are widely recognized as the most important problems hampering the success of national screening programmes in western countries.

These problems are considerably augmented when one examines the situation in developing countries (reviewed by I. Stjernswärd and P. Naud). Dr Herrero pointed out that, in Costa Rica, despite high coverage of the screening programme, very limited impact on cervical cancer rates has been observed in the last 12 years. One of the main reasons for the failure of mass screening is probably the absence of cytopathology quality control, as indicated by a population-based study. Given the limited financial resources and the high proportion of advanced cancers in developing countries, I. Stjernswärd has proposed a policy of downstaging – mass screening by cervical visual inspection during clinical examination as a means of detecting early-stage invasive cancers before they become untreatable. He has also advocated the strategy of empowering women by educating them about the disease and the advantages of their active involvement in cancer control. Trials are now underway in nine countries to assess the relative impact of these two strategies compared with cytology screening. Although promising, the cervical visual inspection approach suffers from low sensitivity and specificity for detecting invasive cancers and preinvasive lesions (reviewed by R. Sankaranarayanan).

In the session on limitations and optimization of cytology, L.G. Koss presented a historical overview of Papanicolaou (Pap) cytology as a screening tool for cervical cancer. In spite of its success, cytology has important limitations, false-negative results being the most important among them. About one-third of false-negative diagnoses are attributable to slide interpretation errors and two-thirds to poor sample collection and slide preparation. The solution to minimize errors in cytology is to improve the quality of smear-taking, slide processing and overall diagnostic performance of cervical cytology.

To help achieve this end, the Bethesda system of cytological diagnoses was developed to provide uniformity in terminology based on current understanding of cervical disease (reviewed by A. Ferenczy). This system has gained popularity, particularly in North America, but not without some drawbacks. It has failed to provide morphological criteria for defining borderline satisfactory

('satisfactory but limited by . . .' category) smears and equivocal smears (the atypical squamous/gland cells of undetermined significance (ASCUS/AGUS) categories). The end-result has been an increase in the number of repeat cytologies and unnecessary colposcopies due to an excessive frequency of equivocal smears, with the attendant financial burden on the health care system.

M. Sherman reviewed the situation in the USA and the impact of the Clinical Laboratory Improvement Act of 1988 (CLIA), which instituted mandatory proficiency testing and quality control. CLIA guidelines limit to 100 the number of cervical cytology slides to be screened by a cytotechnologist per day – a number that should be considered excessive. Also, CLIA's practice of rescreening 10% of negative smears can only provide marginal assurance that false-negative results will not be substantial. False-negative diagnoses have important medical, financial and legal implications, the last case being a particularly acute problem in North America, where false-negative cytologies are among the most frequent reasons for medical malpractice litigation. E. McGoogan showed that cervical cancers can arise after negative smears, with rates varying from 24% to 40%, depending on the time since the last negative Pap smear (3–5 years). Few and small-sized abnormal cells are probably the most common cause of readers' failure in detecting invasive carcinoma and high-grade precursors in these cases.

The advantages and disadvantages of screening for cervical cancer in an organized system (reviewed by M. Hakama) and on a voluntary (also called opportunistic) basis (reviewed by J. Monsonego) were presented during session IV. The decision to screen or not to screen revolves around the effect of screening on the length of life, the quality of life and the cost. The first issue is well known, whereas there is a paucity of data concerning the latter two variables. In France, where voluntary screening has been the norm, J. Monsonego voiced a concern that a proposed change in recommendations for screening intervals from annual to 3 years (following two successive negative smears 1 year apart) may lead to screening failure because of inadequate quality assurance in taking cervical smears and processing them.

In the session on automated screening devices, E. McGoogan reviewed the pros and cons of automation as used in cervical cytopathology. Automation has mainly focused on the following areas of laboratory work: clerical, specimen preparation, microscopic assessment, quality assurance and training. There are several automated systems being marketed, ranging from robotic devices that process the cervical sample to prepare standardized thin smears to computerized slide scanners to detect abnormal cells, thereby allowing appropriate selection of those slides that contain suspect objects for subsequent conventional microscopy by a cytotechnologist. Comparative trials, mostly funded by the commercial sector, are ongoing in many laboratories in North

America and in Europe to answer questions related to screening efficacy and cost-effectiveness of automated devices. The general requirements for an automated screening device include sensitivity and specificity at least equal to conventional methods; relatively low cost as compared to the conventional approach; and relatively shorter time to obtain a diagnosis.

J. Linder reviewed the trial results with the ThinPrep 2000 system (Cytyc Co., Boxborough, MA), a liquid-based alternative to the conventional Pap smear preparation, showing that thin-layer slides can improve detection of abnormal cells, precursor lesions and cancer by producing evenly distributed cells on slides, free of debris and cell clumps that often interfere with microscopic assessment. One attractive feature of this system is the ability to use the remaining cell suspension for subsequent HPV testing.

L.G. Koss gave an overview of historical developments in the technology of computer-assisted slide readers and presented the experience of his laboratory with the Papnet system (Neuromedical Systems, Inc., Suffern, NY), a device that utilizes neural network technology to 'learn' to recognize relevant cellular abnormalities. Fields with the most representative abnormalities are selected for inclusion in a gallery displayed on the computer screen for assessment by a cytotechnologist. M.E. Boon complemented this overview with a personal account of the participation of engineers and pathologists involved with the development and validation of PAPNET.

In the USA two devices have received Food and Drugs Administration approval for review of negative smears in a quality control capacity, not as primary screening devices: the PAPNET and the AutoPap® 300QC (Neopath, Inc., Redmond, WA) systems. The latter device uses high-speed imaging to compute the likelihood of the presence of abnormal cells in any particular smear. Slides can then be selected for rescreening by choosing a sampling fraction based on a suitable cut-off value for the likelihood score. Use of these two devices in the USA is primarily intended to substitute for the 10% random rescreening of negative smears as mandated by CLIA. M.E. Sherman presented data in support of the effectiveness of the two automated systems in identifying cervical smears containing abnormal cells that had been missed by conventional screening. R. Richart presented cost scenarios based on a variety of assumptions, comparing the latter two systems in both quality control and screening capacities.

In the session about HPV testing, speakers focused on the role of HPV assays as an adjunctive or primary screening test for cervical lesions. A. Lorincz presented an overview of HPV-testing methods in the context of clinical and screening practices, emphasizing the superiority of polymerase chain reaction (PCR) and of the Hybrid Capture (a liquid hybridization assay using immuno-capture of DNA–RNA hybrids) techniques. New developments in this area have brought gains in sensitivity and specificity, quantitation of viral burden in cervical cells and easy group-typing of high-oncogenic-risk viruses.

A few speakers documented the value of HPV testing as an adjunct to cytology in triaging women with abnormal smears. A. Ferenczy presented the experience of his laboratory in performing HPV testing coupled to liquid-based cytology in diagnosing low-grade and high-grade CIN in the secondary (alternate) triage of women with a first abnormal smear. By performing the HPV test on the remainder of the cell suspension used for preparing the thin-layer slide there is a potential advantage in eliminating an extra visit by the patient whose cytology contains minor-grade atypia. The addition of HPV testing brought appreciable gains in specificity for detecting lesions. A. Singer discussed the value of HPV testing by Hybrid Capture technology in the diagnostic triage of low-grade lesions, indicating that issues of cost, technology transfer and scepticism as to the relevance of HPV in cervical carcinogenesis have delayed the introduction of HPV testing in clinical practice. M. Sherman presented data illustrating the use of HPV testing for oncogenic types to aid in the quality assurance of cytological diagnoses. The rationale for this strategy is the strong correlation between the presence of oncogenic HPV types and lesion spectrum.

The potential role of HPV testing as a screening tool was discussed by C.J. Meijer, J. Cuzick and A. Lorincz in the context of large-scale screening in the Netherlands, in the UK and in Costa Rica, respectively. The Dutch screening project is assessing the value of HPV testing by PCR as a mass screening tool combined with cytology using an age-stratified approach. The preliminary results have been encouraging in terms of cost and effectiveness in detecting high-grade lesions. The UK team has calculated a number of cost-benefit scenarios evaluating HPV testing alone versus cytology-based screening. Under varying assumptions of HPV prevalence, diagnostic performance and screening intervals, both tests were comparable with respect to the number of referrals for colposcopy. However, the HPV testing programme projected relative savings because of increased spacing of screening intervals among HPV-negative, cytologically normal women. In discussing the UK situation, J. Cuzick presented data to support the notion that HPV testing coupled with quantitation of viral DNA in cervical cells improves the predictive value with respect to persistence of viral infection and presence of high-grade lesions.

E.L. Franco gave an overview of statistical issues affecting epidemiological studies of the natural history of HPV infection and cervical cancer and clinical trials of screening test combinations. Greatest emphasis was placed on the role of measurement errors of HPV status and CIN in the interpretation of epidemiological relations and on the fallacy of claiming gains in sensitivity when combining screening tests serially, as is the case when HPV testing is combined with cytology screening. Any such evaluations must be corrected for the inherent gain in sensitivity expected by chance alone when adding a second test. A study of HPV–cytology combination was presented to show that the real gain in diagnostic yield is in the specificity of the dual test approach, despite a misleading increase in joint sensitivity that did not differ from that expected by chance assuming an equal HPV prevalence scenario.

In the session about adjunct screening tests, R. Barrasso reviewed the role of colposcopy proposing that it should not be used as a screening or diagnostic method but as an adjuvant in combination with cytology or biopsy to assess the nature and extent of a cervical epithelial abnormality in women with an abnormal smear. The traditional approach of referring for colposcopy any instances of high-grade lesions and persistent low-grade lesions has been in effect in most western countries and should not be modified as screening programmes are geared to accommodate new technologies.

A. Singer discussed the value of cervicography, a technique in which a photograph of the cervix is obtained after application of 5% acetic acid and evaluated by a specialist at a remote site for the presence of lesions. The potential of cervicography as a screening tool was discussed based on a variety of small-scale studies and a population-based study in Costa Rica. The major drawbacks are low sensitivity for CIN II–III and low specificity, leading to overreferral for colposcopy.

A. Singer also discussed the value of the polar probe, a device that uses electrical and optical stimulation of the cervical tissue to distinguish between malignant and non-malignant areas. Normal, precancerous and cancerous cervical tissue reflect the light and the voltage in characteristic patterns which are detected by the tip of the probe and analysed by a computer. Limited studies with the polar probe have shown promising results but they need to be confirmed by formal comparative studies before it can be recommended as a screening tool in cervical cancer.

E. Franco discussed the value of molecular variant analysis as a tool to identify cases of persistent HPV infection in longitudinal studies. This method also has the potential to identify particular molecular signatures of oncogenic HPVs that may be correlated with lesion development or progression. Molecular variant analysis is being used in the Ludwig–McGill cohort study of HPV infection and cervical neoplasia in Brazil, with the objective of distinguishing cases of transient infection by different molecular variants of the same HPV type from those of persistent detection of the same variant of a given type. Most cases of presumably persistent infection by HPVs 16 and 18 have had the same variant isolated from the cervix in multiple visits. Persistent HPV infection is also associated with a greater probability of CIN than transient infections.

A key issue discussed in the meeting was whether or not the novel approaches to cervical cancer screening are feasible in developing countries. R. Herrero presented the preliminary results from the large population-based

Costa Rican study which is evaluating multiple screening techniques such as automated cytology, cervicography and HPV testing. There is an indication that the combination brings substantial gains in sensitivity but it remains to be seen whether these are not offset by the losses in specificity, leading to overreferral for colposcopy.

A paper by A. Ferenczy discussed the current guidelines for management of cervical cancer precursors. High-grade epithelial lesions and those with endocervical canal involvement should be excised by cold-cone or loop electrosurgical excision procedures. Small ectocervical high-grade lesions can be treated by local ablation using carbon dioxide laser or cryotherapy. Small-volume (area) low-grade lesions in the ectocervix that have been documented colposcopically and histologically may be managed conservatively in young women (< 25 years) by close cytological surveillance alone or, preferably, by combining HPV testing for oncogenic types. In older women the lesion is best treated with cryotherapy.

In the session on HPV vaccines, N. Muñoz reviewed the progress to date in the field. The recognition that persistent cervical infection by certain HPV types is the central cause in cervical cancer has spawned interest in immunization against HPV as the most promising strategy for preventing this neoplastic disease. Immunization may have greatest value in developing countries, where 80% of the global burden of half a million cases of cervical cancer occur each year and where screening programmes have been largely ineffective. Two main types of vaccines are currently being developed: prophylactic vaccines to prevent HPV infection and consequently the various HPV-associated diseases, and therapeutic vaccines to induce regression of precancerous lesions or remission of advanced cervical cancer.

F. Breitburd reviewed the evidence for the efficacy of HPV vaccines in animal models DNA-free virus-like particles (VLPs) synthesized by self-assembly of fusion proteins of the major capsid antigen L1 induce a strong humoral response with neutralizing antibodies. VLPs are thus the best candidate immunogen for vaccine trials. Protection seems to be type-specific, which will require the production of VLPs for a variety of other oncogenic types besides HPV 16. Many companies are now engaged in production of candidate VLP vaccines adequate for use in human trials.

L. Borysiewicz gave an overview of the bases for various immunotherapeutic approaches for treating HPV-associated lesions. The rationale for the development of therapeutic vaccines lies in the fact that the E6 and E7 viral oncoproteins are present in the majority of cervical cancer cells. Since neither protein is in the cell surface, the most effective mechanism for tumour cell destruction is likely to be cytotoxic T lymphocyte (CTL) responses which recognize intracellularly processed peptides presented with major histocompatibility complex antigens. Experimental studies suggest that E6 and E7 oncoproteins can act as tumour-rejection antigens. Small phase I therapeutic trials have been conducted in Australia and in the UK in women with advanced cervical cancer with no significant side-effects due to vaccination. In the case of studies with recombinant vaccinia encoding E6/E7 antigens, appropriate immune responses to the vaccination were observed, including CTL. L. Qiao discussed another promising approach, namely, the use of genetically modified cervical cancer cells to induce humoral and CTL responses specific to HPV antigens present in carcinomas.

The meeting's final session was devoted to public health aspects, with A. Meheus discussing the role of education and prevention on sexual behaviour and R. Sankanarayanan addressing the practicality of prevention measures in developing countries. Primary prevention of cervical cancer can be obtained through prevention and control of genital HPV infection. Health promotion strategies geared at a change in sexual behaviour targeting all sexually transmitted infections of public health significance can be effective in preventing genital HPV infection. Although there is consensus that symptomatic HPV infection (genital warts) should be managed via treatment, counselling and partner notification, active case finding of asymptomatic HPV infection is currently not recommended as a control measure. Further research is needed to determine the effectiveness of such a strategy.

Organized cytology screening programmes have been successful in industrialized countries but are not practical in many developing countries. In the Third World these programmes lack coverage, accessibility, effectiveness and acceptability – conditions that are not likely to change in the near future due to competing public health priorities. The cost-effectiveness of low-intensity cytology (e.g. one Pap smear every 10 years after age 35) requires evaluation, as does the approach to screening based on visual inspection alone (the so-called downstaging strategy). Detection of cervical infection by oncogenic HPVs using standardized commercial kits based on sensitive and specific non-amplified techniques has great potential as a screening tool in developing countries. These tests are less technically demanding and less labour-intensive than Pap cytology. With the cost of HPV testing being reduced by standardization of reagents and by the adoption of microplate techniques, wide-scale viral testing will become an attractive proposition in developing countries.

A general improvement in socioeconomic status and educational level of the population tends to have a positive impact on the risk of cervical cancer by altering some of the known risk factors, such as age at marriage, parity and health care-seeking behaviour. Perhaps the best hope in developing countries is primary prevention by immunization against genital HPV infection. There is already a widespread commitment by the scientific and clinical community as well as by funding agencies to bring HPV vaccines to the fore in the battle against cervical cancer.

# 53: Highlights and Consensus

## E. L. Franco

The World Health Organization (WHO)–European Research Organization on Genital Infection and Neoplasia (EUROGIN) Geneva meeting was not geared to collect consensus recommendations in each of its sessions because of the large number of presentations (62) during a relatively brief 3-day meeting. The emphasis was mostly on obtaining a sampler of new developments in existing technologies and of emerging and promising tools for cervical cancer control. Many of the sessions had presentations about competing technologies. To reach a consensus in some of the sessions would have required an extensive discussion of the tissues involved in the application of such technologies and of their advantages and disadvantages *vis-à-vis* other approaches. The brief discussion periods that ensued in each session revealed the complexity of the decisions concerning the development and application of different screening technologies.

During the epidemiologically oriented sessions, participants generally agreed that there has been considerable progress in our understanding of the natural history of cervical neoplasia and its precursors. The role of cervical human papillomavirus (HPV) infection seems to be the central element in the aetiology of the disease, given the results from many powerful epidemiological studies published in recent years. There are other questions concerning the dynamics of HPV infection and on how it influences the risk of cervical neoplasia that cannot be answered by case-control studies. Questions addressing the role of viral burden, viral persistence and molecular markers of pathogenicity will be best answered by large-scale prospective studies. These are ongoing in many populations in both high- and low-risk countries for cervical cancer.

The recognition of HPV infection as a central cause in cervical cancer by previous consensus panels convened by the International Agency for Research on Cancer (IARC) and WHO has paved the way for the design of strategies for primary prevention, by immunization and for secondary prevention, using HPV testing as a screening tool. Despite the lack of uniform agreement on whether or not cytology-based cervical cancer screening programmes are ready for a change by bringing in HPV testing, the discussion indicated that the focus of the research on the use of HPV as a screening tool seems to be on the right objectives and that the experience obtained thus far is very promising in terms of cost-effectiveness and in the gains in more accurately detecting clinically relevant lesions.

The experience with computer-assisted devices that automate cytology screening is also very positive in all populations and settings that were presented. These devices seem to be ready to occupy an important niche in quality assurance in cytopathology laboratories. Much of the discussion and rationale for the application of these technologies is driven by the realities of public health practice and the environment of legal liabilities in medicine in the USA. Although participants felt that these technologies were important, there was some concern for the possibility that the problem of quality assurance in cervical cancer screening was being tackled from only one of its fronts, namely, the false negatives due to reader's errors. Many participants insisted that, while we should advance on the development of automated technologies, quality assurance in cytopathology must be dealt with in all of its phases, ranging from specimen collection to cytology reporting.

There was also some discussion on the validity of studies of automated devices conducted or funded by stakeholders. The group was clearly divided between those who felt that the private sector is capable of funding, designing and conducting unbiased studies and those who would prefer to learn about these technologies in the context of peer-reviewed research carried out independently or with increased scrutiny. Those willing to accept the results from privately conducted trials claim the stringent research guidelines for the conduct and auditing of clinical trials established by ministries of health and governmental agencies before a medical device can be sold for its intended purposes. In fact, most of the private companies have to contend with the complexity in obtaining approval by the Food and Drugs Administration in the USA.

There was general enthusiasm about the progress made with the development of vaccines to prevent or control HPV infection. In addition to the promising results of studies using HPV infection as end-point, some pilot studies have indicated the potential for some immunogen preparations to induce tumour regression. As with the development of screening technologies, where the private sector is involved in diagnostics and cytology automation, there are a number of pharmaceutical companies committing large resources in research and development of HPV vaccines. During the final discussion there was a useful exchange between participants who are experts in immunity mechanisms and design of vaccines and those who study the epidemiology of cervical cancer. This discussion revealed the complexity of the issues involved in bringing a candidate vaccine for field evaluation, such as target population, specificity of the desired immune response that is to be induced, choice of lesion end-points, trial size and criteria for effectiveness.

Unlike meetings in which the focus is on a single cancer control technology, the WHO–EUROGIN meeting brought to the fore all competing technologies, old and new. It became clear to all participants that cervical cancer screening and prevention has many facets. There is also much greater commitment now by governmental and private funding agencies to sponsor research on new technologies that may result in changes in current conventional cytology screening programmes and in cervical cancer prevention, in general. The intense research on the application of HPV testing in screening and on the development of HPV vaccines has the potential to bring changes in practices that could have an impact on the public health of peoples in both developed and developing countries. Other technologies are also undergoing extensive testing and are likely to become more popular among those practising cervical cancer control.

WHO would be well-advised to adopt a policy of active engagement in fostering research on all competing cervical cancer-control strategies. Many of the available technologies have just emerged and, before a consensus can be reached, it is imperative that the data in support of or against a particular approach should be appropriately collected and analysed. WHO and other agencies can play a valuable role in providing the stimulus and the subsidies for such studies. Given the current state of the art displayed by the participants in the meeting, one can only expect that the road ahead will show a dynamic and exciting brand of research on cervical cancer prevention.

# Index